Next-Generation Medical Devices and Robotics

Ben Othman Soufiene
King Faisal University, Saudi Arabia

IGI Global
Scientific Publishing
Publishing Tomorrow's Research Today

Vice President of Editorial — Melissa Wagner
Director of Acquisitions — Mikaela Felty
Director of Book Development — Jocelynn Hessler
Production Manager — Mike Brehm
Cover Design — Jose Rosado

Published in the United States of America by
IGI Global Scientific Publishing
701 East Chocolate Avenue
Hershey, PA, 17033, USA
Tel: 717-533-8845 | Fax: 717-533-7115
Website: https://www.igi-global.com E-mail: cust@igi-global.com

Library of Congress Cataloging-in-Publication Data

LCCN: 2025003894 (CIP Data Pending)
ISBN13: 9798337315140
Isbn13Softcover: 9798337315157
EISBN13: 9798337315164
British Cataloguing in Publication Data
A Cataloguing in Publication record for this book is available from the British Library.

Table of Contents

Detailed Table of Contents

research directions and the potential of SSL to transform clinical decision-making through more accessible and robust AI-driven tools.

The adoption of robotics and artificial intelligence (AI) in healthcare is driving significant advancements in patient care, diagnosis, and treatment. AI enables data-driven decision-making, enhances diagnostic accuracy, and supports personalized medicine, while robotics improves surgical precision and procedural efficiency. Despite these benefits, integrating these technologies presents ethical, legal, and social challenges. Key concerns include patient autonomy, data privacy, algorithmic bias, and transparency, causing the development of robust regulatory frameworks. Legal accountability and liability issues related to AI-driven healthcare solutions require careful consideration. This chapter examines these critical aspects, emphasizing the need for ethical AI implementation, informed consent, and interdisciplinary collaboration with healthcare experts, policymakers, and technology developers. Responsible innovation and ethical principles in AI and robotics enhance healthcare accessibility, equity, and patient-centered care while ensuring trust and safety.

The convergence of machine learning (ML) and artificial intelligence (AI) with medical devices is the giant leap for healthcare technology. These smart systems are planned to improve decision-making, diagnostics, and automate clinical workflows to improve patient outcomes. Medical devices are capable of providing real-time analysis and predictive analysis through advanced methods like bi-stacked gated recurrent units (GRU) that are capable of effectively handling sequential and time-series data. This work focuses on the use of AI and ML in medical devices as regards data collection, preprocessing, feature extraction, and model construction. Use of algorithms such as particle swarm optimization (PSO) for feature selection guarantees that information-rich and useful features are used to train the model. From wearable health monitoring to diagnostic imaging, AI-based medical devices hold the potential to transform patient care by minimizing the possibility of human error and allowing for more accurate treatment plans.

The sensing mechanisms have significant applications in healthcare. Integrating nanomaterials in sensing enhances the sensor and target molecule interaction helping analyte detection at minimal concentration which is crucial in early diagnosis and health monitoring. Owing to their special properties, the use of nanomaterials empowers excellent features in healthcare. In this chapter, the concept of nanobiosensors are introduced with background information on their use in wearable devices and disease identification by dint of detecting analytes from biofluids. Moreover, it presents a holistic overview of recent technologies like machine learning (ML), deep learning (DL), internet of things (IOT) and tiny machine learning (TinyML) to enhance personalized health care by remotely monitoring the patient's health status as well as making on-site informed decisions. The integration of nanosensors with TinyML is set to revolutionize personalized healthcare offering a significant advancement in robotic healthcare systems through enhanced sensor-driven autonomy and adaptive intelligence.

Medical robots are sophisticated machines designed to assist healthcare professionals in performing complex medical procedures with precision, accuracy, and minimal invasiveness. Medical robots utilize cutting-edge technologies such as artificial intelligence, machine learning, and sensor systems to enhance surgical outcomes, reduce recuperation periods, and ultimately enhance patient care and happiness. Medical robots are adept at handling even the most delicate jobs. Thus, the use of medical robots in a variety of surgical specialties has grown, including cardiology, urology, neurology, and orthopedics. The real-time data and visualization capabilities of medical robots help surgeons to make more educated decisions, lower the risk of complications, and ultimately improve patient outcomes. This chapter explains different kinds of medical robots, their parts, surgical uses, advantages, challenges, and upcoming developments in surgical medical robots. Lastly, the authors present a case study of Narayana Health in Bangalore, India, where every day robotic procedures are carried out.

Lack of medication and dehydration are major health problems among older people living alone. Often, these problems result in unnecessary hospital visits. Sometimes these problems worsen chronic diseases and reduce the quality of life. As the elderly population grows rapidly, innovative solutions to support their independent living have become important. This chapter presents a robotic system designed to deliver medication (medicines) and water to older people in a home environment. The system integrates robotic systems, various sensing technologies, and the internet of things (IoT). It consists of a wheeled robot that delivers pills and water directly to users, a robot unit that stores, organizes, and prepares medications, and a user-friendly smartphone app for remote monitoring and management. The robotic system ensures accurate and timely delivery of medication and water using a navigation system, infrared sensors, and vision-based person detection algorithms. The robot is connected to an IoT-cloud, which provides personalized schedules, timely reminders to users.

This chapter examines the role of the Internet of Things (IoT) in healthcare, focusing on hospital settings. It begins with a brief overview of IoT and its growing relevance in the healthcare industry. The chapter introduces key technologies such as sensors, remote connectivity, and data processing. It then discusses important hospital applications, including wearable devices, remote patient monitoring, and smart beds. Other use cases include patient tracking, asset management, room automation, and telemedicine. Each example shows how IoT supports hospital operations and patient care. The benefits of IoT integration are also addressed. These include improved quality of care, improved efficiency, and data-driven decision-making. Challenges are also outlined. Several key challenges include data security, patient privacy, system integration, and implementation costs. To support these topics, the chapter presents real-world case studies. These examples demonstrate measurable gains in both patient outcomes and hospital performance. The chapter concludes with a summary of the findings and a forward-looking perspective. It emphasizes the potential of IoT to support efficient, responsive, and patient-centered healthcare systems.

The complexity of next-gen med devices that combine AI with IoT, robotics, and analytics makes regulatory challenges inevitable. It is critical to achieve this safety, efficacy, and compliance in addressing data privacy and cybersecurity concerns. Bold innovations can quickly transcend the boundaries of established regulatory paradigms, demanding that policies evolve and that oversight remains vigilant. The challenge comes from the adaptive nature of machine learning algorithms present in such devices, which make validation and certification processes more involved. Automation in the medical field is transforming workforce dynamics. Although automating these routine tasks such as diagnostics, imaging, and administrative tasks increases efficiency and reduces human error, it does give rise to concerns of personnel displacement of some roles. The challenge in harnessing the full potential of automation lies in balancing innovation with ethical and workforce considerations to cultivate a sustainable and equitable healthcare ecosystem.

Robot system advances have been followed by the rise in usage of artificial intelligence and cloud processing, and this has been followed by some of the most critical issues of data privacy. Data processing of robot systems with secure data is strongly in demand so as to prevent unauthorized access, data leakage, and cyber attacks. The chapter suggests a new lightweight algorithm for data privacy with security while maintaining computational efficiency for robot systems. The new approach combines data anonymization and obfuscation techniques. It is performed with fewer chances of privacy leakage. In comparison, most other privacy-preserving approaches, which have a high computational burden, can manage such data sets in real time on fewer resources and hence are far more suitable in robots' environments of limited resource availability. Experimentation based on theoretical calculation sets the performance of the algorithm to ensure data privacy without degradation in system performance.

Preface

Next-Generation Medical Devices and Robotics explores the transformative convergence of advanced engineering, artificial intelligence (AI), robotics, and biomedical sciences to revolutionize healthcare delivery, diagnosis, treatment, and patient outcomes. This field represents a paradigm shift from traditional medical tools to intelligent, minimally invasive, and highly precise technologies that enhance both clinical efficacy and patient safety.

The subject matter encompasses a broad range of innovations, including robotic surgical systems, wearable and implantable medical devices with real-time monitoring capabilities, smart prosthetics and exoskeletons, micro- and nanorobots for targeted drug delivery, and AI-integrated diagnostic platforms. These technologies leverage breakthroughs in machine learning, sensor miniaturization, wireless communication, biocompatible materials, and human-machine interfaces.

The target audience for Next-Generation Medical Devices and Robotics includes biomedical engineers, healthcare professionals, medical researchers, robotics specialists, and technology innovators who are actively involved in or seeking to advance the development and implementation of cutting-edge medical technologies. It is also tailored for graduate students and academic researchers in engineering, computer science, and clinical medicine who aim to deepen their understanding of intelligent medical systems. Additionally, industry professionals in medical device manufacturing, regulatory affairs, and healthcare innovation will find the content valuable for its insights into emerging trends, technical challenges, and future opportunities at the intersection of robotics, AI, and medicine.

Coverage:

The many academic areas covered in this publication include, but are not limited to:

- AI-Driven Diagnostics
- Robotic Surgery Systems
- Wearable Health Monitors
- Implantable Devices

- Micro- and Nanorobotics
- Rehabilitation Robotics
- Soft Robotics in Medicine
- Teleoperated and Remote Surgery
- Closed-Loop (Smart) Medical Devices
- Human-Robot Collaboration
- Medical Internet of Things (IoMT)
- Neural Interfaces and Brain-Machine Integration
- Regulatory and Ethical Challenges
- Clinical Translation and Validation
- Future Trends and Converging Technologies

CHAPTER OVERVIEW

Chapter 1: Impact of AI in Patient Engagement: Smart Revolution in Health Sector

This chapter examines how artificial intelligence (AI) is revolutionizing patient engagement in healthcare. It highlights AI-driven tools like chatbots, virtual assistants, and personalized apps that empower patients through real-time support and education. By analyzing behavior and preferences, AI enhances medication adherence, chronic disease management, and mental health. The chapter showcases successful applications in remote monitoring and post-treatment care, reducing hospitalizations. It also addresses challenges including data privacy, algorithmic bias, and digital equity. Emphasis is placed on designing inclusive, transparent AI systems. Natural language processing enables more human-like interactions, improving user experience. The integration of AI fosters proactive, preventive care models. Ultimately, this chapter underscores AI's role in transforming patients into active partners in their health journey.

Chapter 2: Generative Artificial Intelligence and Vedic Scripture Enabled Physiotherapy Management System

This chapter introduces a novel physiotherapy system combining generative AI with principles from Vedic scriptures. It leverages AI to create personalized rehabilitation plans based on patient data and real-time feedback. The system integrates traditional knowledge from Ayurveda, Yoga, and holistic healing practices like asanas and pranayama. Generative AI dynamically adapts exercises, lifestyle advice, and wellness strategies for optimal recovery. The approach promotes physical, mental, and energetic balance, aligning modern technology with ancient wisdom. Wearable sensors and biometrics enable continuous monitoring and plan refinement. Emphasis is placed on cultural sensitivity and holistic well-being in rehabilitation. The chapter explores ethical considerations and validation of traditional practices through clinical data. It represents a pioneering model of integrative, AI-driven healthcare. This fusion offers a unique, inclusive pathway for global physiotherapy and digital wellness innovation.

Chapter 3: Future Trends and Opportunities Personalized Medicine Through Next Gen Devices and Robotics

This chapter explores the transformative potential of next-generation medical devices and robotics in advancing personalized medicine, shifting from a one-size-fits-all model to highly tailored, patient-specific care. It examines how wearable sensors, implantable monitors, and AI-driven diagnostics enable continuous, real-time collection of physiological, genetic, and behavioral data, forming the foundation for individualized treatment plans. Robotics plays a key role in precision interventions, from AI-guided surgical systems that adapt to anatomical variations to micro-robots delivering drugs to specific cells based on genomic profiles. The chapter highlights emerging technologies such as organ-on-a-chip, 3D-bioprinted tissues, and closed-loop systems that automatically adjust therapies for conditions like diabetes or epilepsy. It also discusses the integration of multi-omics data with robotic platforms to predict disease progression and optimize interventions.

Chapter 4: Expansion of Self-Supervised Learning in Computer Vision for Medical Image Analysis

This chapter focuses on the growing role of self-supervised learning (SSL) in advancing computer vision for medical image analysis, addressing one of the most critical challenges in AI-driven healthcare: the scarcity of large, annotated medical datasets. Unlike traditional supervised learning, which relies heavily on manually labeled images, a time-consuming and costly process in clinical settings, self-supervised learning leverages vast amounts of unlabeled medical data (e.g., X-rays, MRIs, CT scans) to pre-train deep learning models by creating intrinsic learning tasks, such as predicting image rotations, solving jigsaw puzzles, or masking and reconstructing regions. The chapter details how these pre-trained models can then be fine-tuned with small labeled datasets to achieve high accuracy in tasks like tumor detection, organ segmentation, and disease classification. It presents recent SSL frameworks, such as contrastive learning (e.g., SimCLR, MoCo) and masked autoencoders, adapted for medical imaging, demonstrating their superior performance across diverse modalities and pathologies. Case studies highlight applications in radiology, pathology, and ophthalmology, where SSL reduces dependency on expert annotations while improving generalization across institutions and equipment.

Chapter 5: Ethical Considerations in the Use of Robotics and AI in Healthcare

This chapter provides a comprehensive examination of the ethical challenges arising from the integration of robotics and artificial intelligence into healthcare systems. As intelligent machines assume roles in diagnosis, treatment, surgery, and patient care, critical questions emerge regarding accountability, transparency, bias, and the preservation of human dignity. The chapter explores key issues such as algorithmic bias in AI models that may lead to disparities in care for underrepresented populations, the "black box" nature of deep learning systems that undermines clinical trust, and the potential erosion of the patient-provider relationship when robots replace human interaction. It also addresses concerns around informed consent, how patients understand and agree to AI-driven decisions, and the moral responsibility when autonomous systems cause harm. The role of data privacy, surveillance, and ownership of health information collected by smart devices and robots is analyzed in depth, particularly in the context of evolving cybersecurity threats.

Chapter 6: AI-Enhanced Medical Devices for Smarter Healthcare A Leap Towards Precision Healthcare

This chapter highlights the transformative impact of artificial intelligence (AI) in evolving medical devices from passive tools into intelligent, decision-supportive systems that enable precision healthcare. It explores how AI is embedded directly into diagnostic, therapeutic, and monitoring devices, such as smart ultrasound machines, AI-powered ECG analyzers, radiology workstations, and insulin pumps, to enhance accuracy, speed, and personalization of care. By analyzing vast datasets in real time, these devices can detect subtle anomalies, predict disease progression, and recommend context-aware interventions, often surpassing human performance in specific tasks. The chapter presents real-world applications, including AI-enabled point-of-care devices in rural settings, closed-loop neuromodulation systems for epilepsy, and robotic endoscopes with real-time polyp detection. It emphasizes the shift from reactive to proactive and preventive medicine, where continuous learning algorithms adapt to individual patient profiles for truly personalized treatment. The integration of edge computing allows on-device AI processing, reducing latency and improving data privacy. However, the chapter also addresses critical challenges, including clinical validation, regulatory compliance, interoperability, and the need for human-in-the-loop oversight.

Chapter 7: A Review on Nanosensor-Based Body Fluids Monitoring for Next-Generation Medical Devices and Robotics

This chapter provides a comprehensive review of nanosensor technologies designed for real-time, non-invasive, or minimally invasive monitoring of body fluids, such as blood, sweat, saliva, urine, and interstitial fluid, and their critical role in advancing next-generation medical devices and robotic healthcare systems. It explores the design, fabrication, and functionalization of nanomaterials that enable ultra-sensitive detection of biomarkers like glucose, lactate, electrolytes, hormones, proteins, and pathogens at extremely low concentrations. The chapter highlights how integration of nanosensors into wearable patches, implantable devices, and robotic diagnostic platforms allows continuous physiological tracking with high spatial and temporal resolution. Special emphasis is placed on their application in personalized medicine, early disease detection (e.g., cancer, diabetes, sepsis), and closed-loop therapeutic systems were real-time data drives automated interventions. The review also covers advances in wireless data transmission, energy-efficient nanoelectronics, and biocompatibility to ensure long-term safety and reliability. Challenges such as signal interference, calibration drift, mass manufacturing, and regulatory approval are critically examined. Furthermore, the chapter discusses the convergence of nanosensors with AI and robotics, where robotic systems use nanosensor data to adjust drug delivery or perform microsurgeries with precision.

Chapter 8: Medical Robots Applications in Surgery

This chapter provides a comprehensive overview of the role and evolution of medical robots in surgical practice, highlighting their transformative impact on precision, safety, and patient outcomes. It details the design, functionality, and clinical applications of robotic surgical systems such as the da Vinci Surgical System, Senhance, and next-generation autonomous platforms used in minimally invasive procedures across specialties including urology, gynecology, cardiothoracic, neurosurgery, and general surgery. The chapter explains how robotic systems enhance surgeon capabilities through high-definition 3D visualization, tremor filtering, motion scaling, and wristed instruments that surpass human dexterity, enabling delicate maneuvers in confined anatomical spaces. It explores the benefits of robotic surgery, including reduced blood loss, smaller incisions, shorter hospital stays, and faster recovery times. The integration of AI and machine learning for preoperative planning, intraoperative guidance, and real-time tissue recognition is also discussed, paving the way for semi-autonomous and intelligent surgical assistants. Case studies illustrate successful implementations and comparative outcomes versus traditional laparoscopic and open techniques.

Chapter 9: Robotic Medication and Water Delivery: A Solution for Independent Living in Seniors

This chapter explores the development and implementation of robotic systems designed to assist seniors in managing medication adherence and hydration, two critical factors in maintaining health and enabling independent living. As the global elderly population grows, so does the need for smart, reliable solutions to support aging in place. The chapter presents a specialized assistive robot capable of autonomously dispensing prescribed medications at scheduled times, verifying dosage accuracy, and delivering water to ensure proper intake, thereby reducing the risk of medication errors and dehydration-related hospitalizations. Equipped with AI-driven scheduling, voice reminders, facial recognition for user authentication, and IoT connectivity for remote monitoring by caregivers or healthcare providers, the robot adapts to individual routines and health conditions. The system integrates with electronic health records and telehealth platforms to provide real-time alerts in case of missed doses or anomalies. The chapter discusses hardware design considerations, including safety mechanisms, ease of use for individuals with limited dexterity or cognitive decline, and intuitive human-robot interaction through voice and touch interfaces. Case studies from pilot programs in senior homes and private residences demonstrate improved medication compliance, reduced caregiver burden, and enhanced quality of life. Ethical and privacy concerns, such as autonomy, surveillance, and data security, are also addressed.

Chapter 10: Smart Hospitals: The Role of IoT in Modern Healthcare

This chapter examines the transformation of traditional healthcare facilities into smart hospitals through the integration of the Internet of Things (IoT), where interconnected devices, sensors, and data systems work in unison to optimize patient care, operational efficiency, and clinical decision-making. It explores how IoT enables real-time monitoring of patients via wearable and ambient sensors, automated tracking of medical equipment and inventory, intelligent environmental controls (e.g., temperature, lighting, air quality), and seamless communication between staff, devices, and electronic health records (EHRs). The chapter highlights key applications such as smart beds that detect patient movement and vital signs, RFID-tagged assets for efficient logistics, and AI-powered analytics platforms that predict patient deterioration or hospital-acquired infections. By creating a fully connected ecosystem, IoT reduces human error, streamlines workflows, and enhances responsiveness in critical care settings like ICUs and emergency departments. The chapter also discusses infrastructure requirements, including robust Wi-Fi 6/5G networks, edge computing for low-latency processing, and cloud-based data integration. Cybersecurity, data privacy, interoperability standards, and regulatory compliance are critically analyzed as essential components for safe and scalable deployment. Case studies from leading smart hospitals around the world illustrate measurable improvements in patient satisfaction, staff productivity, and resource utilization. Ethical considerations around surveillance and patient consent are also addressed.

Chapter 11: Regulatory Challenges for Next-Generation Medical Devices Impact of Automation on Medical Workforce

This chapter addresses two interconnected and critical dimensions of the digital healthcare revolution: the evolving regulatory landscape for next-generation medical devices and the profound impact of automation on the medical workforce. As AI-driven diagnostics, robotic surgery systems, autonomous monitoring tools, and adaptive implants become increasingly prevalent, regulatory bodies such as the FDA, EMA, and other global agencies face unprecedented challenges in ensuring safety, efficacy, and ethical deployment. The chapter examines the limitations of traditional regulatory frameworks when applied to adaptive, self-learning AI systems that evolve post-approval, highlighting emerging concepts like predetermined change control plans (PCCPs), real-world performance monitoring, and software-as-a-medical-device (SaMD) classifications. It discusses the need for agile, risk-based, and lifecycle-oriented regulatory pathways that accommodate continuous innovation without compromising patient safety. Parallel to this, the chapter investigates how increasing automation in clinical settings affects healthcare professionals, from physicians and nurses to radiologists and technicians. It analyzes job displacement fears, shifts in skill requirements, and the transformation of roles into more supervisory, interpretive, and patient-centered functions. While automation reduces repetitive tasks and diagnostic errors, it also raises concerns about deskilling, over-reliance on technology, and erosion of clinical judgment. The chapter presents case studies on AI in radiology, robotic assistants in surgery, and virtual nursing agents, illustrating both efficiencies gained, and tensions introduced. It emphasizes the need for proactive workforce reskilling, interdisciplinary training, and human-centered design in technology integration.

Chapter 12: A Lightweight Enhanced Security Approach for Data Privacy in Robotic Systems

This chapter presents a novel, lightweight security framework designed to protect sensitive data in robotic systems used in healthcare, where privacy, real-time performance, and resource constraints are critical concerns. As medical robots, such as surgical assistants, rehabilitation devices, and telepresence systems, collect and transmit vast amounts of personal health information (PHI), they become attractive targets for cyberattacks, including data breaches, spoofing, and remote hijacking. Traditional encryption methods often impose high computational overhead, making them unsuitable for resource-limited robotic platforms with limited processing power and battery life. To address this, the chapter introduces an optimized, lightweight cryptographic approach that combines secure key exchange protocols, efficient symmetric encryption (e.g., AES-128 with reduced-round variants), and blockchain-inspired integrity checks to ensure confidentiality, authenticity, and data integrity without compromising system responsiveness. The proposed model integrates role-based access control (RBAC) and secure boot mechanisms to prevent unauthorized access and firmware tampering. It also employs dynamic authentication for human-robot interaction, ensuring that only authorized clinicians or patients can access or command the robot. The framework is tested in simulated hospital environments, demonstrating low latency, minimal energy consumption, and resilience against common threats like man-in-the-middle and replay attacks.

Chapter 13: Privacy-Aware Modeling of Healthcare IoT With Deep Neural Networks

This chapter addresses the critical challenge of preserving patient privacy in Healthcare Internet of Things (IoT) systems that leverage deep neural networks (DNNs) for intelligent data analysis and decision support. As wearable sensors, smart implants, and connected medical devices generate vast streams of sensitive health data, the use of powerful deep learning models for disease prediction, anomaly detection, and personalized treatment raises significant privacy concerns, particularly when data is processed in the cloud or shared across institutions. This chapter presents a privacy-aware modeling framework that integrates advanced techniques such as federated learning, differential privacy, homomorphic encryption, and edge AI to enable robust model training and inference without exposing raw patient data. It demonstrates how DNNs can be trained locally on devices or within secure hospital networks, with only model updates, rather than personal data, transmitted to central servers, minimizing data breach risks. The chapter evaluates trade-offs between privacy protection, model accuracy, and computational efficiency across various architectures, including CNNs for medical imaging and RNNs/LSTMs for time-series physiological data. Case studies illustrate applications in remote cardiac monitoring, epilepsy prediction, and chronic disease management using real-world IoT datasets.

Chapter 14: Understanding Perceived Risks and Drivers of Health Technology Adoption From User and Physician Perspectives

This chapter investigates the psychological, social, and practical factors that influence the adoption of next-generation health technologies, from wearable devices and AI diagnostics to robotic assistants and telehealth platforms, by examining the perspectives of both end users (patients) and healthcare providers (physicians). It explores the dichotomy between the rapid advancement of medical technology and the often-slow pace of real-world implementation, identifying key drivers such as perceived usefulness, ease of use, improved health outcomes, time efficiency, and enhanced access to care. Conversely, it delves into the perceived risks that hinder adoption, including concerns about data privacy, loss of human touch, algorithmic errors, over-reliance on automation, and fear of misdiagnosis. The chapter presents findings from empirical studies, surveys, and focus groups that reveal significant differences between patient and physician attitudes: while patients often value convenience and continuous monitoring, physicians prioritize clinical accuracy, integration with workflows, regulatory validation, and liability implications. Trust in technology, digital literacy, age, and prior experience with digital tools are analyzed as critical moderating variables.

CONCLUSION

Next-Generation Medical Devices and Robotics stands at the forefront of a transformative era in healthcare, offering a comprehensive, interdisciplinary exploration of how cutting-edge technologies are redefining diagnosis, treatment, and patient care. By bringing together advancements in artificial intelligence, robotics, nanotechnology, IoT, and data science, this book not only showcases the immense potential of intelligent medical systems but also addresses the critical challenges that accompany innovation, ethical dilemmas, regulatory complexity, cybersecurity risks, and equitable access. Each chapter contributes a vital piece to the evolving puzzle of modern medicine, from AI-driven diagnostics and robotic surgery to privacy-preserving algorithms and human-centered design in eldercare. What sets this book apart is its balanced focus: it celebrates technological breakthroughs while grounding them in real-world applicability, clinical safety, and societal responsibility. It bridges the gap between engineers, clinicians, policymakers, and patients, fostering a collaborative vision for the future of healthcare. By highlighting both the promises and pitfalls of automation and intelligence in medicine, this publication serves as an essential reference, a catalyst for research, and a guide for responsible innovation. Ultimately, Next-Generation Medical Devices and Robotics does not merely document the state of the art, it helps shape the ethical, technical, and human-centered trajectory of healthcare for generations to come.

Acknowledgment

This work was supported by the Deanship of Scientific Research, Vice Presidency for Graduate Studies and Scientific Research, King Faisal University, Saudi Arabia.

Chapter 1
Impact of AI in Patient Engagement:
Smart Revolution in Health Sector

Leena Jenefa
https://orcid.org/0000-0002-1324-7083
Hindustan Institute of Technology and Science, Chennai, India

M. Jayakumar
https://orcid.org/0009-0006-4569-495X
Vel Tech Rangarajan Dr. Sagunthala R&D Institute of Science and Technology, Chennai, India

ABSTRACT

The healthcare sector is always evolving, but keeping ahead of the curve necessitates more than simply new medical procedures and technologies. Artificial intelligence (AI) is a fast emerging field that will have an impact on both individual patient care and the healthcare system. As the sector grows, so does the demand for efficient marketing tactics that target the appropriate audience at the right time. AI improves patient education by selecting trustworthy, tailored material and offering rapid responses via chatbots. This increases patient awareness, fosters confidence, and establishes healthcare institutions as reliable providers of information and assistance. This paper will look at the acceptance, advantages, and limitations of AI in the healthcare business, focusing light on AI's potential to revolutionize healthcare while also emphasizing the importance of cautious deployment and ethical consideration.

DOI: 10.4018/979-8-3373-1514-0.ch001

INTRODUCTION

Health care systems must assess their policies and procedures in order to improve quality and safety, increase productivity, and encourage employee happiness. Advancements in technology, particularly Artificial Intelligence (AI) and patient engagement efforts, are driving a fundamental transformation in healthcare in the 21st century (Aggarwal et al., 2023). These advanced technologies powered by Artificial Intelligence enable patients to interact with their doctors and overall healthcare applications in such a localized and efficient manner that the communication gap between patients and healthcare practitioners is eliminated, particularly for regular appointments, check-ups, and simple questions and answers (Bacha & Shah, 2025).

The combination of artificial intelligence (AI) and sensor technology has ushered in a new age in healthcare, dramatically altering patient care, diagnostic, and treatment techniques. This abstract investigates the revolutionary potential of AI-powered sensors in a variety of healthcare fields (Bhamidipaty et al., 2025). Recognize the changing dynamics of patient care as we approach a healthcare revolution. Pharmaceutical and medical device companies use patient engagement to improve adherence to treatment protocols during clinical trials and care operations. This approach involves the entire healthcare system (Jenefa et al., n.d.).

Patient involvement and satisfaction are crucial indicators of hospital administration. Patient participation involves cognitive, behavioral, and emotional components, as well as transparency (Xiang, 2021). Effective patient engagement requires active participation and collaboration. Empowering patients to manage their own healthcare can increase outcomes and satisfaction. Integrating AI technology into current systems can improve efficiency and functionality. Artificial intelligence systems are computer models that employ machine learning techniques to function alone or with human aid (Jayakumar et al., 2025; Topol, 2018).

AI chatbots and virtual assistants simplify interactions between patients and providers. They provide patients quick access to resources and help. Chatbot-based symptom checkers (CSCs) identified important difficulties such as restricted input, limited medical history, confusing probing inquiries, and insufficient illness coverage (Siddiqui et al., 2025). Users suffer with limited symptom input, complicated medical vocabulary, and a lack of follow-up treatment. The study underlines the importance of flexible input, better diagnostics, and AI-driven flexibility. CSCs lack a complete medical history, follow-ups, and adaptive questioning. Users encounter input limitations, perplexing questioning, and limited disease identification.

Predictive analytics detect high-risk patients and recommend proactive therapies, whilst AI-powered solutions optimize operations, increasing efficiency and patient satisfaction. Furthermore, AI-powered robotics automate jobs and improve healthcare delivery, notably in rehabilitation and surgery (Koehler, 2018).

AI, particularly machine learning, and its applications in healthcare have received a lot of interest for detecting and forecasting high-risk groups for unfavorable health consequences, as well as developing public health treatments that are employed in the public health sector (McLean, 2021). AI can reduce analytical and behavior mistakes in human healthcare practice by employing machine learning to investigate processor algorithms that improve task presentation based on previous knowledges (Soomro et al., 2022). For example, it is feasible to forecast negative hemodynamic events and other disasters in patients following surgery, which is a realism in many intensive care units.

AI has various and diverse uses in healthcare, including as enhancing enduring involvement and outcomes, delivering value, increasing quality and safety, enabling evidence-based choice making, and optimizing health system performance (Kumar et al., 2023).

Medical mistakes, or avoidable bad outcomes occurring from medical care, are a major public health problem and one of the top causes of mortality (Kavitha et al., 2023). Health practitioners can make a variety of mistakes, including incorrect blood transfusions, misdiagnosis, under and overtreatment, surgical injuries, self-inflicted damage, and deaths. However, difficulties such as data excellence, interpretability, bias, and legal outlines must be solved in order to adopt responsible AI.

The references emphasize the need for strong ethical and legal frameworks, human-AI collaboration, safety authentication, education, and thorough regulation to enable AI's ethical and successful incorporation into healthcare. This analysis offers useful insights on AI's troublesome possible in healthcare, while also calling for accountable deployment to guarantee patient safety and effectiveness (Nayyar et al., 2021).

Furthermore, the healthcare business is undergoing fast technological development, resulting in the creation of massive volumes of data in various health databases, yet little effort is being made to use this knowledge to prevent illness (Catherine et al., 2025). Moving from manual to automated healthcare systems is critical for improving patient care and maximizing medical resource use. Modern technology, such as AI for data processing, are required to meet this difficulty.

CHALLENGES OF AI IN HEALTHCARE

The healthcare business is shifting from a hospital-centric to a patient-centric perspective, allowing patients to have more influence over their health. Although AI has the potential to transform the sector by increasing diagnostics, operational efficiency, and tailored therapy, its implementation is hampered by many barriers.

Data privacy, security problems, high costs, ethical dilemmas, legislative complications, and the need for workforce adaption are among the key challenges.

The change is being realized and aided by coming disruptions in artificial intelligence (AI), the Internet of Things (IoT), big data, and assisted fog and edge networks. In a nutshell, digital health includes smart sensors that provide real-time prediction models and commercial data (Umapathy et al., 2023).

Despite significant development in healthcare, deep learning presents several obstacles and drawbacks. Deep learning necessitates a significant quantity of data to function well. A neural network requires a significant amount of data to accurately calculate its parameters. Typically, neural networks require ten times as many parameters as samples (Al-Dhaen et al., 2023).

Due to privacy concerns, patients in the health care area are typically reluctant to submit data. Understanding illness diversity across individuals is more complex than other disciplines in AI (Jenefa et al., 2024). Healthcare data is unclear, noisy, and incomplete, unlike other domains in AI such as vision, voice, and language, which often contain clean and structured data (Jayakumar et al., 2024). While deploying AI in healthcare is more challenging than in other disciplines, we have made significant progress in recent years.

Cancer kills millions of people each year, making it one of the world's most serious public health challenges. Despite breakthroughs in research and therapy, cancer diagnosis and care remain complex and diverse, usually necessitating interdisciplinary collaboration and personalized methods (Al Kuwaiti et al., 2023). AI-based screening algorithms can evaluate medical pictures or biomarker data to detect worrisome lesions or patterns that indicate cancer, allowing for early intervention and improving prognosis (Alhashmi et al., 2019). Early identification and diagnosis is one of the key issues in cancer care since many malignancies are asymptomatic in their early stages, making prompt diagnosis challenging. AI-based screening algorithms have unique possibilities for addressing these critical concerns (McCurdie et al., 2012).

Figure 1. Challenges of AI in Healthcare

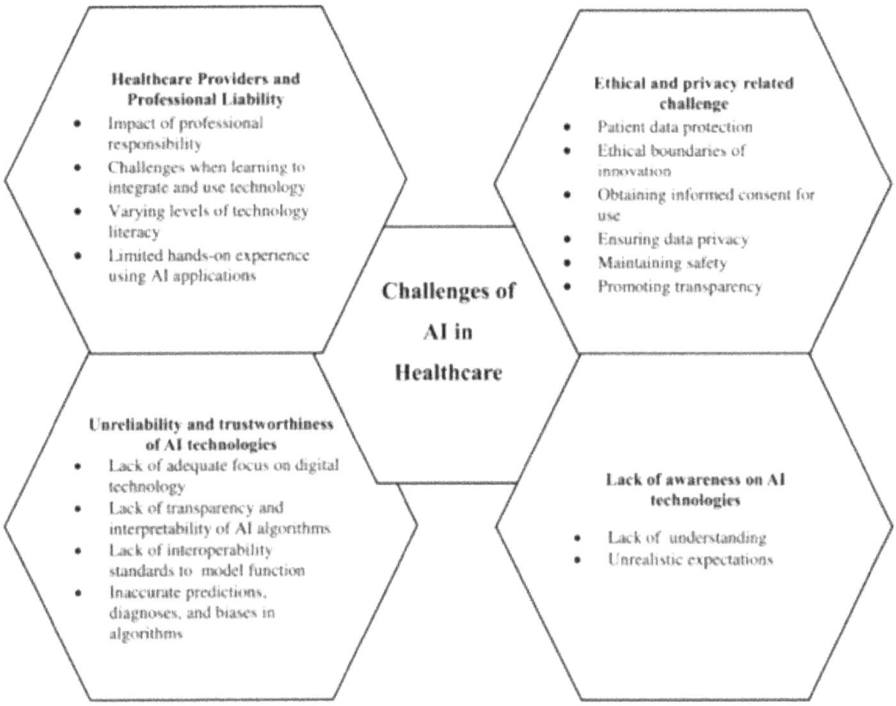
Healthcare Providers and Professional Liability
Impact of professional responsibility
Challenges when learning to integrate and use technology
Varying levels of technology literacy
Limited hands-on experience using AI applications
Ethical and privacy related challenge
Patient data protection
Ethical boundaries of innovation
Obtaining informed consent for use
Ensuring data privacy
Maintaining safety
Promoting transparency
Challenges of AI in Healthcare
Unreliability and trustworthiness of AI technologies
Lack of adequate focus on digital technology
Lack of transparency and interpretability of AI algorithms
Lack of interoperability standards to model function
Inaccurate predictions, diagnoses, and biases in algorithms
Lack of awareness on AI technologies
Lack of understanding
Unrealistic expectations

Legal & Ethical Challenges

The moral and confidentiality issues are critical in the healthcare profession, which needs stringent adherence to laws, regulations, and norms (Alanazi, 2022). The addition of AI in medication poses a wide range of obstacles in terms of secrecy and ethics, including issues with patient data defense, ethical bounds of invention, and the real influence of technology on both physicians and patients.

Protecting patient privacy and the security of sensitive medical data is one of the most pressing challenges concerning AI in healthcare. To address these issues, strict data protection methods such as encryption, anonymization, and access controls for patient confidentiality must be implemented (Jenefa & Ravikumar, 2024; Ramanathan et al., 2024).

Lack of Awareness on AI Technologies

Health systems will play critical roles in the research and development of new AI technologies for clinical treatment, which requires regulatory approval. Healthcare organizations and medical practices will not only use industry-developed AI platforms, but will also lead the creation of new AI platforms. For example, healthcare systems may create autonomous AI for many aspects of its operations, such as billing (Rodziewicz & Hipskind, 2020).

Because health systems will be involved in both adopting and developing new AI platforms, organizations should think about the many issues that each choice may provide (Jeshuram et al., 2019).

Collaboration and openness with suppliers will be important for successfully using industry-developed AI, given the potential liability that healthcare systems face when using AI technology for patient care. Furthermore, the AI industry is continuously changing, making it difficult to identify prominent AI suppliers in the early stages. Individual enterprises have the difficulty of determining how to evaluate various AI platform suppliers (Mohanta et al., 2019). Notably, the absence of established AI providers may expose healthcare to startups that exaggerate their services and have a weak knowledge of how to apply AI's capabilities to healthcare demands. Early AI solutions may lack characteristics like interoperability and interaction with current electronic infrastructures and electronic health record (Wachter, 2010).

Trustworthiness of AI Technologies

Technological constraints impede the move from traditional computer systems to AI architectures, since the introduction of visuals computers, field-programmable and special-purpose AI circuits necessitates improved computing and storage devices to provide AI applications (Pham et al., 2012). Basis for healthcare practitioners to determine whether to use the algorithm's results in their practices (Pisarchik et al., 2019). Only after validating the link between AI algorithms' judgment logic and their output can one determine whether the output is the result of a clinically unimportant characteristic or a simple error. Understanding the rationales behind algorithms' results is critical for reaching a final choice, especially when there are discrepancies between healthcare practitioners' and AI's judgments (Salman et al., 2017). Furthermore, if the AI algorithm's conclusion is true, healthcare providers may learn the AI judgment process to help them advance professionally. Otherwise, if the healthcare provider's assessment is right, it might give an opportunity to determine how to retrain the algorithm.

However, installing these infrastructures and storages can be complicated and costly for healthcare institutions.

Furthermore, certain healthcare professionals, such as physicians, nurses, and assistant nurses, may not devote enough time to digital technology, which can impede AI's adoption in healthcare (Bartoletti, 2019). Additional major topic is the lack of openness and interpretability of AI procedures, especially when dealing with formless data (Alarie et al., 2018). These technology-related anxieties are common between hospital managers and clinicians, posing a hurdle for AI systems. Also, adopting an AI prototypical needs interoperability values that allow for easy incorporation with statistics from diverse electrical health archives (Murdoch, 2021).

Medical records contain information that may be used to identify individuals, such as social security numbers and birth dates, as well as sensitive information that may jeopardize personal privacy, such as medical histories. Introducing medical AI technology may jeopardize the privacy protections offered by medical records. The training dataset may be recreated using just the final output and the AI model (Lehne et al., 2019). When medical data is acquired at scale in the course of constructing training datasets, a leak of personal data can have a large societal impact.

These problems must be solved in healthcare to ensure that AI technology is seamlessly integrated and widely used. Aside from that, in an AI system, algorithms are used, but there is also a model deployment step (Holm, 2019).

Healthcare Providers and Professional Liability

Clinical decision has continuously been the responsibility of educated and accredited healthcare practitioners. However, growing usage of AI choice support systems to aid with clinical duties may have an influence on healthcare personnel' professional responsibilities to their patients (Zhang & Dafoe, 2020). One issue is that health care workers may grow overly reliant on AI technology and be less ready to question mistakes or insure results.

TECHNOLOGICAL ADVANCEMENTS

AI-enabled health specialist care technology can aid the elderly by assuring timely delivery of treatment, allowing healthcare practitioners to expand patient care efforts separate of office hours, and encouraging self-management (Sun & Medaglia, 2019). AI-based approaches use computer algorithms for a variety of medical diagnostic tasks such as illness prediction, treatment, and disease diagnosis. Machine Learning (ML) and Deep Learning (DL) are sophisticated AI approaches that can help with the process. ML is a learning approach that involves preprocessing of the input data to prevent incorrect predictions and outcomes, whereas DL is a strategy for developing ML that requires the building of a deep data structure with numerous processing layers (Vollmer et al., 2020).

There are three basic categories of diagnostic tools used in medicine: imaging tools, pathology tools, and prediction tools. The use of AI in these applications can assist healthcare providers in making better decisions. However, the healthcare professional would need to integrate a number of data sets in order to acquire a more thorough picture of the patients' indications and symptoms. This sort of data allows the healthcare professional to track the evolution of a patient's disease over time. AI would also produce patient-specific treatment regimens, lifestyle adjustments, and so on, assuming relevant data is available, resulting in better patient results. However, the application of AI in healthcare-based decision making requires ethical, regulatory, and technological advances (Iliashenko et al., 2019).

Figure 2. Opportunities of AI in Healthcare

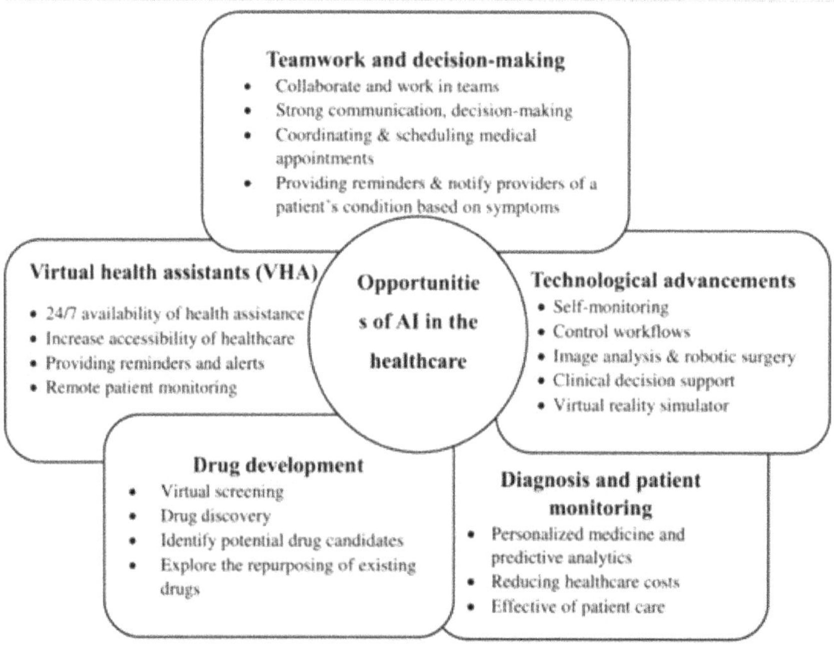

Virtual Health Assistants

The Internet of Things (IoT) is expected to benefit several businesses, including manufacturing, retail, and government. The Internet of Things (IoT) has led to the resurgence of artificial intelligence (AI), which can perceive, learn, and behave based on their surroundings and goals (Papernot et al., 2016).

Chat Generative Pre-Trained Transformer (ChatGPT) has the potential to improve patient care by serving as a virtual healthcare assistant. Inadequate patient care within healthcare systems is a major concern, resulting in reduced satisfaction and medical mistakes. Virtual healthcare assistants, such as ChatGPT, have emerged as a viable answer to these difficulties (Singh et al., 2020; Moosavi-Dezfooli et al., 2016). A thorough literature analysis compares the advantages and disadvantages of deploying virtual healthcare assistants to those of actual healthcare practitioners in order to determine their usefulness in improving patient care (Liyanage et al., 2019).

Sensor networks play a crucial role in designing, developing, and implementing healthcare applications, which are further explored in this study. Wireless device networks to test IoT models during design phase. Sensors improve design and challenging processes, reducing the need for costly revisions after launch. New designs for sensor networks address security and privacy concerns (Licci et al., 2020).

Healthcare chatbots (also known as virtual assistants) provide users with services, tools, and interactions that include guidance, aid, support, and illness management. Users of these chatbots may include patients, caregivers, and healthcare professionals, all of whom have various wants and requirements. Patients with chronic conditions who must take many drugs throughout the day may struggle to remember their medication intakes. This condition might have a detrimental impact on treatment efficacy (Hill et al., 2020).

A technology that assists the end user in completing a task faster and more efficiently than normal (Kaushik et al., 2021). In recent years, IVAs have grown in importance in everyday life, due to major investment in resources by huge worldwide corporations and the ability to enhance them with intelligent behavior (Mehra et al., 2022). Natural language engagement with these technologies has become simpler and more successful as a result of machine learning methods.

Implementing patient care technology may enhance the quality of care in hospitals, which prioritizes patient care. Smart hospitals would leverage integrated technology, an ecosystem of platforms, and staff to reinvent treatment and better meet patient requirements (Yang & Xu, 2018).

Currently, the platform gives the user entire authority over the insertion, modification, and deletion of her personal information, such as demographic information, therapies, symptoms, and biometric measures (Rayan et al., 2021). For the platform's assessment with real users, we obtained their consent to collect, alter, and publish their data in aggregated and anonymized form. Real-world solutions, on the other hand, will necessitate more complex privacy management (Zhao et al., 2021).

Robotic Surgery

Robotic surgery has transformed the medical sector by increasing precision, minimizing invasiveness, and improving patient outcomes. Surgical intervention has evolved from open procedures to minimally invasive approaches, thanks to advances in imaging, equipment, and robots (Devi et al., 2019). Artificial Intelligence (AI) is set to revolutionize robotic surgery, transforming its capabilities and outcomes.

Over the last two decades, breakthroughs in artificial intelligence (AI), machine learning, and robotic-assisted technologies have had a substantial impact on the development of robotic surgery.

CONCLUSION

AI's use in healthcare has increased in current years, with several advantages. This study revealed numerous issues and opportunities for the use of AI in the healthcare industry. The introduction of AI-powered patient interactions is a big milestone in medicine. As AI evolves and plays a larger role in healthcare, appropriate regulation and utilization become increasingly important.

This technological revolution has the potential to improve long-term experiences by allowing for more personalized action, improved clinical judgment, and efficient resource management. AI has the potential to improve medicine and create a healthier society for all.

Ethical problems, such as data privacy and discrimination, were among the most critical challenges we faced while using AI in healthcare. The protection of patient data and the avoidance of societal prejudices are crucial for the responsible and equitable implementation of AI in healthcare. Furthermore, patients and the general public lack information and understanding of artificial intelligence, which may lead to resistance and mistrust.

REFERENCE

Aggarwal, A., Tam, C. C., Wu, D., Li, X., & Qiao, S. (2023). Artificial Intelligence–Based Chatbots for Promoting Health Behavioral Changes: Systematic Review. *Journal of Medical Internet Research, 25*, e40789.

Al-Dhaen, F., Hou, J., Rana, N. P., & Weerakkody, V. (2023). Advancing the Understanding of the Role of Responsible AI in the Continued Use of IoMT in Healthcare. *Information Systems Frontiers, 25*(6), 2159–2178.

Al Kuwaiti, A., Nazer, K., Al-Reedy, A., Al-Shehri, S., Al-Muhanna, A., Subbarayalu, A. V., Al Muhanna, D., & Al-Muhanna, F. A. (2023). A Review of the Role of Artificial Intelligence in Healthcare. *Journal of Personalized Medicine, 13*(6), 951.

Alanazi, A. (2022). Using machine learning for healthcare challenges and opportunities. *Informatics in Medicine Unlocked, 30*, 100924.

. Alarie B, Niblett A, Yoon AH (2018) How artificial intelligence will affect the practice of law. Univ Toronto Law J 68(s1):106±124

Alhashmi, S., Salloum, S. A., & Mhamdi, C. (2019). Implementing artificial intelligence in the United Arab Emirates healthcare sector: An extended technology acceptance model. *International Journal of Information Technology and Language Studies, 3*(3), 27–42.

Bacha, A., & Shah, H. H. (2025). AI-Powered Virtual Health Assistants: Transforming Patient Care and Engagement. *Global Insights in Artificial Intelligence and Computing, 1*(1), 15–30.

Bartoletti, I. (2019). AI in healthcare: Ethical and privacy challenges. In *Artificial Intelligence in Medicine: 17th Conference on Artificial Intelligence in Medicine, AIME 2019, Poznan, Poland, June 26–29, 2019* [Springer International Publishing.]. *Proceedings, 17*, 7–10.

. Bhamidipaty, V., Bhamidipaty, D. L., Guntoory, I., Bhamidipaty, K. D. P., Iyengar, K. P., Botchu, B., & Botchu, R. (2025). Revolutionizing Healthcare: The Impact of AI-Powered Sensors. *Generative Artificial Intelligence for Biomedical and Smart Health Informatics*, 355-373.

Catherine, S., Suresh, N. V., Mangaiyarkarasi, T., & Jenefa, L. (2025). Unveiling the Enigma of Shadow: Ethical Difficulties in the Field of AI. In *Navigating Data Science: Unleashing the Creative Potential of Artificial Intelligence* (pp. 57-67). Emerald Publishing Limited.

Devi, S., Merchant, Z. A. M., Siddiqui, M. S., & Lobo, M. (2019). Artificial intelligence based personal assistant. *Asian J. Converg. Technol.*, *5*(1), 1–4.

Hill, M. G., Sim, M., & Mills, B. (2020). The quality of diagnosis and triage advice provided by free online symptom checkers and apps in Australia. *The Medical Journal of Australia, 212*(11), 514–519.

Holm, E. A. (2019). In defense of the black box. *Science, 364*, 26–27.

Iliashenko, O., Bikkulova, Z., & Dubgorn, A. (2019). Opportunities and challenges of artificial intelligence in healthcare. In *E3S Web of Conferences* (Vol. 110, p. 02028). EDP Sciences.

Jayakumar, M., Jenefa, L., Dulloo, R., Jose, J. S., & Kumar, A. (2025, March). Smart and Sustainable Tourism Development: Contention convenience and accessibility using Artificial Intelligence, Internet of Things, Augmented Reality and Virtual Reality Technologies. In *2025 International Conference on Data Science, Agents & Artificial Intelligence (ICDSAAI)* (pp. 1-6). IEEE.

Jayakumar, M., Jenefa, L., Mishra, N., Kumar, A., & Sumitha, S. (2024, December). Artificial Intelligence In Digital Marketing Platform: Impact In Consumer Buying Behaviour. In *2024 International Conference on Emerging Research in Computational Science (ICERCS)* (pp. 1-6). IEEE.

Jenefa, L., Jayakumar, M., Catherine, S., Kumar, S. A., Tripathi, R., & Jeevitha, M. The Application of Artificial Intelligence and Robotics in Healthcare Services. In *Revolutionizing Healthcare Services* (pp. 27–45). CRC Press.

Jenefa, L., Kanchana, K., Jayakumar, M., & Kumar, A. (2024, December). The Impact of Artificial Intelligence for Developing Supply Chain Collaboration Performance: An Empirical Investigation. In *2024 International Conference on Emerging Research in Computational Science (ICERCS)* (pp. 1-4). IEEE.

Jenefa, L., & Ravikumar, S. (2024, September). Improving Diagnosis and Classification of Severity in Diabetic Retinopathy Using Transfer Learning. In *2024 International Conference on Integration of Emerging Technologies for the Digital World (ICIETDW)* (pp. 1-5). IEEE.

Jeshuram, S. B., Ebenzer, K., & Jenefa, L. (2019). An Empirical Study on satisfaction towards selected herbal medicines. *History Research Journal, 5*, 30–36.

Kaushik, K., Dahiya, S., & Sharma, R. (2021). Internet of things advancements in healthcare. In *Internet of things* (pp. 19–32). CRC Press.

. Kavitha, M., Roobini, S., Prasanth, A., & Sujaritha, M. (2023). Systematic view and impact of artificial intelligence in smart healthcare systems, principles, challenges and applications. *Machine learning and artificial intelligence in healthcare systems*, 25-56.

. F. Koehler. (2018). Telemedical Interventional Management in Heart Failure II (TIM-HF2), a randomized, controlled trial investigating the impact of telemedicine on unplanned cardiovascular hospitalizations and mortality in heart failure patients: Study design and description of the intervention.

Kumar, Y., Koul, A., Singla, R., & Ijaz, M. F. (2023). Artificial intelligence in disease diagnosis: A systematic literature review, synthesizing framework and future research agenda. *Journal of Ambient Intelligence and Humanized Computing*, *14*(7), 8459–8486.

Lehne, M., & Sass, J. (2019). Essen wanger A, Schepers J, Thun S. Why digital medicine depends on interoperability. *Digital Medicine*, *2*, 1–5.

Licci, M., Thieringer, F. M., Guzman, R., & Soleman, J. (2020). Development and validation of a synthetic 3D-printed simulator for training in neuroendoscopic ventricular lesion removal. *Neurosurgical Focus*, *48*(3), E18.

. Liyanage, H., Liaw, S. T., Jonnagaddala, J., Schreiber, R., Kuziemsky, C., Terry, A. L., & de Lusignan, S. (2019). Artificial intelligence in primary health care: perceptions, issues, and challenges. *Yearbook of medical informatics, 28*(01), 041-046.

McCurdie, T., Taneva, S., Casselman, M., Yeung, M., McDaniel, C., Ho, W., & Cafazzo, J. (2012). mHealth consumer apps: The case for user-centered design. *Biomedical Instrumentation & Technology*, *46*(s2), 49–56.

McLean, G. (2021). Alexa, do voice assistants influence consumer brand engagement? Examining the role of AI-Powered voice assistants in influencing consumer brand engagement,

Mehra, P. S., Goyal, L. M., Dagur, A., & Dwivedi, A. K. (Eds.). (2022). *Healthcare Systems and Health Informatics: Using Internet of Things*. CRC Press.

Moosavi-Dezfooli, S. M., Fawzi, A., & Frossard, P. (2016). DeepFool: a simple and accurate method to fool deep neural networks. In: *Proceedings of the IEEE Conference on Computer Vision and Pattern Recognition*; 2016 Jun 27–30; Las Vegas, NV. p. 2574–82.

Murdoch, B. (2021). Privacy and artificial intelligence: Challenges for protecting health information in a new era. *BMC Medical Ethics*, *22*, 1–5.

. Nayyar, A., Gadhavi, L., & Zaman, N. (2021). Machine learning in healthcare: review, opportunities and challenges. *Machine learning and the internet of medical things in healthcare*, 23-45.

Papernot, N., McDaniel, P., Jha, S., Fredrikson, M., Celik, Z. B., & Swami, A. (2016). The limitations of deep learning in adversarial settings. In: Proceedings of 2016 IEEE European Symposium on Security and Privacy (EuroS&P); Saarbruecken, Germany. p. 372–87.

Pham, J. C., Aswani, M. S., Rosen, M., Lee, H., Huddle, M., Weeks, K., & Pronovost, P. J. (2012). Reducing medical errors and adverse events. *Annual Review of Medicine*, *63*(1), 447–463.

Pisarchik, A. N., Maksimenko, V. A., & Hramov, A. E. (2019, October). From Novel technology to novel applications: Comment on "An Integrated Brain-Machine Interface Platform With Thousands of Channels" by Elon Musk and Neuralink. *Journal of Medical Internet Research*, *21*(10).

Ramanathan, K., Jenefa, L., & Radhi, A. R. A. H. (2024). Redesigning of Marketing Mix Elements Affecting Medical Tourism Through Artificial Intelligence (AI). In *Reskilling the workforce for Technological Advancement* (pp. 222–240). IGI Global.

. Rayan, R. A., Tsagkaris, C., & Iryna, R. B. (2021). The Internet of things for healthcare: applications, selected cases and challenges. *IoT in healthcare and ambient assisted living*, 1-15.

Rodziewicz, T. L., & Hipskind, J. E. (2020). *Medical error prevention. StatPearls*. StatPearls Publishing.

Salman, M., Ahmed, A. W., Khan, A., Raza, B., & Latif, K. (2017). Artificial intelligence in biomedical domain an overview of ai based innovations in medical. *International Journal of Advanced Computer Science and Applications*, *8*, 319–327.

. Siddiqui, R., Tariq, A., Mariyam, F., Singh, A., & Khan, N. (2025). Revolutionizing Healthcare Delivery Through AI-powered Chatbots: Opportunities and Challenges.

Singh, R. P., Hom, G. L., Abramoff, M. D., Campbell, J. P., & Chiang, M. F. (2020). Current challenges and barriers to real-world artificial intelligence adoption for the healthcare system, provider, and the patient. *Translational Vision Science & Technology*, *9*(2), 45–45.

Soomro, T. A., Zheng, L., Afifi, A. J., Ali, A., Yin, M., & Gao, J. (2022). Artificial intelligence (AI) for medical imaging to combat coronavirus disease (COVID-19): A detailed review with direction for future research. *Artificial Intelligence Review*, **•••**, 1–31.

Sun, T. Q., & Medaglia, R. (2019). Mapping the challenges of Artificial Intelligence in the public sector: Evidence from public healthcare. *Government Information Quarterly*, *36*(2), 368–383.

Topol. E. J. (2018). High-performance medicine: The Convergence of human of human and artificial intelligence.

Umapathy, V. R., Raj, R. D. S., Yadav, S., Munavarah, S. A., Anandapandian, P. A., Mary, A. V., & Mary, V. (2023). Perspective of artificial intelligence in disease diagnosis: A review of current and future endeavours in the medical field. *Cureus*, *15*(9).

. Vollmer, S., Mateen, B. A., Bohner, G., Király, F. J., Ghani, R., Jonsson, P., ... & Hemingway, H. (2020). Machine learning and artificial intelligence research for patient benefit: 20 critical questions on transparency, replicability, ethics, and effectiveness. *bmj, 368.*

Wachter, R. M. (2010). Patient safety at ten: Unmistakable progress, troubling gaps. *Health Affairs*, *29*(1), 165–173.

. Xiang. D. (2021). Privacy Protection and Secondary use of Health Data: Strategies and Methods, doi: .DOI: 10.1155/2021/6967166

Yang, P., & Xu, L. (2018). The Internet of Things (IoT): Informatics methods for IoT-enabled health care. *Journal of Biomedical Informatics*, *87*, 154–156.

Zhang, B., & Dafoe, A. U. S. (2020). Public opinion on the governance of artificial intelligence. In: *AIES 2020—Proceedings of the AAAI/ACM Conference on AI, Ethics, and Society*. New York, NY, USA: Association for Computing Machinery, Inc; 187–193.

Zhao, M., Hoti, K., Wang, H., Raghu, A., & Katabi, D. (2021). Assessment of medication self-administration using artificial intelligence. *Nature Medicine*, *27*(4), 727–735.

Chapter 2
Generative Artificial Intelligence and Vedic Scripture–Enabled Physiotherapy Management System

Sachin Sharma
https://orcid.org/0000-0002-7821-3685
Amity University Punjab, Mohali, India

ABSTRACT

This chapter presents a novel physiotherapy management system based on generative artificial intelligence (AI) and Vedic scriptures. In healthcare, especially in recovery, personalized and effective treatment approaches are fundamental to optimize insights. The use of generative AI provides an energetic system to tailor physiotherapy interventions to human understanding needs. This study explores potential applications of generative AI in physiotherapy administration, sports medicine assessment, treatment management, and pre-screening. Through hypothetical research and experimental case reflections, the paper demonstrates how generative AI computing can analyze persistent information, calculate recovery trajectory, development plans, and treatment responses to create personalized recovery programs. By explaining the synergy between generative AI and physiotherapy delivery, this research promotes personalized approaches to recovery, promotional experiences for physical therapists, healthcare professionals, and innovators seeking to improve silent care and recovery outcomes.

DOI: 10.4018/979-8-3373-1514-0.ch002

I. INTRODUCTION

Innovation improvements and an expanding accentuation on all encompassing wellness strategies are driving a quick advancement of the healthcare segment. Among these advancements, Generative Artificial Intelligence (GAI) has become a game-changer, opening the door to custom-made, data-driven healthcare arrangements. Within the setting of physical treatment in specific, the antiquated information of the Vedic sacred writings when combined with this approach gives an interesting system for improving quiet care, empowering all encompassing mending, and optimizing treatment results (Sharma et al., 2025b). Progressed machine learning calculations that can deliver modern information, experiences, and suggestions based on preexisting information sets are alluded to as generative AI. When it comes to physical treatment, GAI can look at tremendous volumes of quiet information to discover patterns, estimate treatment comes about, and plan individualized recuperation programs. Physical advisors can utilize prescient analytics to more accurately survey quiet issues and improve determination since to GAI's control. By making interesting treatment programs based on complex understanding profiles, physical specialists may personalize care. By robotizing regulatory obligations, physical advisors can streamline operations and free up specialists to concentrate more on giving coordinate persistent care. The Vedic scriptures begin from antiquated India and give significant knowledge into the interface between intellect, body, and soul. For ideal wellbeing, these works push the noteworthiness of concordance and adjust (Sharma et al., 2024). One of the most thoughts of Vedic reasoning is all encompassing wellbeing, which sees well-being as a multifaceted idea enveloping mental, enthusiastic, physical, and otherworldly perspectives. Personalization, which acknowledges that each person is particular and might require distinctive strategies to reach adjust (e.g., the varieties of doshas in Ayurveda), may be a portion of Vedic philosophy. Preventive care, which emphasizes dietary and way of life choices that support long-term wellbeing as restricted to as it were treating indications, may be a component of the Vedic reasoning. By consolidating GAI with Vedic concepts into a physiotherapy management system (PMS), a powerful, all-encompassing understanding care methodology is delivered. Utilizing GAI to evaluate persistent information, this technique looks for to personalize treatment regimens and create customized restoration programs that incorporate Vedic hones like yoga, meditation, and dietary exhortation. By utilizing all encompassing strategies that improve both physical and mental mending, this show looks for to extend persistent support, which advances a closer relationship between patients and their care. By utilizing information analytics and progressing criticism, this demonstrate looks for to maximize treatment comes about by permitting real-time treatment arrange alterations and guaranteeing that mediations are proficient and adjust to desires of patients. By utilizing AI-based robotization to optimize authoritative strategies and documentation, this methodology looks for to boost proficiency and free up physical therapists' time to lock in with and care for patients. The burgeoning scene of advanced healthcare is progressively characterized by the integration of advanced advances and a recharged intrigued in all encompassing, individualized care. Inside this advancing worldview, the conceptualization of a Generative Artificial Intelligence (AI) and Vedic Scripture Empowered Physiotherapy Management System speaks to a pioneering intrigue endeavor, looking for to synthesize the prescient and imaginative control of progressed AI with the timeless intelligence implanted in ancient Indian Vedic traditions (R. Rawat et al., 2024b). This presentation will delineate the center components of such a framework, investigate the theoretical underpinnings of their convergence, and talk about the significant suggestions, as well as the inborn challenges, in actualizing this yearning vision for personalized physiotherapy. At its innovative vanguard lies Generative Artificial Intelligence. Unlike discriminative AI, which basically classifies or predicts based on existing information, generative models are planned to deliver novel data yields that resemble their preparing information but are entirely modern creations. This capability stems from structures such as Generative Adversarial Networks (GANs), Variational Autoencoders (VAEs), and more recently, large language models (LLMs) like Transformers. In a healthcare setting, Generative AI holds immense potential. It can synthesize practical medical images for preparing purposes, create personalized drug compounds, create synthetic persistent datasets for investigate, and most applicably for this talk, plan exceedingly customized treatment plans. For physiotherapy, this implies an AI able of analyzing a endless cluster of patient information – counting therapeutic history, current physical confinements, torment profiles, biomechanical appraisals, and indeed way of life variables – to powerfully produce work out regimens, restoration conventions, and instructive substance custom-made to the individual's advancing needs, instead of depending on standardized approaches. The AI's capacity to learn intricate designs and connections from complex physiological information makes it extraordinarily suited to distinguishing ideal pathways for recuperation and execution improvement, continually adjusting as the understanding advances. Complementing this innovative ability is the significant philosophical and viable system advertised by Vedic Scriptures. These ancient Indian writings, enveloping the Vedas, Upanishads, and united writing like Ayurveda, speak to a holistic understanding of life, wellbeing, and infinite arrange. Unlike a absolutely reductionist biomedical demonstrate, Vedic conventions emphasize the complicated interaction between the individual (Purusha) and the universe (Prakriti), viewing wellbeing not just as the absence of disease but as a state of adjusted well-being over physical, mental, enthusiastic, and spiritual measurements. Key Ayurvedic concepts such as Prakriti (individual structure based on the five elements),

Doshas (Vata, Pitta, Kapha – the three crucial psycho-physiological energies), Agni (digestive fire), and Dhatus (body tissues) give a nuanced system for understanding person inclinations to wellbeing and illness. Moreover, Vedic wisdom amplifies to standards of Dinacharya (day by day schedule), Ritucharya (seasonal routine), dietary guidelines, yoga asanas (postures), Pranayama (breathing techniques), and meditation, all of which contribute to maintaining balance and advancing healing. The integration of these standards into physiotherapy administration would move the center from symptomatic help to tending to the root causes of imbalance, cultivating a more sustainable and comprehensive recovery. For occurrence, a Vedic viewpoint might propose that certain physical afflictions are exacerbated by particular dietary habits or mental stressors, directing the AI to prescribe not just works out but also way of life modifications adjusted with the patient's special constitutional profile. The merging of these two distinct spaces forms the center of the Vedic Scripture Empowered Physiotherapy Management Framework. Here, Generative AI acts as the brilliantly engine, not fair preparing information but effectively making bespoke administration plans, with the parameters and considerations for era significantly impacted by Vedic principles. The framework envisions a continuous criticism circle where the AI learns from a patient's reactions to produced mediations, refining future suggestions. For case, on the off chance that a persistent with a 'Vata' dominant Prakriti (inclined to dryness, anxiety, and fluctuating energy) presents with joint torment, the AI, educated by Vedic insights, might produce a physiotherapy arrange that prioritizes tender, warming exercises, suggests particular herbal poultices, and proposes calming reflective hones, nearby routine physiotherapy methods. This contrasts with a 'Pitta' dominant person (inclined to inflammation, intensity) who might receive proposals for cooling works out and stress-reduction procedures. The AI's generative capability would amplify to crafting personalized guidelines recordings, sound guides for reflection, and indeed textual clarifications of how particular Vedic principles relate to the patient's condition and treatment arrange, thereby enabling patients with a deeper understanding of their claim healing journey. The potential benefits of such a framework are multifold and transformative. Firstly, it guarantees unparalleled personalization, moving past generic treatment conventions to offer care absolutely tailored to an individual's interesting physiological, psychological, and protected makeup as caught on through both advanced diagnostics and Vedic insights (Kapruwan et al., 2025). Besides, it cultivates all encompassing approach to recovery, acknowledging the interconnectedness of physical symptoms with mental, enthusiastic, and lifestyle variables. By coordination dietary counsel, mindfulness practices, and every day schedules nearby physical works out, the framework addresses the patient's well-being comprehensively. Thirdly, it offers the potential for social resonance and improved persistent engagement, especially for people who distinguish with or discover comfort in conventional Indian intelligence. Understanding their wellbeing through a recognizable philosophical lens can improve adherence to treatment plans and cultivate a more dynamic part in their possess healing. Besides, the framework might give data-driven insights into the viability of coordination conventional practices with present day physiotherapy, opening modern roads for inquire about and evidence-based complementary medication. By analyzing results over a differing persistent population, the AI might iteratively refine its understanding of which Vedic standards, when combined with particular physiotherapy methods, surrender the foremost useful comes about for different conditions. Be that as it may, the way to realizing such a advanced framework is full with significant challenges. A primary concern spins around information integration and standardization. Translating nuanced Vedic concepts into quantifiable parameters that an AI can handle requires fastidious exertion and cross-disciplinary collaboration between Ayurvedic professionals, Sanskrit researchers, and AI engineers. There is no existing standardized dataset that maps Vedic standards to advanced physiological reactions or physiotherapy results. Moreover, the ethical suggestions are significant. Ensuring that the AI's translations of Vedic scriptures are exact, respectful, and free from misrepresentation is foremost. The potential for misapplication or distortion of antiquated shrewdness, or generating exhortation that's not evidence-based from a present day scientific perspective, must be thoroughly mitigated. Approval and clinical viability are too basic. Any generative yield from the AI, particularly concerning wellbeing proposals, would require rigid clinical trials and master oversight to guarantee security and viability. Regulatory systems would have to be advance to suit such novel AI-driven, intrigue healthcare arrangements. At last, user acknowledgment and openness will be key. Patients and healthcare suppliers alike must be taught on the system's capabilities and impediments, cultivating believe and encouraging consistent integration into existing clinical workflows. The complexity of the system also raises questions approximately its evenhanded get to over different financial foundations. The concept of a Generative Artificial Intelligence and Vedic Scripture Empowered Physiotherapy Management Framework stands at the energizing wilderness of healthcare development. By synergistically mixing the creative control of progressed AI with the immortal, all encompassing wisdom of Vedic traditions, it holds the guarantee of introducing in a time of really personalized, socially touchy, and comprehensive restoration. Whereas the specialized, moral, and clinical obstacles are significant, the potential for reclassifying understanding care by tending to wellbeing not fair as a physical state but as a holistic adjust of existence makes this a compelling and significantly significant range for future investigation and advancement within the advanced age of medicine, especially in regions like India where both the ancient intelligence and the modern technological ability coexist.

II. LITERATURE REVIEW

Zhang et al. (2022) gives a comprehensive survey of Explainable Artificial Intelligence (XAI) applications inside cybersecurity. It highlights that whereas AI and Machine Learning (ML) have altogether progressed cyber defense instruments, progressing discovery and reaction against advancing dangers, numerous AI models work as “black boxes.” This need of transparency undermines client believe and hampers security experts' capacity to get it and confirm AI-driven choices, particularly in basic security assignments like intrusion discovery, malware investigation, and spam sifting. The authors emphasize the need of integrating XAI into cybersecurity models to cultivate transparency and interpretability whereas keeping up tall precision. They contend that XAI arrangements offer human-friendly clarifications for complex AI choices, permitting security experts to comprehend, believe, and effectively oversee next-generation cyber defense frameworks. The survey categorizes XAI strategies, talks about existing challenges (like data predisposition and the trade-off between exactness and explainability), and recognizes inquire about holes, focusing the significance of creating strong XAI systems for a more reliable and productive cybersecurity scene. Roppelt, Kanbach, and Kraus (2023) conducted a systematic writing audit to recognize components affecting Artificial Intelligence (AI) selection in healthcare teach. Recognizing the fracture of existing investigate in spite of AI's promising potential to address challenges like maturing populaces and inveterate illnesses, their survey synthesized 130 studies to propose a comprehensive framework: the “Adoption of AI within the Healthcare Industry Model.” This demonstrate categorizes affecting components into five measurements. They contend that macro-economic, administrative, and innovative status serve as outside predecessors, forming the environment for AI adoption. Inside, organizational and person preparation are crucial antecedents. The authors emphasize that understanding these coordinates variables is crucial for both AI suppliers and healthcare teach, advertising practical direction to cultivate AI appropriation and use its esteem in healthcare for a more economical and productive future. Aldoseri et al. (2023) examines the significant part of information within the victory of Artificial Intelligence (AI) applications over different businesses, counting healthcare, finance, and transportation. They emphasize that whereas AI thrives on large datasets, the successful utilization of this information presents various challenges. The authors altogether survey these challenges, categorizing them into key zones: information quality (accuracy, completeness, timeliness, integrity, relevance), information volume, security and security, bias and fairness, interpretability and explainability, moral concerns, and the accessibility of specialized ability and abilities. For each challenge, the paper delves into the specifics and offers proposals for organizations to address them. The center message is that for companies to really saddle the control of AI and gain a competitive advantage within the advanced age, an essential re-thinking of their information techniques and integration approaches is basic. This includes proactive measures in information administration, quality control, and moral considerations. Hirani et al. (2024) offers a comprehensive investigation of Artificial Intelligence (AI) in healthcare, following its historical advancement, current developments, and future potential. The paper highlights AI's transformative part in improving clinical decision-making and operational effectiveness, leveraging advances like machine learning, deep learning, characteristic language processing, and mechanical mechanization. The authors detail AI's current applications over different healthcare domains, including accuracy pharmaceutical, drug development, restorative imaging and diagnostics, and open wellbeing activities like immunization. They too discuss how the COVID-19 widespread quickened AI's appropriation in telemedicine and chatbots, progressing openness and medical instruction. Urgently, the review addresses the significant ethical and societal considerations going with AI's extension, especially concerning data utilization, patient protection, and the potential to exacerbate wellbeing disparities. The paper emphasizes the require for advancing rules to administer AI's application, supporting for its dependable improvement to advance understanding security, openness, and inclusivity in healthcare. Bowers and Cheer (2017) investigate the developing phenomenon of yoga tourism, centering on its commodification and Western embrace of what originated as an Eastern spiritual practice. They recognize the expanding worldwide popularity of yoga, especially its integration into wellness tourism, yet raise basic questions around its change from a significant spiritual discipline to a marketable product. The authors examine how the commercialization of yoga, particularly in Western settings, frequently leads to a de-emphasis or dilution of its otherworldly and transformative principles, moving center towards physical wellbeing, wellness, and wellness. They highlight the paradox of this broad acceptance, where the fundamental Sanskrit meaning of "union" is frequently overshadowed by consumerism. The paper investigates the inherent pressures between keeping up yoga's deep conventional roots and its advancement into modern shapes for broader purposes, prompting discourses around social assignment and the secularization of sacred practices inside the tourism industry. Martins et al. (2025) investigate the transdisciplinary crossing point of awareness, otherworldly existence, physics, and healing, proposing a worldview move in understanding restorative practices. The paper extends on past work concerning integrator medication, pointing to highlight the pivotal part of awareness and spirituality in both the physical world and recuperating forms. The authors examine classical recuperating strategies, particularly referencing the therapeutic effectiveness of Chinese pharmaceutical for different illnesses. They also dig into modern recuperating phenomena, such as "spontaneous healing," exemplified by Sister Bernardette Moriau, which resists ordinary restorative clarification. The paper presents concepts like morphogenic areas as a potential component to clarify the viability of Chinese medication and investigates modified states of awareness as a conceivable clarification for "spontaneous healing." Ultimately, it interfaces the concept of biofields with a proposed modern mending worldview established within the integrator medication demonstrate, proposing a more profound exchange between intellect, matter, and mending results. Charnysh et al. (2024) explored the impact of workplace genetic testing (wGT) on employee health behaviors and healthcare utilization inside a large US healthcare framework. The inquire about pointed to get it the wellbeing implications of wGT, which is frequently advertised as a wellness advantage covering risks for cancer, heart disease, and pharmacogenomics (PGx). Analyzing overview reactions from workers who received wGT comes about, the study found that people accepting "increased risk" (IR) comes about for cancer and/or heart infection showed essentially higher rates of wellbeing behavior changes (e.g., diet, exercise) and expanded healthcare utilization (e.g., seeking restorative follow-up). Specifically, those with IR comes about were 3.23 times more likely to alter health behaviors and 8.60 times more likely to extend healthcare utilization. Enlightening PGx comes about were also related with medicine changes. The discoveries propose that wGT can successfully prompt employees to require proactive steps towards their wellbeing, contributing to the understanding of the ethical and social measurements of such workplace wellness activities.

III. GENERATIVE ARTIFICIAL INTELLIGENCE IN HEALTHCARE

Healthcare is seeing critical progressions in generative artificial intelligence (AI), which is changing a few aspects of the industry. The appearance of Generative Artificial Intelligence (AI) marks a essential minute in the advancement of healthcare, promising to revolutionize about every feature of the industry, from medicate disclosure and personalized medicine to diagnostics, operational efficiency, and understanding engagement (Sharma et al., 2025a). Unlike conventional AI frameworks that basically analyze and classify existing information, generative models have the remarkable capacity to form novel, reasonable yields, be it content, images, atomic structures, or indeed simulated persistent scenarios. This transformative capability is presently being harnessed to address a few of healthcare's most complex and tireless challenges, driven by advancements in designs like Generative Adversarial Networks (GANs), Variational Autoencoders (VAEs), and especially Large Language Models (LLMs) such as the Generative Pre-trained Transformer (GPT) series. One of the foremost significant impacts of Generative AI is being felt in drug revelation and advancement, customarily a protracted, cosmically costly, and frequently uncertain handle. Generative AI can quicken this by independently planning novel atomic structures with desired helpful properties. By learning from endless datasets of chemical compounds, biological targets, and clinical results, these AI models can foresee how a potential drug will associated with organic frameworks, optimize its adequacy, and indeed distinguish potential side impacts before expensive research facility synthesis begins. For occasion, generative models are being utilized for de novo drug design, making entirely modern particles from scratch, or for lead optimization, refining existing candidates to upgrade their execution and security profiles. They can also encourage medicate repurposing by recognizing novel applications for existing, endorsed compounds, significantly decreasing improvement timelines and costs (R. Rawat et al., 2025b). Companies are leveraging generative AI to predict drug-target intelligent with high accuracy, recognize promising biomarkers for illness movement or treatment reaction, and indeed simulate preclinical trials with engineered information, vastly streamlining the early stages of pharmaceutical inquire about. This increasing speed is significant for handling infections with high unmet needs, counting uncommon infections and certain types of cancer, where traditional revelation strategies are regularly as well slow or resource-intensive. In the realm of personalized medication and treatment arranging, Generative AI is clearing the way for genuinely individualized patient care. By analyzing broad datasets including a patient's genetic information, electronic health records (EHRs), lifestyle components, medical images, and indeed real-time wearable gadget information, generative AI can make highly tailored treatment plans. For oncology patients, this seem mean an AI framework creating a customized immunotherapy regimen based on the interesting genetic transformations of their tumor. In unremitting disease administration, AI can give personalized suggestions for way of life alterations, medicine adherence, and early mediation techniques, continuously adjusting as the patient's condition advances. Past producing treatment conventions, generative AI can moreover create personalized instructive substance for patients, clarifying complex restorative conditions and treatment alternatives in an understandable language, in this way enabling them to require a more dynamic part in their claim health management (Kohli & Sharma, 2025b). The ability to generate realistic 3D models of understanding anatomy from imaging data assist changes surgical arranging and preparing, allowing surgeons to practice complex strategies in a risk-free virtual environment and anticipate potential complications some time recently real surgery, driving to more secure and more successful results. Medical imaging and diagnostics are too experiencing a significant change with Generative AI. These models can upgrade the quality of medical checks (e.g., X-rays, MRIs, CT checks) by generating missing data, diminishing noise, or changing over low-resolution images into high-resolution ones, subsequently improving demonstrative accuracy. Generative AI can robotize the location of abnormalities, segment organs and injuries, and indeed anticipate pathological conditions by analyzing inconspicuous designs in medical pictures that can be intangible to the human eye. This not as it were upgrades diagnostic exactness but too essentially decreases the workload for radiologists and pathologists, permitting them to center on more complex cases. The capacity to generate synthetic images of rare conditions or assorted patient populations can too expand preparing datasets for other AI models, progressing their strength and generalizability without compromising understanding protection. The era of synthetic data is an especially capable application of Generative AI in healthcare. Real-world patient information is regularly rare, particularly for rare diseases, and its utilize is intensely confined by security directions like HIPAA and GDPR. Generative AI can make synthetic patient information that mimics the factual properties and complexities of real information but contains no actual patient data (Dangi et al., 2025b). This engineered information can then be utilized for preparing modern AI models, developing and testing hypotheses, simulating clinical trials, and conducting research, all without the security concerns related with real understanding information. This quickens inquire about and advancement, fosters development, and democratizes access to valuable datasets for analysts and designers. Beyond coordinate clinical applications, Generative AI is also essentially improving operational effectiveness and organization inside healthcare frameworks. It can automate mundane however time-consuming assignments such as restorative coding, earlier authorization demands, claims handling, and appointment planning. By summarizing unstructured clinical documentation from EHRs, producing draft clinical notes from physician-patient discussions (with consent), and streamlining medical report generation, Generative AI can ease the administrative burden on healthcare experts, decreasing clinician burnout and freeing up more time for direct patient care. In contact centers, AI-powered virtual wellbeing associates can handle routine patient questions, give fundamental wellbeing data, and direct patients through authoritative forms, improving understanding fulfillment and operational stream. In spite of these immense openings, the widespread selection of Generative AI in healthcare is went with by significant challenges and ethical considerations. A primary concern is information quality and predisposition. Generative AI models are as it were as great as the information they are prepared on. In case the preparing information contains inherent biases (e.g., underrepresentation of certain demographic groups or skewed medical results from particular populations), the AI may perpetuate or indeed open up these inclinations in its produced yields, driving to inaccurate analyze or inequitable treatment suggestions for certain quiet groups. Ensuring interpretability and transparency is another jump. Numerous generative AI models are "black boxes," meaning their decision-making forms are murky. In healthcare, where choices can have life-or-death results, clinicians need to get it why an AI generated a specific suggestion to guarantee believe and responsibility. Regulatory and legal systems are still advancing to capture up with the quick headways in Generative AI. Clear rules are required for the validation, arrangement, and ongoing checking of AI as a medical device or demonstrative instrument. Questions of obligation, obligation, and mental property for AI-generated substance too need to be tended to. Patient protection and information security remain foremost. Whereas synthetic data offers an arrangement, the handling of genuine patient information for preparing purposes requires strong cybersecurity measures and strict adherence to protection controls. The potential for malicious utilize, such as producing deepfakes of medical experts or fabricating medical records, moreover poses a critical hazard. At last, the integration into existing clinical workflows can be challenging. Healthcare frameworks are complex, and introducing unused AI apparatuses requires careful arranging, preparing, and a change administration technique to guarantee seamless appropriation by healthcare suppliers and patients alike. There's moreover the chance of depersonalization of care on the off chance that AI totally replaces human interaction in certain viewpoints, possibly disintegrating the significant patient-provider relationship. Looking ahead, the future of Generative AI in healthcare is balanced for proceeded exponential development. We are able expect the improvement of more advanced multimodal AI models able of joining and creating experiences from different information sorts (text, images, genomics, real-time physiological signals) at the same time, driving to indeed more comprehensive and exact applications. Expanded center on ethical AI governance, explainable AI (XAI), and bias mitigation strategies will be significant to building believe and ensuring impartial results. Collaborations between AI engineers, clinicians, ethicists, and policymakers will be basic to explore the complex scene and establish responsible sending procedures. As Generative AI develops, it guarantees to not as it were improve clinical decision-making, quicken investigate, and streamline operations but too fundamentally rethink the quiet involvement, making healthcare more available, personalized, and proactive. The travel is still in its early stages, but the transformative potential of Generative AI to progress human wellbeing on a worldwide scale is verifiable, speaking to one of the foremost energizing frontiers in medical science within the 21st century. Among the most zones of utilize are:

- Medicate improvement and revelation: Generative AI models are able to assess colossal datasets in arrange to discover conceivable medicate candidates, figure their viability, and optimize their chemical structure. This speeds up the discharge of novel medicines onto the showcase.
- Personalized medication: By analyzing hereditary information, medical histories, and way of life factors, AI helps within the creation of individual-

ized treatment regimens. This makes it conceivable to supply more patient-specific, more successful treatments.

- Therapeutic imaging: Generative AI calculations can move forward restorative picture preparing to produce high-quality pictures or find anomalies, thus upgrading the recognizable proof and determination of illnesses such as cancer, cardiovascular illnesses, and neurological clutters.
- Clinical choice support: AI advances can help therapeutic professionals in making way better choices by anticipating quiet results, assessing clinical information, and advertising evidence-based recommendations.
- Persistent instruction and engagement: By creating instructive materials and wellbeing exhortation that are particularly customized to a patient's affliction, generative AI can progress quiet engagement and adherence to treatment plans.
- Virtual restorative associates: Chatbots and virtual collaborators driven by fake insights (AI) can offer patients round-the-clock help by settling health-related request, setting up arrangements, and reminding patients to require their drugs.
- Prescient analytics: Generative AI can estimate the event of infections, quiet hospitalizations, and other critical measurements by assessing past quiet information. This makes a difference healthcare organizations apportion assets as productively as conceivable
- Natural Language Processing (NLP): To produce insightful information and boost the effectiveness of healthcare documentation and research, generative AI may process and evaluate research papers, clinical notes, and patient records.

IV. VEDIC SCRIPTURE IN HEALTHCARE

The ancient Indian manuscripts known as Vedic traditions provide a comprehensive approach to health and well-being. Their emphasis on the unity of the mind, body, and spirit has influenced many traditional medical treatments, especially yoga and Ayurveda. Here are some essential characteristics of how Vedic concepts might be implemented in healthcare [Fig. 1]:

Figure 1. Vedic scriptures in healthcare

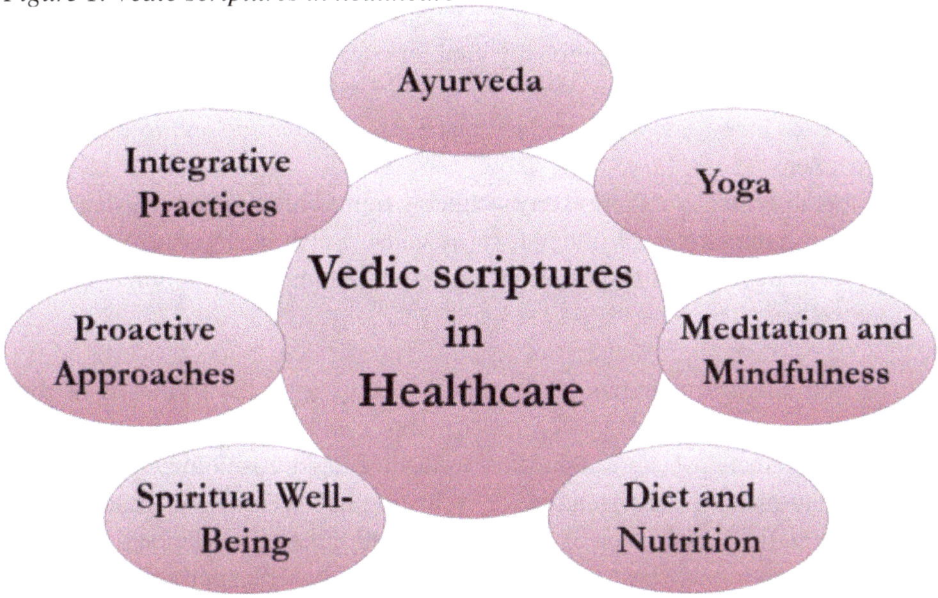

- Ayurveda: Ayurveda sees health as a state of equilibrium between the body, mind, and spirit and is based on Vedic texts. It places a strong emphasis on preventive care and natural remedies specific to each person's dosha (or constitution). Ayurvedic treatment is based on the use of natural ingredients and medicinal plants with the goal of promoting well-being and restoring balance. Based on Vedic lessons, suggestions for every day schedules (dinacharya) and regular schedules (ritucharya) emphasize living in agreement with the common world.
- Yoga: Combining stances, breathing works out, and reflection, yoga draws its philosophical roots from the Vedas and may be a implies to progress common wellbeing. Normal yoga hone increments mental clarity and passionate steadiness whereas bringing down push and uneasiness.
- Mindfulness and Meditation: Conventional Indian contemplation strategies cultivate passionate grit and mental clarity, both of which are basic for common well-being. Vedic practices energize self-reflection and mindfulness, which back mental wellbeing.
- Nutrition and Diet: Concurring to Vedic lessons, a sattvic (clean) count calories that emphasizes entirety, new nourishments is suggested in arrange to feed the body and intellect and advance more noteworthy vitality and clarity.

- Spiritual Well-Being: Agreeing to Vedic convictions, having a reason and a sense of association can improve both physical and mental wellbeing. Otherworldly hone is additionally vital for common wellbeing.
- Proactive approach: The Vedic perspective advances way of life choices that back long-term wellbeing and places an accentuation on avoidance over treatment.
- Integrative practice: Present day wellbeing frameworks are progressively recognizing the esteem of integrator medicines, which incorporate Vedic concepts nearby standard medication and empower a more all encompassing see of wellbeing.

The rich tapestry of Indian civilization is deeply joined with the significant experiences contained inside the Vedic scriptures, a endless corpus of old writings that expands remote past devout doctrine to include logic, cosmology, morals, and a remarkably modern understanding of wellbeing and well-being. Remote from being a insignificant collection of otherworldly songs, these foundational writings, nearby their subordinate branches, lay the basis for a holistic approach to life that intrinsically joins the person to the infinite arrange, seeing wellbeing not simply as the absence of illness but as a state of adjusted agreement over physical, mental, passionate, and otherworldly measurements. The impact of Vedic intelligence on conventional Indian healthcare frameworks, most eminently Ayurveda and Yoga, is evident and proceeds to offer important viewpoints for modern worldwide wellbeing challenges. At the heart of this old intelligence are the Vedas themselves – the Rigveda, Yajurveda, Samaveda, and Atharvaveda. Whereas the Rigveda, the oldest, fundamentally comprises of songs and supplications, it contains embryonic references to different maladies and restorative herbs, implying at early perceptions of human physiology and the mending properties of nature. The Atharvaveda, in specific, is frequently considered the most punctual store of medical information, highlighting numerous hymns devoted to recuperating different sicknesses, charms to ward off illnesses, and depictions of anatomical parts and essential surgical strategies. It subtle elements medications for fever, leprosy, dropsy, and indeed mental sicknesses, frequently intertwining magical and ritualistic components with what appear to be experimental perceptions of medicinal plants and their applications (Devgan et al., 2025b). These early Vedic texts emphasize a worldview where wellbeing is affected by both physical and non-physical variables, counting planetary positions, divine intercession, and the individual's karmic activities, establishing a psychosomatic approach to ailment that predates advanced understanding. Streaming from the Vedas, the Upanishads dive deeper into philosophical concepts, emphasizing the interconnecting of the person soul (Atman) with the universal consciousness (Brahman). This significant metaphysical understanding has coordinate suggestions for wellbeing, setting that genuine well-being emerges from a concordant relationship between the body, mind (Manas), intellect (Buddhi), and ego (Ahamkara), ultimately established in otherworldly liberation. Concepts like Prana (life force energy) are extensively discussed, seen as the imperative breath that quickens the body and intellect, and its adjusted flow is considered vital for wellbeing. Disturbances in Prana are linked to illness, laying a philosophical establishment for practices that control breath, such as Pranayama, to restore wellbeing. The Upanishadic emphasis on self-realization and mental tranquility specifically informs the stress-reduction and mindfulness techniques presently broadly recognized in cutting edge medicine. The foremost coordinate and comprehensive restorative framework stemming from Vedic information is Ayurveda, meaning "the science of life." Ayurveda is not just a framework of medication but a way of life, predicated on the rule that the universe, and by expansion the human body, is composed of five great elements or Panchamahabhutas: earth (Prithvi), water (Jala), fire (Agni), air (Vayu), and ether (Akasha). These elements combine to form the three fundamental psycho-physiological energies or Doshas: Vata (air and ether), Pitta (fire and water), and Kapha (earth and water). Every person has a unique constitutional outline, or Prakriti, determined by the predominant Doshas at the time of conception. Health is understood as a state of balance among these Doshas, whereas disease could be a result of their imbalance. Ayurvedic conclusion includes surveying a person's Prakriti, the state of their current Doshas (Vikriti), the strength of their Agni (digestive fire), the presence of Ama (toxins), and the health of their Dhatus (body tissues) and Mala (waste products). Ayurvedic healthcare interventions are highly personalized and point to reestablish Dosha balance. These incorporate:

- Ahara (Dietary Principles): Food is considered medicine. Ayurvedic dietetics centers on taste (Rasa), potency (Virya), post-digestive effect (Vipaka), and special properties (Prabhava) of foods, suggesting diets based on an individual's Prakriti and current imbalances. For case, a person with excess Pitta might be advised cooling, sweet, and bitter foods, whereas somebody with Vata imbalance might require warm, sleek, and establishing nourishments.
- Vihara (Lifestyle Routines): This encompasses Dinacharya (daily routines like waking time, oil massage, exercise, meditation) and Ritucharya (seasonal routines), designed to harmonize the body with natural cycles and prevent disease. These practices advance physical and mental hygiene, robust digestion, and stress decrease.
- Oushadhi (Herbal Medicine): Ayurveda utilizes a vast pharmacopoeia of single herbs and complex polyherbal formulations, carefully selected based on their energetic properties to balance specific Doshas and address disease

pathways. Examples incorporate Ashwagandha for stress, Turmeric for irritation, and Triphala for digestive wellbeing.

- Panchakarma (Detoxification Therapies): These five therapeutic procedures (Vamana, Virechana, Nasya, Basti, Raktamokshana) are designed for deep cleansing and rejuvenation, systematically eliminating accumulated toxins (Ama) from the body and restoring Dosha balance. They are highly individualized and performed under master supervision.

Integral to Vedic health reasoning is Yoga, meaning "union," signifying the integration of body, mind, and spirit. Originating in ancient India, though codified later by Patanjali within the Yoga Sutras, its roots are deeply implanted in Vedic thought. Yoga's contribution to healthcare is multifaceted:

- Asanas (Physical Postures): These exercises improve flexibility, strength, balance, and circulation, directly impacting musculoskeletal health and organ function.
- Pranayama (Breath Control Techniques): Regulating the breath is believed to directly influence the flow of Prana, calming the nervous system, reducing stress, and enhancing vital energy.
- Dhyana (Meditation): Meditation practices cultivate mental clarity, emotional regulation, and deep relaxation, significantly impacting mental health conditions like anxiety, depression, and stress-related disorders. It advances self-awareness and helps people detach from negative thought designs.
- Yama and Niyama (Ethical Disciplines): These moral and ethical guidelines foster positive social behavior and personal discipline, contributing to mental peace and overall well-being.

Beyond Ayurveda and Yoga, other subordinate Vedic sciences too contribute to wellbeing. Jyotisha (Vedic Astrology), for instance, gives insights into an individual's planetary impacts at birth, which are accepted to incline them to certain physical or mental qualities and vulnerabilities. Whereas not a direct medical framework, it can educate preventive methodologies and lifestyle choices to moderate potential imbalances. So also, Vastu Shastra (ancient Indian architecture) offers standards for planning living spaces that advance positive vitality flow and well-being, indirectly affecting health. The utilize of Mantra chanting and sound vibrations is additionally accepted to have therapeutic impacts, affecting mental states and energy areas inside the body. The holistic perspective is the overarching theme connecting all Vedic contributions to healthcare. It emphasizes the interconnectedness of all viewpoints of presence and recognizes that health isn't a fragmented state but a dynamic balance. Illness is seen as an expression of imbalance, regularly emerging from a disharmony between the person and their environment, their lifestyle choices, or indeed their spiritual arrangement. This comprehensive see energizes a proactive approach to health (Swasthavritta – the regimen for wellbeing) rather than merely reactive treatment of disease, focusing on prevention, self-care, and the development of inner harmony. Within the context of modern healthcare, Vedic scriptures and their derived systems like Ayurveda and Yoga are gaining expanding recognition, fundamentally as Complementary and Alternative Medicine (CAM). Their emphasis on preventive healthcare and wellness adjusts perfectly with contemporary public health objectives, offering non-pharmacological interventions for stress administration, constant disease anticipation, and generally lifestyle improvement. The concept of Prakriti in Ayurveda resonates strongly with the burgeoning field of personalized medicine, suggesting an exceedingly individualized approach to wellbeing that considers hereditary predispositions, environmental factors, and unique physiological responses. Research is increasingly exploring the efficacy of Ayurvedic herbs, yoga poses, and meditation techniques for different conditions, aiming to provide evidence-based approval for these ancient practices. However, integrating Vedic knowledge into mainstream modern healthcare presents challenges. The need of standardized research techniques, troubles in conducting randomized controlled trials for highly individualized Ayurvedic medicines, and the require for thorough scientific validation for particular claims are critical obstacles. There's moreover the challenge of bridging the conceptual hole between a holistic, energetic understanding of wellbeing and a reductionist, molecular-based biomedical demonstrate. Ethical considerations regarding the capability of practitioners, ensuring item quality in herbal medicines, and avoiding misinterpretation or commercial abuse of ancient shrewdness are foremost. In spite of these challenges, the persevering intelligence of Vedic scriptures offers invaluable experiences into the art and science of living a healthy, adjusted, and satisfying life. Their emphasis on natural remedies, personalized approaches, the mind-body association, and preventive strategies gives a rich asset that can profoundly improve and humanize modern healthcare, cultivating a more total and sustainable approach to global well-being.

V. PHYSIOTHERAPY MANAGEMENT SYSTEM

The reason of a PMS is to move forward and speed up the arrangement of physiotherapy administrations. It encourages more viable persistent care, arrangement planning, invoicing, and documentation administration for physiotherapists. These are the basic components and characteristics of a fruitful physiotherapy administration framework [Fig. 2]:

Figure 2. Components of PMS

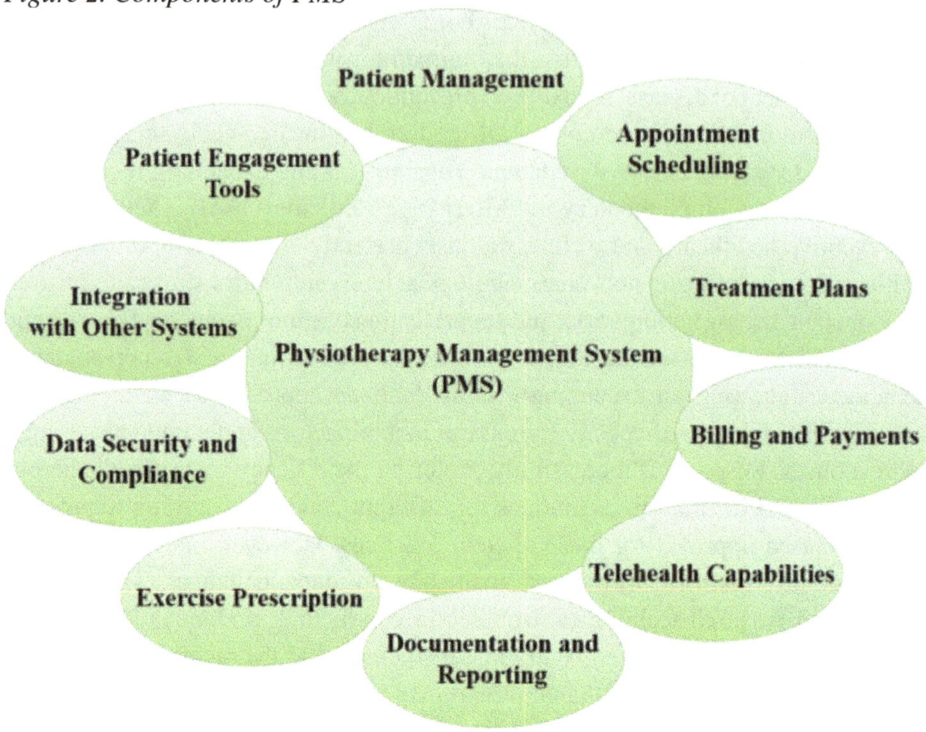

- Patient management: This incorporates keeping track of each patient's total Electronic Health Records (EHR), which incorporate their restorative history, treatment arrange, advance reports, and other points of interest. It comprises of computerized shapes for quiet enrollment and therapeutic history gathering in expansion to admissions shapes.
- Appointment Scheduling: This include empowers patients to plan arrangements online through online booking. In addition, it has calendar integration, which permits arrangements to be synchronized with person calendars and to trigger mail or SMS updates naturally.
- Treatment Plans: These are made up of editable, standardized treatment formats that can be customized to meet the necessities of particular patients. This incorporates advance following, which records a patient's headway over time utilizing reports and visual charts.
- Billing and Payments: This segment covers protections administration, which is vital to viably handle claims and oversee quiet protections information. This incorporates the capacity to charge, create receipts and solicitations, and acknowledge an assortment of installment choices.

- Telehealth Capabilities: Offers video conferencing alternatives for inaccessible interviews through virtual meetings. licenses the utilize of computerized instruments and programs for inaccessible observing to take after a patient's improvement.
- Documentation and reporting: Subjective, Objective, Evaluation, and Arranging (Cleanser) notes are made and put away for each session as portion of the documentation and detailing handle. Reports on quiet results, participation, and the adequacy of treatment can be created utilizing announcing frameworks.
- Exercise Prescription: This include comprises of a work out library with recordings and enlightening that patients can be doled out to perform. Furthermore, it grants the creation of personalized domestic workout regimens that patients can follow to in between sessions.
- Data Security and Compliance: Guarantees that understanding information is put away securely which the framework adjusts with healthcare enactment. This incorporates HIPAA compliance. This includes overseeing client authorizations through client access control to defend private information.
- Integration with other systems: This alludes to the capacity to consistently trade information and give way better quiet care by coordination with other wellbeing frameworks (such as EHRs).
- Patient engagement tools: One such device is the understanding entry, an extraordinary site where patients may make arrangements, see their restorative data, and get in touch with physiotherapists. In arrange to raise the caliber of administrations, it too features a criticism framework for gathering understanding input.

The utilize of a PMS has various points of interest and components to require under consideration. When utilized accurately, a PMS can incredibly increment your physical treatment practice's operational adequacy whereas moreover improving understanding care and treatment comes about:

- Enhanced productivity: By automating administrative duties, physical therapists can concentrate more on treating patients.
- Better patient experience: Patients benefit from easier access and better communication thanks to streamlined procedures.
- Higher quality of care: Providing individualized care is made possible by accurately monitoring patient progress and treatment results.
- Better financial management: Better revenue cycle management is the result of more effective billing and insurance processing.

- User training: Ensure that your staff members are properly taught to operate the system.
- Customization: Select a framework that will be custom-made to your practice's interesting necessities.
- Technical support: Having get to tried and true client benefit is significant for instantly settling any issues.

The advancing scene of healthcare within the 21st century, especially inside rehabilitation sciences, increasingly requires advanced advanced arrangements to optimize quiet care, streamline regulatory forms, and upgrade clinical results. At the forefront of this advanced change lies the Physiotherapy Management System (PMS), a comprehensive program stage designed to manage the multifaceted operations of a physiotherapy clinic or office. Far from being a mere planning device, a modern PMS coordinating a wide cluster of functionalities that support each arrange of the patient travel, from starting contact and appraisal to treatment conveyance, advance checking, charging, and long-term follow-up. Its execution is vital for improving effectiveness, data accuracy, patient engagement, and eventually, the quality of physiotherapy administrations delivered. At its center, a robust PMS centralizes basic persistent and operational information, disposing of the inefficiencies and errors related with paper-based records or different advanced frameworks (Devliyal et al., 2025b). A foundational component is Patient Registration and Demographics, which captures fundamental data such as individual details, contact data, insurance specifics, and referral sources. This module guarantees that every patient's section into the framework is smooth and accurate, making a unique identifier for longitudinal following. Seamlessly coordinates with this is Appointment Scheduling and Management, a sophisticated highlight that permits clinics to effectively oversee specialist plans, book arrangements, send automated updates (via SMS or e-mail), and handle rescheduling or cancellations. This decreases no-shows, optimizes clinic capacity, and upgrades the patient involvement by giving comfort and convenient communication. The backbone of any effective PMS is its Electronic Health Records (EHR) / Electronic Medical Records (EMR) for Physiotherapy. This module digitizes and organizes all clinical documentation, counting detailed understanding histories, chief complaints, current medicines, allergies, and past restorative records. Crucially, it gives specialized areas for Assessment and Diagnosis Tools unique to physiotherapy. This incorporates standardized shapes for objective evaluations (e.g., extend of motion measurements, muscle strength tests, pain scales, utilitarian outcome measures like WOMAC or Oswestry Disability Index), postural examination, neurological assessments, and extraordinary tests. Specialists can input discoveries, create differential analyze, and report their clinical thinking specifically inside the framework, guaranteeing comprehensive and neat records that are effectively available and auditable. Building upon the evaluation information, the PMS facilitates comprehensive Treatment Planning and Protocol Management. Based on the diagnosis and individualized patient needs, advisors can make detailed treatment plans, outlining particular interventions, exercise medicines, manual treatment methods, modalities to be utilized, and the recurrence and term of treatment sessions. Many advanced systems permit for the capacity of pre-defined treatment conventions for common conditions, which can then be customized for each patient, saving valuable time whereas guaranteeing consistency and adherence to best practices (D. Rawat et al., 2025b). As therapy advances, the Progress Tracking and Outcome Measurement module gets to be imperative. Therapists can frequently record patient advance utilizing follow-up evaluations, visual helps (e.g., photo/video comparison), and re-administration of result measures. The framework then automatically produces charts and reports outlining advance over time, giving objective prove of treatment adequacy for both the clinician and the persistent, and helping in clinical decision-making with respect to release or adjustment of the arrange. Beyond direct persistent care, a PMS essentially optimizes the administrative and financial aspects of a physiotherapy practice. Billing and Invoicing capabilities mechanize the era of bills, coordinated with insurance suppliers for coordinate claims submission, track installments, and oversee accounts receivable. This reduces administrative overhead, minimizes charging errors, and quickens income cycles. Comprehensive Reporting and Analytics functionalities give clinic owners and administrators with valuable insights into different operational measurements. These reports can incorporate patient demographics, referral designs, advisor caseloads, treatment results, financial execution, and arrangement patterns. Such data-driven insights are indispensable for strategic arranging, identifying areas for enhancement, assessing showcasing effectiveness, and guaranteeing clinic benefit. Effective communication is foremost in healthcare, and a modern PMS regularly incorporates robust Communication Tools. A Patient Portal engages patients to access their arrangement plans, see their treatment plans, review instructive materials, and indeed communicate safely with their specialists. Secure messaging highlights enable encrypted communication between advisors, referring doctors, and other healthcare suppliers, cultivating a collaborative care environment whereas ensuring patient data privacy. For clinics that offer supportive devices, braces, or other related items, Inventory Management inside the PMS makes a difference track stock levels, manage procurement, and monitor sales, guaranteeing that fundamental supplies are continuously accessible. Referral Management streamlines the method of accepting and recognizing referrals from specialists, specialists, or other healthcare offices, encouraging smooth moves of care and strengthening professional systems. The rapid advancements in innovation have extended the scope of PMS to incorporate specialized functionalities that upgrade patient care delivery.

Tele-rehabilitation Integration has ended up especially basic, particularly within the post-pandemic time, enabling advisors to conduct virtual discussions, evaluate patients remotely, and direct them through works out via video conferencing. This amplifies access to care, especially for patients in remote areas or those with versatility confinements. Besides, integration with committed Exercise Prescription Software allows specialists to generate personalized work out programs with detailed instructions, recordings, and progression rules, which can be shared specifically with patients through the patient entrance or a committed app, upgrading adherence and self-management. Ensuring Compliance and Regulatory Adherence, particularly with protection controls like HIPAA (globally recognized standards) or India's upcoming Data Protection Act, and billing controls, is another basic aspect of a modern PMS, giving audit trails and secure information taking care of. The benefits of executing a comprehensive PMS are far-reaching and affect all partners. For patients, it implies improved access to care, greater comfort through online planning and updates, improved understanding of their condition and treatment via patient entrances, and eventually, way better clinical results due to steady and personalized care. For physiotherapists, a PMS diminishes authoritative burden, freeing up more time for direct quiet interaction and clinical thinking. It gives prompt access to total persistent histories, helps in exact documentation, supports evidence-based hone through result following, and encourages inter-professional communication. For clinic owners and chairmen, it interprets into expanded operational effectiveness, optimized asset utilization, decreased authoritative costs, improved income cycle administration, valuable commerce insights through analytics, and improved patient fulfillment, driving to a stronger notoriety and development. Looking towards the future Physiotherapy Management Systems are set to advance dramatically, driven by developing innovations and a greater accentuation on personalized, predictive, and preventive care. Greater AI and Machine Learning Integration will be a significant trend. AI algorithms seem analyze vast sums of patient information to foresee treatment results, identify patients at risk of poor adherence, or indeed suggest ideal treatment pathways based on similar persistent profiles. Generative AI, as discussed already, could personalize exercise plans with unparalleled exactness, making energetic schedules that adjust in real-time to a patient's advance and indeed emotional state. Enhanced Tele-rehabilitation Capabilities will incorporate more advanced remote monitoring utilizing wearable sensors that track development, posture, and physiological parameters, giving advisors with objective information indeed when patients are not within the clinic. The integration of Wearable Innovation and IoT (Internet of Things) gadgets will become consistent, allowing PMS to collect persistent, real-time information on quiet movement levels, rest designs, run of movement, and work out adherence, giving a more holistic see of a patient's everyday life and how it impacts their recovery. Virtual Reality (VR) and Augmented Reality (AR) are poised to convert therapy delivery, making works out more engaging, interactive, and gamified. VR situations can recreate real-world challenges for adjust and gait preparing, whereas AR can overlay digital enlightening or criticism onto a patient's physical developments. Predictive Analytics for Treatment Results will move past straightforward following to estimating, permitting therapists to intercede proactively if a patient's advance deviates from anticipated directions. Moreover, concepts like Blockchain for Data Security and Interoperability may revolutionize how understanding information is safely shared over diverse healthcare providers, upgrading care coordination whereas keeping up robust security. Finally, future PMS will put an indeed greater center on quiet engagement and self-management, giving more intuitive interfacing, gamified approaches, and AI-driven coaching devices to enable patients to require a driving part in their claim recovery travel, amplifying the reach of care past the clinic dividers. Physiotherapy Management System is not an extravagance but an indispensable apparatus for cutting edge physiotherapy practices. As technology proceeds its relentless march forward, PMS will progressively incorporate advanced AI, remote observing, and immersive helpful advances, fundamentally reshaping how physiotherapy is delivered, making it more personalized, accessible, and effective for patients across the globe.

VI. PROPOSED METHODOLOGY

The proposed calculation for a PMS utilizing GAI and Vedic sacred writings contains a few key components. The calculation ought to coordinated quiet information, treatment suggestions, and the by and large standards of Vedic sacred texts to guarantee personalized care. The proposed model consists of the following phases: The input phase consists of patient data collection such as demographic information (age, gender, etc.), medical history (past injuries, surgeries, chronic diseases), assessment of current health status (symptoms, pain levels), and lifestyle factors (diet, exercise, stress levels) are recorded. The next stage is the Vedic assessment, where the patient's dosha (Vata, Pitta, Kapha) is determined using a questionnaire. At this stage, mental and spiritual well-being is also assessed (meditation practices, stress levels). The next phase is the data processing phase. In the data pre-processing phase, data is cleaned and normalized to ensure consistency, and categorical variables (e.g. dosha type) are encoded for the machine learning model. The feature extraction phase identifies key features that influence treatment outcome (age, health status, dosha). Additional features are generated based on historical data and treatment response. In the treatment recommendation phase, the generative model training uses past patient data to train a generative model (e.g., neural network), which includes treatment outcomes related to different doshas and diseases. In the recommendation generation phase, the processed data is fed into the trained model for the new patient. It generates a personalized treatment plan that includes physiotherapy exercises, duration and frequency of sessions, home exercise recommendations, and Vedic practices (e.g., yoga, meditation, dietary suggestions). In the progress tracking phase, monitoring and feedback is performed to collect continuous patient feedback after treatment (pain levels, improvement in mobility). It integrates the patient's self-assessment of dosha and mental health. Dynamic Adjustment uses feedback to continually refine treatment recommendations. Reassess dosha balance based on changes in the patient's condition. Reporting and Analysis stage analyzes the effectiveness of treatment using data analytics (success rate, patient satisfaction, etc.). Generates a report for the physiotherapist to review and discuss with the patient. Holistic insights include insights from the Vedic scriptures regarding overall health and well-being, emphasizing the connection between physical and mental health.

The following is the proposed model Pseudocode:

```
function PhysiotherapyManagementSystem(patientData):
//Phase I
patientProfile = CollectPatientData()
doshaProfile = AssessVedicFactors(patientProfile)
// Phase II
cleanedData = PreprocessData(patientProfile)
features = ExtractFeatures(cleanedData, doshaProfile)
// Phase III
model = TrainGenerativeModel(historicalData)
treatmentPlan = GenerateTreatmentPlan(model, features)
// Phase IV
while patientIsActive:
feedback = CollectPatientFeedback()
UpdatePatientProfile(feedback)
AdjustTreatmentPlan(treatmentPlan, feedback)
// Phase V
outcomeReport = AnalyzeOutcomes(treatmentPlan)
Return outcomeReport
```

VII. RESULT ANALYSIS AND DISCUSSION

Analysis of the results of the proposed PMS using GAI and Vedic scriptures included evaluation of various indicators regarding patient outcomes, system performance and overall effectiveness. To measure clinical efficacy, the following parameters were evaluated: Symptom improvement was measured by pain reduction, improvement in mobility and general health status before and after treatment. Functional assessment used standardized tools (e.g. SF-36, Oswestry Disability Index) to evaluate improvement in activities of daily living. Adherence to the treatment plan was assessed using exercise compliance to track patient adherence to the prescribed home exercise program and Vedic practices (e.g. yoga, meditation). Follow-up rate analyzed patient follow-up appointment rates and adherence to treatment plans. Quality of life was assessed using patient satisfaction surveys and feedback on overall treatment experience, including holistic practice integration. Vedic well-being assessment assessed changes in mental and emotional health using subjective measures such as stress and happiness surveys. Algorithm accuracy evaluates how accurately the GAI model predicts effective treatment plans based on patient data. Outcome correlation analyzes the correlation between the created treatment plans and actual patient outcomes to determine effectiveness. Processing efficiency measures the time it takes from entering patient information to creating an individualized treatment plan. Data processing speed represents the assessed speed of data processing and analysis, minimizing delays in patient care. User experience focuses on interface and functionality and is measured through a usability evaluation to gather feedback from healthcare professionals on the ease of use of the PMS. Requirements for training assess how much time employees need to spend learning how to utilize the system efficiently. The overall insights measure the frequency with which patients apply Vedic aspects like meditation and dietary adjustments, thereby integrating Vedic principles with patient engagement. Culture Sensitivity evaluated patient input on the relevance and acceptability of Vedic principles in treatment. Utilizing longitudinal wellbeing following, one may evaluate the long-term adequacy of joining Vedic and GAI strategies by observing changes in patients' wellbeing over time. Populace Wellbeing Experiences looks at combined information to spot designs in wellbeing results concurring to different dosha sorts and helpful approaches. A comprehensive appraisal of understanding results, framework execution, and the consolidation of Vedic standards ought to be the most targets of a result investigation of a physiotherapy administration framework built on generative manufactured insights and Vedic sacred writings. Healthcare specialists will be able to distinguish the system's qualities and regions for advancement by measuring the clinical viability, client fulfillment, and precision of AI-driven suggestions. This will offer assistance to guarantee that the framework provides meaningful, high-quality care that's in line with both ordinary and present day restorative hones. This careful examination not as it were affirms your system's viability but moreover offers proposals for assist improvement and upgrade.

VIII. ADVANTAGES

There are a few preferences to joining GAI and Vedic principles into a PMS for physical treatment, which upgrade understanding care and operational viability:

- Treatment regimens: These are particularly custom-made to each patient's needs, inclinations, and advance can be recommended utilizing generative AI, which can assess persistent information. Employing all encompassing Vedic approach to tailor a technique that considers the patient's physical, mental, and otherworldly well-being is another way to form utilize of Vedic thoughts.
- Upgraded persistent engagement: GAI may deliver updates, guidelines materials, and personalized informing for patients, keeping them educated and included. Advisors can progress understanding adherence by advancing mindfulness and all encompassing hone through the application of concepts from Vedic writings.
- Successful investigation and documentation: Helps within the programmed note-generation prepare. GAI can give total Cleanser notes and treatment rundowns, diminishing the documentation burden. Counting Vedic lessons gives quiet evaluations more noteworthy setting, which empowers more in-depth recording and examination.
- Telehealth and inaccessible checking: Based on understanding input and information, GAI may offer real-time appraisals and suggestions, as well as virtual meetings. Consolidating breathing works out and reflection, two Vedic conventions, into telemedicine sessions can bolster mental wellbeing in expansion to physical treatment.
- Information analytics: Utilizing information bits of knowledge, GAI can look at persistent movement patterns and prescribe changes to treatment approaches. Physical advisors can superior identify non-physical components impacting restoration by centering on the mind-body connect. GAI's result expectation instrument helps therapists in making well-informed treatment choices by utilizing past information to estimate persistent results. Avoidance is emphasized in Vedic lessons. By incorporating these discoveries, proactive understanding care strategies can be coordinated.
- Superior quiet instruction: Contributes to the advancement of energetic substance. GAI creates instructive assets that are customized to each patient's needs in arrange to progress comprehension of their condition. By conferring thoughts from the Vedic compositions, patients are able to see wellbeing from a more extensive point and are empowered to seek after all encompassing wellness.

- Streamlined authoritative strategies: GAI increments operational effectiveness by streamlining the charging and planning methods. Joining Vedic concepts gives a more patient-centric climate and moves forward the in general understanding encounter
- Combining conventional information with modern innovation: Combining advanced AI with age-old Vedic information comes about in a particular care system that respects both customary and present day helpful modalities. Vedic concepts can upgrade the system's social competency and increment its appropriateness to different persistent populaces.

IX. CHALLENGES

Whereas joining Vedic texts and GAI into a PMS has various advantages, there are downsides as well.

- Private data almost patients: Dealing with private wellbeing data brings up issues with protection and following to laws like HIPAA.
- Cybersecurity dangers: It's pivotal to create beyond any doubt frameworks are protected against interruptions and illicit access.
- Algorithmic predisposition: GAI systems may display inclinations characteristic within the preparing set, which might lead to proposals for treatment that are not evenhanded for certain quiet populaces.
- Reliance on information quality: The completeness and quality of the information utilized to prepare GAI have a critical affect on its adequacy.
- Compatibility with other systems: There can be specialized troubles and a got to make significant changes to current strategies when incorporating GAI and Vedic concepts into an already-existing PMS.
- Interoperability: It can be troublesome to form beyond any doubt the modern framework can associated with other healthcare innovation in a productive way.
- Information of Vedic standards: A few therapeutic professionals may not be acquainted with or open to actualizing Vedic ideas, which seem lead to resistance.
- Acknowledgment by patients: Persistent interest is affected by patients' skepticism around combining routine information with modern innovations.
- Staff instruction: To function the modern framework efficiently, healthcare professionals may have to be total preparing, especially within the zones of AI apparatuses and Vedic concepts.

- Continuing instruction: In arrange to remain current with advancements in all encompassing hones and AI innovation, proceeding instruction is fundamental.
- Non-compliance: It can be troublesome and time-consuming to explore the regulatory landscape for both fake insights and ordinary strategies.
- Moral suggestions: It is essential to supply clarification on issues relating to the ethical application of AI in healthcare, especially the decision-making handle.
- Monetary speculation: A complex PMS that coordinating Vedic principles with GAI may require a sizable whole of cash to create and actualize.
- Return on speculation: It can be challenging to gage a system's adequacy and ROI, especially in its early stages. Keeping up the human component of physiotherapy whereas consolidating AI arrangements is fundamental for building understanding associations and believe.

X. FUTURE PERSPECTIVES

Energizing openings lie ahead for PMS that utilize Vedic thoughts and GAI. This combination has the control to alter persistent care, operational adequacy, and common wellbeing as healthcare changes. Imperative lessons for long-standing time incorporate:

- Custom fitted treatment plans: GAI is still refining its capacity to utilize huge datasets and patient-specific data to supply amazingly customized programs.
- Holistic health models: Based on the standards of yoga, a more careful information of wellbeing is conceivable, taking into consideration not fair physical care but moreover mental, enthusiastic, and otherworldly measurements.
- Anticipating results: Within the future, PMS may estimate treatment comes about utilizing advanced prescient models, permitting for preemptive medicines.
- Population wellbeing insights: Specialists can have improved understanding of the in general wellbeing affect of Vedic hones by analyzing patterns among different bunches.
- Consistent telecare: Expanding telehealth capacity will permit for progressing perception, farther physiotherapy sessions, and GAI integration for in-the-moment adjustments.
- Intuitively instruments: Up and coming frameworks might have intelligently stages where patients can donate input and inclinations to customize their care and take a dynamic part in it.

- Gamification: Including components of gamification grounded in Ayurvedic standards might boost understanding inspiration and treatment arrange adherence.
- International trade of information: When specialists from distinctive foundations work together, the comprehension and utilization of different therapeutic modalities are upgraded.
- Virtual reality and reenactment: State-of-the-art preparing innovations can combine evidence-based practice with Vedic thoughts for persistent care by utilizing VR to show understanding scenarios.
- Interoperable frameworks: The most focus of future PMS will be interoperability, which is able empower easy data sharing over different healthcare stages and might indeed improve care coordination.
- Data-driven bits of knowledge: Leveraging enormous information analytics can give critical insights into the victory of coordinates approaches and help progress hone over time.
- Patient-centric AI: Planning AI with the welfare of the understanding in intellect ensures that innovation improves instead of takes the put of the human component in healthcare.

XI. CONCLUSION

This inventive approach to healthcare combines cutting-edge development with age-old insights to advance holistic repairing, move forward determined wellness, and advance the quality of care by uniting generative manufactured insights and Vedic scripture standards into a physiotherapy organization system. The utilize of such cutting-edge frameworks will be essential to guaranteeing compelling, individualized, and compassionate care as the healthcare division makes. The meeting of Generative Artificial Intelligence and Vedic Scripture Enabled Physiotherapy Management Frameworks represents a captivating and possibly transformative wilderness in healthcare, especially in India. As we have investigated the distinct yet complementary capabilities of these two spaces, it becomes evident that their keen integration holds the guarantee of a genuinely holistic, personalized, and socially resounding approach to physical well-being. Generative AI, with its capacity to synthesize novel information and make bespoke arrangements, moves past insignificant data examination to effectively plan individualized restorative pathways. Within the context of physiotherapy, this deciphers into an AI that can learn from a vast repository of patient information – enveloping detailed biomechanical assessments, physiological responses, pain profiles, and indeed patient-reported results – to dynamically craft tailored exercise regimens, manual therapy protocols, and rehabilitation strategies. This goes past inactive layouts, permitting the framework to adjust in real-time to a patient's advance, adherence, and advancing needs, possibly driving to more efficient recovery directions and superior useful picks up. The capacity of generative models to create profoundly practical visual and auditory instructions for exercises, personalized instructive substance, and indeed simulated situations for recovery (e.g., via VR/AR) could significantly enhance patient engagement and comprehension. Simultaneously, the significant intelligence implanted in Vedic scriptures, especially through the lens of Ayurveda and Yoga, offers a foundational system for understanding health not in isolation, but as a complex interaction of physical, mental, emotional, and spiritual dimensions. Concepts like Prakriti, Doshas, Agni, and Prana provide a sophisticated blueprint for individualized assessment, recognizing that each person's unique constitution dictates ideal approaches to wellbeing and healing. By consolidating these standards, the Generative AI system would be able to transcend purely symptomatic treatments, instead generating physiotherapy plans that consider a patient's inherent bio-energetic balance, dietary habits, lifestyle rhythms, and mental mien. This could show in AI-generated suggestions that incorporate not as it were specific exercises but too complementary dietary advice, mindfulness practices, and every day routines tailored to adjust an individual's Doshas, in this manner addressing the root causes of musculoskeletal imbalances and advancing systemic well-being. The amalgamation of these two powerful domains aims to form a physiotherapy management framework that's unparalleled in its personalized and all encompassing scope. It envisions an AI that, educated by the deep, time-tested insights of Vedic wisdom, can generate highly nuanced and versatile therapeutic mediations. Such a framework seem offer significant benefits, especially in a differing nation like India, where traditional wellbeing practices hold significant social esteem. It might lead to improved quiet adherence, as treatment plans resound with their social understanding of wellbeing; improved long-term results by tending to multifactorial perspectives of well-being; and greater effectiveness for clinicians by computerizing personalized arrange era. Besides, it opens avenues for evidence-based approval of coordinates care models, possibly illustrating how old intelligence, when intelligently connected through advanced innovation, can lead to superior patient comes about. In any case, the realization of such a framework isn't without significant challenges. First among them is the complex assignment of precisely and morally deciphering the subjective, philosophical, and frequently allegorical concepts of Vedic sacred writings into quantifiable parameters that an AI can prepare and produce proposals from. This demands thorough interdisciplinary collaboration among Ayurvedic researchers, AI engineers, and clinical physiotherapists to avoid misinterpretation or oversimplification of ancient knowledge. Ensuring information quality, relieving algorithmic inclination implanted in preparing information (which seem inadvertently propagate health disparities), and establishing clear ethical guidelines for AI-generated wellbeing advice are vital. Administrative systems will need to advance to certify and oversee such novel hybrid frameworks, especially concerning responsibility and clinical safety. The system's viability will too hinge on robust clinical approval through experimental studies, illustrating that AI-generated, Vedic-informed physiotherapy in fact yields prevalent and secure results compared to routine approaches. Eventually, the Generative Fake Insights and Vedic Scripture Enabled Physiotherapy Management System represents a bold step towards a future where innovation amplifies wisdom, instead of supplanting it. It looks for to bridge the chasm between ancient, all encompassing wellbeing standards and cutting-edge advanced development, advertising a vision for physiotherapy that's deeply personalized, culturally delicate, and comprehensively adjusted to the human being. Whereas the travel from concept to widespread execution is arduous, the potential for this synergistic approach to revolutionize persistent care and cultivate a more coordinates understanding of wellbeing and mending makes it a compelling and crucial range for continued investigate, improvement, and mindful application, especially in districts like India, where the roots of this antiquated wisdom run deep.

REFERENCES

Aldoseri, A., Al-Khalifa, K. N., & Hamouda, A. M. (2023). Re-Thinking Data Strategy and Integration for Artificial intelligence: Concepts, opportunities, and challenges. *Applied Sciences (Basel, Switzerland), 13*(12), 7082. DOI: 10.3390/app13127082

Bowers, H., & Cheer, J. M. (2017). Yoga tourism: Commodification and western embracement of eastern spiritual practice. *Tourism Management Perspectives, 24*, 208–216. DOI: 10.1016/j.tmp.2017.07.013

Charnysh, E., Pal, S., Reader, J. M., Uhlmann, W. R., McCain, S., Sanghavi, K., Blasco, D., Brandt, R., Feero, W. G., Ferber, R., Giri, V. N., Hendy, K., Prince, A. E. R., Lee, C., & Roberts, J. S. (2024). Health care utilization and behavior changes after workplace genetic testing at a large US health care system. *Genetics in Medicine, 26*(8), 101160. DOI: 10.1016/j.gim.2024.101160 PMID: 38733246

Dangi, S., Ghanshala, K., & Sharma, S. (2025b). LIFT: Lightweight incremental and federated techniques for live memory forensics and proactive malware detection. *International Journal of Advanced Computer Science and Applications, 16*(4). Advance online publication. DOI: 10.14569/ijacsa.2025.0160445

Devgan, K., Sharma, S., Jangra, D., & Sharma, S. (2025b). Artificial Intelligence-Enabled Apple Disease Monitoring System for environmental protection and resource conservation. In Advances in computational intelligence and robotics book series (pp. 271–300). https://doi.org/DOI: 10.4018/979-8-3373-3246-8.ch011

Devliyal, S., Goyal, H. R., & Sharma, S. (2025b). ICDRET: A dynamic cyber risk estimation technique for intelligent Cyber-Physical Systems in PCS. *The Open Bioinformatics Journal, 18*(1). Advance online publication. DOI: 10.2174/0118750362380269250502062754

Hirani, R., Noruzi, K., Khuram, H., Hussaini, A. S., Aifuwa, E. I., Ely, K. E., Lewis, J. M., Gabr, A. E., Smiley, A., Tiwari, R. K., & Etienne, M. (2024). Artificial Intelligence and Healthcare: A Journey through History, Present Innovations, and Future Possibilities. *Life (Chicago, Ill.), 14*(5), 557. DOI: 10.3390/life14050557 PMID: 38792579

Kapruwan, A., Sharma, S., & Goyal, H. R. (2025). ESCBR: Expert System Enabled Case-based Reasoning Approach in IDDCS for CIND. *Recent Patents on Engineering, 19*. Advance online publication. DOI: 10.2174/0118722121336689250116074945

Kohli, P., & Sharma, S. (2025b). EDGE Artificial Intelligence-Enabled 6G communication security system for connected vehicles in revolutionizing urban development and governance. In IGI Global eBooks (pp. 431–462). https://doi.org/DOI: 10.4018/979-8-3373-1375-7.ch015

Martins, P., Matos, L., Moreira, A., Simões, M., & Silva, B. (2025). A transdisciplinary approach of the role of consciousness and spirituality in physics and healing. *Transdisciplinary Journal of Engineering & Science*, *16*. Advance online publication. DOI: 10.22545/2025/00273

Rawat, D., Sharma, S., & Bhadula, S. (2025b). CT Imaging-Based Deep Learning System for Non-Small Cell Lung Cancer Detection and Classification. *International Journal of Advanced Computer Science and Applications*, *16*(5). Advance online publication. DOI: 10.14569/ijacsa.2025.0160561

Rawat, R., Goyal, H. R., & Sharma, S. (2024b). Hofstede's Cultural Dimension Driven Artificial Narrow Intelligence IDFIS for Industry 5.0 Empowered Digital Society. *Recent Patents on Engineering*, *19*. Advance online publication. DOI: 10.2174/0118722121334543241001050846

Rawat, R., Goyal, H. R., Sharma, S., & Kotiyal, B. (2025b). SQRCD: Building Sustainable and Customer Centric DFIS for the Industry 5.0 ERA. *International Journal of Advanced Computer Science and Applications*, *16*(2). Advance online publication. DOI: 10.14569/ijacsa.2025.0160293

Roppelt, J. S., Kanbach, D. K., & Kraus, S. (2023). Artificial intelligence in healthcare institutions: A systematic literature review on influencing factors. *Technology in Society*, *76*, 102443. DOI: 10.1016/j.techsoc.2023.102443

Sharma, S., Tyagi, R., & Mohan, S. (2024). Generative Artificial Intelligence-Enabled climate change and Deep-Sea food webs. In Advances in environmental engineering and green technologies book series (pp. 199–224). https://doi.org/DOI: 10.4018/979-8-3693-6670-7.ch009

Sharma, S., Tyagi, R., & Mohan, S. (2025a). Artificial intelligence and optimized computational modelling against climate crisis. In Elsevier eBooks (pp. 1–14). https://doi.org/DOI: 10.1016/b978-0-443-21905-4.00006-7

Sharma, S., Tyagi, R., & Mohan, S. (2025b). Blockchain-Based Security and Privacy in Digital Healthcare Recommender Systems. In In Healthcare Recommender Systems (pp. 221–237). https://doi.org/DOI: 10.1007/978-3-031-80056-6_10

Zhang, Z., Hamadi, H. A., Damiani, E., Yeun, C. Y., & Taher, F. (2022). Explainable Artificial intelligence Applications in Cyber Security: State-of-the-Art in Research. *IEEE Access : Practical Innovations, Open Solutions*, *10*, 93104–93139. DOI: 10.1109/access.2022.3204051

Chapter 3
Future Trends and Opportunities:
Personalized Medicine Through Next Gen Devices and Robotics

Himadri Sekhar Das
https://orcid.org/0000-0002-3509-3388
Haldia Institute of Technology, Haldia, India

Sudipta Banerjee
https://orcid.org/0000-0003-0150-6794
Symbiosis Institute of Technology, Symbiosis International University, India

Heranmoy Maity
Pailan College of Management and Technology, Kolkata, India

ABSTRACT

Personalized medicine is rapidly evolving, driven by advancements in next-generation medical devices and robotics. These technologies enable real-time monitoring, precise diagnostics, and individualized treatment, transforming healthcare from reactive to proactive. Wearable biosensors, surgical robots, and AI-integrated systems are central to this shift, offering tailored therapies and improving patient outcomes. Robotics enhances surgical precision and rehabilitation, while AI leverages big data for predictive care. Despite challenges in data privacy, equity, and regulation, the future promises smarter, more accessible, and highly personalized healthcare. This chapter explores emerging trends, innovations, and opportunities shaping the next frontier of individualized medicine.

DOI: 10.4018/979-8-3373-1514-0.ch003

INTRODUCTION

Personalized medicine-tailoring medical treatment to the individual characteristics of each patient-is revolutionizing healthcare. At the core of this transformation lies the convergence of advanced technologies, particularly next-generation medical devices and robotics (B S Junaid et al, (2022). These innovations are enabling unprecedented precision in diagnostics, treatment, and patient monitoring. This chapter explores the emerging trends, transformative technologies, and the future opportunities that next-gen devices and robotics present in the realm of personalized medicine (Adib Bin Rashid,(2024).

The future of healthcare is being shaped by a powerful convergence of personalized medicine, next-generation medical devices, and advanced robotics. This triad is driving a paradigm shift from generalized treatment approaches to highly individualized, data-driven care strategies. Personalized medicine, which seeks to customize healthcare based on a person's genetic profile, lifestyle, and environment, is no longer a conceptual ideal—it is becoming a clinical reality. At the heart of this transformation are emerging technologies that are reshaping every facet of healthcare delivery, from diagnostics and treatment to long-term disease management and rehabilitation (L H Goetz et al, (2018).

Next-generation devices, including wearable and implantable biosensors, smart drug delivery systems, and lab-on-a-chip technologies, are central to this change. These devices continuously gather real-time physiological data, enabling early detection of disease, precise monitoring of treatment responses, and dynamic adjustment of care plans (Sushma Dave et al, (2024). With the integration of artificial intelligence and big data analytics, this information is no longer siloed but is used to generate meaningful insights that guide clinical decisions on an individual level. These innovations are fostering a shift from reactive treatment to predictive and preventive care, ultimately reducing healthcare costs while improving outcomes.

Robotics is another critical pillar supporting the advancement of personalized medicine. Surgical robotics, for instance, now offer enhanced precision, smaller incisions, and quicker recovery times, all tailored to the unique anatomy of each patient (M. Iftikhar et al, (2024). Robotic systems are also being used in rehabilitation, where they adapt therapy in real-time based on a patient's physical progress and neurological feedback. Furthermore, social and assistive robots are being introduced into home care settings to support individuals with chronic illnesses, disabilities, or age-related conditions, delivering not only physical assistance but also companionship and mental health support.

The integration of these technologies is accelerated by the rise of interconnected digital health ecosystems. Electronic health records (EHRs), cloud-based platforms, and health data interoperability standards allow for seamless communication among devices, clinicians, and patients (V. Padmavathi,(2025). This ecosystem supports the development of "digital twins"—virtual replicas of patients that can be used to simulate treatment outcomes, forecast disease progression, and optimize care plans without invasive procedures.

The intersection of robotics, artificial intelligence (AI), and wearable technologies is reshaping the terrain of contemporary healthcare. Despite swift advancements in technology, a core challenge persists: the majority of medical devices and robotic systems are not tailored for personalization, accessibility, or sustainable clinical integration. Their extensive use is still hampered by high costs, limited adaptability to various patient needs, and regulatory complexities. This book tackles that gap head-on by examining the development and use of next-generation technologies—from AI-assisted surgical robots to context-aware wearable devices—to foster healthcare solutions that are genuinely patient-centered, scalable, and rooted in ethics.

We investigate developments in surgical robotics, diagnostic algorithms, rehabilitation systems, and bionic interfaces through a multidisciplinary perspective, while critically addressing concerns related to usability, safety, and global equity. The book offers a technical basis and a forward-looking view by anchoring each chapter in real-world use cases, validated performance metrics, and emerging clinical frameworks. We aim not only to record innovation but also to offer a framework for the responsible design and implementation of personalized medical technologies that are both cutting-edge and adaptable. This lays the groundwork for a new age in which machines do not supplant humans, but rather enhance human care.

Despite these advancements, challenges remain. Issues of data privacy, ethical AI deployment, equitable access to technology, and regulatory oversight must be addressed to ensure that the benefits of these innovations are distributed fairly and safely (C Mennella et al,(2024). Moreover, clinicians and healthcare systems must be trained and equipped to integrate these tools effectively into their workflows.

The current literature in medical robotics and personalized healthcare shows significant advancement; however, there remain several important limitations related to cost-efficiency, clinical scalability, data integration, and accessibility. Earlier research has laid the groundwork in fields such as robotic-assisted surgery, AI-driven diagnostics, and wearable health monitoring. Nonetheless, numerous technologies of this kind are confined to affluent medical institutions in developed areas, and frequently do not offer adaptability for varied patient demographics or healthcare systems lacking sufficient resources.

The goal of this chapter is to tackle these shortcomings by presenting new frameworks and device architectures that emphasize cost-effectiveness, modular design, and real-time data integration, thus improving clinical performance and ease of deployment. For instance, although prior research shows that AI models have a high diagnostic accuracy, our approach incorporates explainable AI mechanisms to enhance transparency and clinician trust. Likewise, our creation of adaptive, lightweight systems designed for in-home and outpatient care enhances the progress of robotic rehabilitation.

This work addresses the limitations identified in the literature—like high production costs, limited user-centered design, and lack of demographic inclusivity—thereby building on previous innovations and moving the field forward toward more inclusive, scalable, and patient-personalized solutions. Gap is identified with the methodological innovation shown in Table.1

Table 1. Linking Methodological Innovations to Gaps Identified in Literature

Identified Gap (from Related Work)	Novel Method / Approach Introduced	How the Innovation Addresses the Gap
Limited real-time explainability in AI-guided robotic systems	Integration of interpretable AI (e.g., SHAP/LIME) in decision-support module	Enhances trust and clinical transparency during autonomous or semi-autonomous tasks
High cost and limited scalability of haptic systems	Use of 3D-printed tactile sensors and open-source haptics framework	Reduces production cost and enables wider deployment in low-resource settings
Lack of demographic diversity in wearable-based monitoring trials	Inclusion of diverse patient datasets across geographies and age groups	Improves generalizability and equity in personalized diagnostics
Weak integration between genomics and robotic biopsy tools	Unified interface for real-time genomic marker alignment during robotic targeting	Enables precise, data-driven interventions aligned to molecular profiles
Insufficient long-term durability of soft robotics in pediatric settings	Development of bioresorbable and sterilizable materials for soft actuators	Improves safety, sustainability, and regulatory compliance
Complexity in deploying neuro-rehabilitation systems in outpatient settings	Adaptive calibration protocol using EEG + EMG fusion with mobile interfaces	Makes neuro-rehab robotics feasible in at-home recovery programs

Critical Reflection: Surgical Robotics

Although robotic-assisted surgical systems like the da Vinci Surgical System have greatly enhanced precision and minimized invasiveness, several limitations remain. Due to the high acquisition and maintenance costs, access is restricted to well-funded institutions, leaving smaller or rural hospitals neglected. In addition, existing systems depend significantly on preoperative imaging and provide limited adaptability during surgery, especially in unstructured surgical environments. Challenges for broad implementation are also presented by the need for training and the existence of steep learning curves. Most importantly, genuine autonomy in surgery is still developing, with outstanding issues regarding safety, explainability, and regulatory oversight. The existence of these gaps emphasizes the necessity for systems that are semi-autonomous and cost-effective and that improve usability, adaptability, and accessibility—key aims of the work detailed in this chapter.

Critical Reflection: AI Diagnostics

The literature showcases remarkable advancements in AI-driven diagnostics, especially concerning image-based disease detection and risk prediction models. Nevertheless, a lot of models are created in controlled academic environments and have limited validation in real-world scenarios. Significant worries exist regarding data bias, the absence of clinical interpretability, and inadequate integration with electronic health record (EHR) systems. Moreover, the process of obtaining regulatory approval for AI diagnostics is slow and lacks cohesion, which postpones their clinical deployment. The urgent necessity for explainable, generalizable, and clinically embedded AI tools is underscored by these issues. This book promotes such tools by stressing transparent model design and integration into workflows.

Critical Reflection: Wearable Monitoring

Wearable technology has revolutionized the way individuals monitor their health, serving functions that include cardiac alerts and sleep pattern assessments. Nonetheless, the existing body of work uncovers multiple limitations: the precision of sensors differs greatly depending on skin type, degree of activity, and situational factors. Moreover, proprietary ecosystems and data fragmentation impede interoperability among providers and platforms. From the viewpoint of users, worries about privacy and the practicality of long-term use (such as comfort and battery longevity) still restrict adoption rates. Especially, these devices are not used to their full potential in preventive care and frequently do not have actionable feedback mechanisms. This book presents research that overcomes these limitations by proposing advanced wearable systems that are interoperable, adaptable, and able to provide real-time context-aware, patient-specific insights.

Looking ahead, the synergy between personalized medicine, next-gen devices, and robotics holds immense promise. As these technologies continue to evolve and integrate, they will redefine the standard of care—making it more precise, responsive, and tailored to the unique needs of every individual (G Molla et al,(2024). This chapter explores the emerging trends, technologies, and opportunities that are shaping the future of medicine and outlines how these innovations are not only transforming clinical practice but also empowering patients in unprecedented ways.

1. THE RISE OF PERSONALIZED MEDICINE

1.1 Definition and Importance

Personalized medicine leverages genetic, environmental, and lifestyle data to craft individualized treatment plans. This approach moves away from the "one-size-fits-all" model, offering more effective and targeted interventions.

Personalized medicine, also known as precision medicine, is a healthcare approach that tailors medical decisions, treatments, practices, and products to the individual characteristics of each patient. It integrates a wide range of personal data—including genetic makeup, environmental exposures, biomarker profiles, and lifestyle factors—to design customized treatment strategies. Unlike the traditional "one-size-fits-all" model, personalized medicine recognizes that each patient is biologically unique and may respond differently to the same therapy (L. Marques et al,(2024).

The importance of personalized medicine lies in its potential to increase the efficacy of treatments, reduce adverse drug reactions, and improve overall patient outcomes. By identifying the most suitable interventions based on a patient's specific profile, healthcare providers can deliver more accurate diagnoses, select the best therapeutic options, and even predict disease risks before symptoms appear. This approach not only enhances the quality of care but also supports the development of more efficient healthcare systems by reducing trial-and-error prescribing, minimizing unnecessary procedures, and cutting long-term costs associated with ineffective treatments (L. Marques et al,(2024). As technology continues to advance, personalized medicine is becoming a cornerstone of modern, patient-centered healthcare.

1.2 Driving Forces

The rapid evolution of personalized medicine is fueled by a combination of technological, societal, and systemic factors that are reshaping the landscape of healthcare. Several key drivers are accelerating the development and adoption of personalized approaches:

Advances in Genomics and Biomarker Discovery

The dramatic decrease in the cost and time required for genome sequencing has opened new possibilities in understanding disease at the molecular level (H Satam et al, (2023). Genetic profiling and biomarker discovery now allow for more precise disease classification and the identification of individuals at high risk, paving the way for targeted therapies and preventive strategies.

Integration of Big Data and Artificial Intelligence (AI)

The explosion of health-related data—from electronic health records and genomic databases to wearable devices—has created an opportunity to derive actionable insights through AI and machine learning (Mohd Javaid et al,(2022). These tools can process vast, complex datasets to uncover patterns, predict outcomes, and guide personalized treatment decisions in real time.

Growing Patient Demand for Customized Care

Modern patients are more informed and engaged in their health than ever before. There is a rising expectation for care that reflects individual needs, preferences, and values. Personalized medicine aligns with this demand by offering tailored solutions that improve both clinical outcomes and patient satisfaction (D C Ferreira et al, (2023).

The Shift toward Value-Based Healthcare Systems

Healthcare systems globally are moving away from volume-based care models toward value-based frameworks that prioritize outcomes and cost-efficiency. Personalized medicine supports this shift by improving the effectiveness of interventions, reducing unnecessary treatments, and enabling earlier disease intervention—ultimately leading to better results and more sustainable healthcare delivery.

Together, these driving forces are setting the stage for a healthcare revolution—one that is smarter, more efficient, and truly centered around the individual.

2. NEXT-GEN DEVICES IN PERSONALIZED CARE

Next-generation medical devices are at the forefront of the personalized medicine revolution. These cutting-edge technologies are designed not only to monitor health in real time but also to respond dynamically to the unique physiological needs of each patient. By integrating sensors, artificial intelligence, and wireless connectivity, these devices enable more accurate diagnostics, continuous monitoring, and precise therapeutic delivery tailored to the individual (Sweety Pal et al, (2024).

2.1 Wearable and Implantable Biosensors

Wearable and Implantable Biosensors: Wearable and implantable biosensors are pivotal in advancing personalized medicine by enabling continuous, real-time health monitoring and data collection (D K Vo et al,(2024). These devices bridge the gap between traditional clinical assessments and daily health tracking, allowing for a more holistic and dynamic understanding of a patient's physiological state. By capturing vital signs and biological signals around the clock, they empower healthcare providers to deliver proactive, preventive, and highly individualized care.

Wearables-such as smart watches, fitness trackers, and adhesive patches—are non-invasive and user-friendly, making them ideal for monitoring common health metrics like heart rate, sleep, physical activity, glucose levels, and oxygen saturation. Implantable biosensors, on the other hand, are designed for long-term internal monitoring. Devices such as cardiac monitors, neuro stimulators, and continuous glucose monitors provide deeper insights into critical health conditions without the need for frequent clinical visits. Different key areas in personalized medicine with upcoming device and robotics are shown in Table.2.

Table 2. Key Areas in Personalized Medicine with Next-Gen Devices and Robotics

Key Area	Description	Emerging Trends / Examples
Diagnostics	Use of AI, machine learning, and advanced imaging for early and personalized diagnosis.	AI-powered imaging (e.g., PathAI), wearable biosensors (e.g., Apple Watch ECG).
Surgical Robotics	Robotic systems enhancing precision, minimizing invasiveness, and improving surgical outcomes.	da Vinci Surgical System, Versius Robot, AI-assisted laparoscopic tools.
Rehabilitation	Use of smart prosthetics, robotic exoskeletons, and neuromodulation for recovery and mobility.	Ekso Bionics, ReWalk Robotics, brain-computer interfaces for motor rehab.
Therapeutics	Personalized drug delivery and targeted therapies using nanodevices and smart implants.	Insulin pumps, micro-needle patches, targeted cancer nanocarriers.
Genomic & Omics Tools	Integration of genomics, proteomics, and metabolomics to tailor treatments at molecular levels.	CRISPR-based therapies, 23andMe diagnostics, pharmacogenomics platforms.
Remote Monitoring	Continuous health monitoring using connected devices and AI for chronic disease management.	Telemedicine, RPM devices, AI chatbots for follow-up care.
Data Integration & AI	Leveraging big data and AI to synthesize patient records and guide clinical decisions.	IBM Watson Health (legacy), Tempus, deep learning for EHR analytics.

Key Trends in Biosensor Technology:

Multi-Sensor Integration

Modern biosensors are evolving into multifunctional health platforms. Advanced devices can simultaneously track multiple parameters such as ECG (electrocardiogram), SpO_2 (oxygen saturation), hydration levels, respiration rate, body temperature, and even metabolic activity. This integration enables a more comprehensive view of a patient's health and helps in the early detection of anomalies or disease progression.

Continuous Drug Delivery

Smart biosensors are increasingly being combined with drug delivery mechanisms, such as transdermal patches and implantable pumps, to administer medications in a personalized and timely manner. These systems can respond to real-time biomarker levels, releasing medication as needed—improving treatment adherence and reducing the risk of over- or under-dosing. For example, insulin pumps that adjust doses based on continuous glucose readings are becoming the standard of care in diabetes management.

Biofeedback Loops

One of the most promising trends is the development of closed-loop systems, where biosensors and therapeutic devices work together autonomously. These biofeedback loops allow the device to detect physiological changes and automatically adjust treatment—such as modulating the rate of insulin delivery or adjusting pacemaker rhythms (Z Zheng et al, (2024). This real-time responsiveness ensures more effective management of chronic diseases and reduces the burden on both patients and healthcare providers.

As biosensors continue to become smaller, smarter, and more integrated with digital health ecosystems, their role in personalized medicine will expand. These devices not only offer early warnings and precise monitoring but also enable continuous optimization of therapy, fundamentally changing how care is delivered-putting the patient at the center of a responsive, technology-driven healthcare system.

2.2 Lab-on-a-Chip and Micro-fluidics

Lab-on-a-chip (LOC) and micro-fluidic technologies represent a groundbreaking advancement in personalized medicine, offering compact, efficient, and highly sensitive diagnostic platforms. These devices miniaturize complex laboratory processes—such as sample preparation, biochemical analysis, and detection—onto a single microchip, often no larger than a credit card. By manipulating minute volumes of fluids through microscopic channels, LOC systems enable rapid, accurate diagnostics at the point of care (POC), often requiring only a drop of blood, saliva, or urine (N Azizipour et al, (2020).

These innovations dramatically reduce the time between testing and diagnosis, eliminate the need for large lab infrastructure, and open the door to more frequent, decentralized, and patient-specific testing. As a result, clinicians can make quicker, more informed treatment decisions tailored to the individual's unique physiological and genetic profile.

Key Applications:

Early Cancer Detection

LOC devices can analyze blood or other body fluids to identify cancer biomarkers such as circulating tumor DNA (ctDNA), exosomes, or specific protein markers (H Wang et al, (2024). Early detection is critical in cancer care, as it significantly improves the chances of successful treatment. These devices enable routine screening for at-risk individuals and personalized surveillance for cancer survivors.

Infectious Disease Screening

Microfluidic diagnostics allow for the rapid detection of pathogens such as bacteria, viruses, and fungi directly at the point of care. This is especially vital in remote or low-resource settings and during outbreaks of contagious diseases like COVID-19, influenza, or tuberculosis. Personalized responses can then be crafted based on pathogen type, resistance profiles, and patient risk factors.

Pharmacogenomics Testing

By analyzing a patient's genetic response to drugs, LOC platforms help determine the most effective medication and dosage with minimal side effects. This is particularly valuable in areas like oncology, cardiology, and psychiatry, where drug response varies greatly between individuals. Fast, on-site pharmacogenomic testing allows for real-time optimization of therapeutic regimens (W Sadee et al, (2023).

Lab-on-a-chip and microfluidic technologies are revolutionizing diagnostic medicine by making it faster, more accessible, and more aligned with personalized care goals. As these platforms become more integrated with digital health systems and data analytics tools, they will further enhance the ability to deliver timely, precise, and patient-specific interventions—ushering in a new era of truly individualized healthcare.

3. ROBOTICS IN PERSONALIZED MEDICINE

3.1 Surgical Robotics

Surgical robotics has emerged as a transformative force in modern healthcare, redefining how surgeries are planned, executed, and monitored. Robotic-assisted surgeries enhance a surgeon's capabilities by offering superior precision, improved dexterity, and enhanced visualization-often surpassing the limitations of the human hand. These systems enable minimally invasive procedures with smaller incisions, reduced blood loss, lower risk of complications, and quicker recovery times, making them ideal for a wide range of medical specialties including urology, cardiothoracic surgery, orthopedics, and gynecology (M Fairag et al, (2024).

What sets surgical robotics apart in the context of personalized medicine is their ability to tailor procedures to the unique anatomical and physiological characteristics of each patient. With the integration of advanced imaging, AI, and machine learning, robotic systems are no longer just mechanical tools-they are intelligent platforms capable of delivering highly customized surgical care. Fig.1 shows the different way of Micro/nanorobots in Medicine.

Figure 1. Micro/nanorobots in Medicine

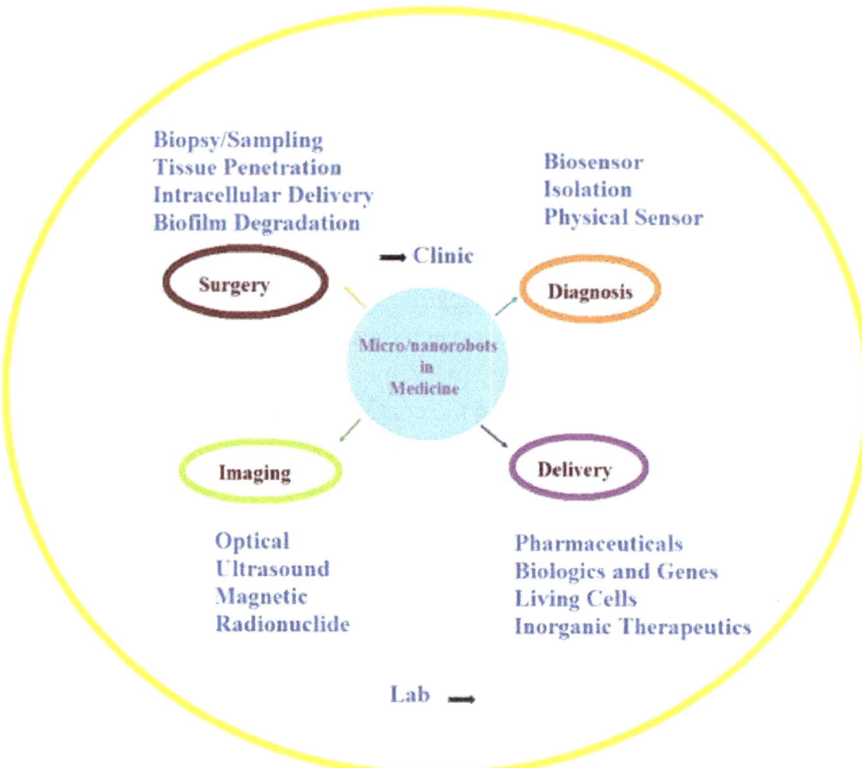

Previous research on medical robotics and gadgets can be categorized thematically into a number of important categories. One group focuses on surgical robotics, investigating human-robot interaction, precision, and minimally invasive techniques. Another focuses on assistive technology and rehabilitation, with the goal of improving patient mobility and recuperation. Robotic endoscopy and image-guided operations are examples of diagnostic and interventional robotics, which constitute a third category. Chronic disease management and real-time monitoring are the focus of wearable and implantable device research. Lastly, research on AI integration and control systems places a strong emphasis on robotic operations' safety, flexibility, and autonomy. The multidisciplinary development of medical robots toward better patient care is shown in Table.3 these concepts taken together.

Table 3. Thematic Grouping of Prior Studies in Medical Robotics and Devices

Theme	Representative Studies (Year)	Key Contributions	Insights / Research Gaps
1. Imaging & Diagnostic Devices	- Apple Heart Study (2021) - Lancet Digital Health (2024) - NEJM (2022)	AI-enhanced wearables; early disease prediction; real-time vital sign tracking	Accuracy varies by demographics; data standardization and integration needed.
2. Robotic-Assisted Surgery	- Nature Biomed Eng (2025) - IEEE TMRB (2024) - da Vinci Case Studies	Real-time navigation; enhanced surgical precision; tactile feedback in laparoscopic tools	Limited explainability in AI, cost-prohibitive systems, regulatory barriers.
3. Rehabilitation Robotics	- Frontiers in Robotics and AI (2024) - Ekso Bionics Trials	Exoskeletons for stroke rehab; brain–machine interface for mobility recovery	High cost, bulkiness, and need for adaptable algorithms per user.
4. Genomics-Integrated Robotics	- J. Personalized Medicine (2025) - Nature Genetics + Robotics (2023)	Robotic biopsy guided by genomic markers; precision targeting in tumor diagnostics	Complexity of data integration and clinical translation remains a challenge.
5. Soft & Miniaturized Robotics	- Science Robotics (2025) - Nature Nanotechnology (2023)	Pediatric-friendly soft actuators; microbots for minimally invasive procedures	Material durability, biocompatibility, and sterilization constraints.
6. AI-Based Therapeutic Systems	- Nature Rev Drug Disc (2024) - Sci Transl Med (2023)	AI and microfluidics for drug screening and personalized treatment plans	Need for clinical validation and standard testing pipelines.

Personalized Applications:

Patient-Specific 3D Surgical Planning

Before surgery, high-resolution imaging technologies such as CT or MRI scans are used to create detailed, three-dimensional models of the patient's anatomy. Surgeons can simulate the procedure virtually, plan the optimal surgical path, and customize the robotic system's movements to fit the patient's unique anatomical structure. This approach reduces intraoperative uncertainty and enhances surgical outcomes (Shreya Shah et al, (2025).

AI-Guided Robotic Arms Adapting to Individual Anatomy

Modern surgical robots are increasingly equipped with AI and machine learning capabilities, allowing them to adapt in real time to subtle differences in tissue structure, positioning, and movement. The system can assist the surgeon by providing dynamic feedback, suggesting optimal cutting paths, and automatically adjusting tool pressure or angles based on the patient's specific anatomy and intraoperative conditions.

Here are some of the most notable recent (2024–2025) advances in medical robotics and personalized medicine Table.4.

- Magnetically-guided miniature robot for bowel cancer screening—about the size of a UK penny, it can 3D-scan and potentially deliver treatment in a single, non-invasive procedure; human trials are planned for 2026 after successful pig studies
- Robotic-assisted endovascular AI systems enhancing vessel navigation with real-time segmentation and reinforcement learning, improving autonomy in catheter guidance
- Robot-assisted knee arthroplasty using CPAK alignment tailoring to each patient's native anatomy, shown to reduce long-term complications.
- AI-driven patient-specific surgical tools and implants, increasingly 3D-printed, are delivering better fit and outcomes in orthopaedic and cranial procedures
- AI-powered personalized mRNA cancer vaccines entering NHS-led trials in 2024, targeting tumor mutations unique to individuals.

Table 4. Recent Studies (2024–2025) in Medical Robotics and Personalized Medicine

Study / Publication	Focus Area	Key Contributions / Findings	Relevance to Chapter
Nature Biomedical Engineering (2025) – "Autonomous Surgical Navigation with AI-Integrated Robotics"	Surgical Robotics	Demonstrated a robotic system using deep reinforcement learning for real-time surgical guidance.	Advances autonomous decision-making in robotic surgery.
IEEE Transactions on Medical Robotics (2024) – "Haptic Feedback in Robotic-Assisted Laparoscopy"	Human-Robot Interface	Improved tactile precision for robotic arms using novel sensors and haptic actuators.	Supports better clinical outcomes through enhanced surgeon control.
Lancet Digital Health (2024) – "AI Wearables for Predictive Oncology Monitoring"	Diagnostics & Remote Monitoring	Wearable biosensors predicted tumor growth patterns with 92% accuracy in clinical trials.	Showcases real-time, AI-driven personalized monitoring.
Journal of Personalized Medicine (2025) – "Genomic-Guided Robotic Biopsies"	Genomics-Integrated Robotics	Robotic system integrated with genomic markers for site-specific tumor sampling.	Merges genomics with robotic intervention for targeted treatment.

continued on following page

Table 4. Continued

Study / Publication	Focus Area	Key Contributions / Findings	Relevance to Chapter
Frontiers in Robotics and AI (2024) – "Rehabilitation Robots Using Adaptive Neuroplasticity Models"	Rehabilitation & Neuro-Robotics	Developed exoskeletons adapting to brain plasticity for stroke recovery.	Innovation in personalized neuro-rehab technologies.
Science Robotics (2025) – "Soft Robotics in Pediatric Minimally Invasive Surgery"	Soft Robotic Systems	Bio-compatible, flexible robots designed for pediatric applications reduced recovery time by 40%.	Introduces new materials and design paradigms.
Nature Reviews Drug Discovery (2024) – "Robotic Microfluidics for Personalized Drug Testing"	Therapeutics / Drug Response	High-throughput micro-robots tested drug responses on patient-derived cells.	Critical for precision pharmacology and personalized medicine.

Real-Time Intraoperative Data Integration

Surgical robots can integrate live data from various sources-such as imaging devices, vital sign monitors, and tissue sensors-during the procedure. This allows surgeons to make informed decisions on the fly, such as adjusting surgical plans based on real-time tumor margins or vascular mapping. The combination of robotic precision and live data ensures a safer, more personalized approach to complex surgeries.

Surgical robotics represents a major leap toward precision and personalization in operative care. As these technologies continue to evolve with the integration of AI, machine vision, and haptic feedback, they will offer even greater levels of customization, safety, and efficiency. In the future, robotic systems may become capable of learning from previous procedures, refining their performance, and autonomously adapting to each new case-bringing us closer to a new standard of personalized surgical excellence (G. Dagnino et al, (2024).

3.2 Rehabilitation Robotics

Rehabilitation robotics is revolutionizing the recovery process for patients with physical impairments, offering tailored therapies that are adaptive to individual needs. Powered by artificial intelligence (AI), these robotic systems are designed to assist patients in regaining motor function, enhancing mobility, and improving overall quality of life. Unlike traditional rehabilitation methods, which often follow a standardized protocol, robotic systems can adjust therapy to the patient's unique recovery trajectory, ensuring a personalized approach to rehabilitation (Spandana Rajendra Kopalli et al, (2025).

These technologies are particularly impactful for patients with neurological injuries or disorders, such as those caused by stroke or spinal cord injuries. Through continuous adaptation to the patient's progress, rehabilitation robotics can help optimize the healing process, reduce recovery times, and increase long-term functional outcomes.

Innovations:

Exoskeletons for Spinal Cord Injuries or Stroke Recovery

Wearable robotic exoskeletons are designed to support and assist patients with spinal cord injuries or severe neurological conditions such as stroke. These devices consist of rigid frames equipped with motors and actuators that assist in standing, walking, or other rehabilitative movements. Using sensors, the exoskeletons can detect a patient's intent to move and provide the necessary mechanical support to carry out the action.

Personalized Benefits:

- Gradual, controlled reintroduction of weight-bearing and walking functions
- Assistance with posture and alignment to prevent further injury
- Continuous feedback that can be used to adapt the rehabilitation plan as the patient progresses

Robotic Limbs with Neural Interface for Custom Motor Control

Robotic limbs equipped with neural interfaces allow patients with lost or impaired motor functions to regain control of prosthetics or exoskeletal devices. These systems interpret neural signals—either from the brain or from residual nerve endings in the muscles—and translate them into motor commands that guide the robotic limb's movement.

Personalized Benefits:

- Real-time adaptation to the patient's motor capabilities and neurological feedback
- Custom motor control tailored to the individual's needs, whether it's for basic movements or fine motor skills
- The potential to retrain neural pathways and improve coordination over time through repetitive, targeted exercises

Rehabilitation robotics is a powerful tool that enhances the precision and personalization of recovery programs, offering patients more than just assistance—it offers a chance to reclaim their independence and functionality. As these technologies evolve, they will continue to break new ground in tailoring therapy to each patient's pace and abilities, ensuring that recovery is not only efficient but also more aligned with the patient's unique needs and goals.

Both technological and clinical aspects are integrated into the methodological framework for assessing robotics and medical devices (Table.5). Bench testing for mechanical performance is usually the first step, and then safety, biocompatibility, and functional reliability are evaluated through in vitro and in vivo preclinical experiments. Human factors engineering is used to assess ergonomics and usability. Clinical studies, frequently using staged methodologies, assess patient outcomes, safety, and efficacy in real-world settings. Throughout, regulatory compliance with standards such as FDA or CE is crucial. Comprehensive validation and adoption readiness are supported by both qualitative input (user happiness, ease of use) and quantitative indicators (e.g., precision, accuracy, operation time).

Table 5. Methodological Framework for Device and Robotics Evaluation

Component	**Description**	**Selection / Design Criteria**	**Justification for Reproducibility**
Technology Selection	Choice of robotic system, wearable device, or AI algorithm.	Clinical relevance, FDA/CE approval, user adaptability, prior clinical evidence.	Ensures real-world relevance and comparability with existing systems.
Hardware/Software Integration	Interfacing sensors, processors, AI models with physical components.	Modularity, scalability, data compatibility, ease of debugging.	Enables repeatable assembly and platform-agnostic deployment.
Patient/Use Case Definition	Clinical or demographic context used for testing (e.g., cardiac rehab, oncology).	Representativeness, age range, disease stage, ethical approvals.	Ensures generalizability and ethical transparency.
Evaluation Protocol	Procedures for system testing—lab tests, simulations, clinical pilots.	ISO/ASTM standards, trial duration, sensor calibration frequency.	Enables peer labs to recreate environment and procedure.
Performance Metrics	Accuracy, latency, user feedback, power consumption, error rate, etc.	Clinically validated benchmarks, statistical thresholds, expert rating.	Establishes replicable outcome measures.

continued on following page

Table 5. Continued

Component	Description	Selection / Design Criteria	Justification for Reproducibility
Validation Approach	How system effectiveness is confirmed (e.g., comparative trials, cross-validation).	Randomized controlled trials (RCTs), k-fold validation, baseline system comparison.	Enhances credibility and eliminates overfitting or anecdotal bias.
Limitations & Constraints	Known limitations in scope, performance, or ethical deployment.	Disclosed assumptions, controlled variables, hardware dependencies.	Aids researchers in refining or improving the methodology.

3.3 Companion and Care Robots

Companion and care robots are transforming the landscape of elderly care and chronic disease management by providing personalized support to patients in need of both physical and emotional assistance. These robots are designed to enhance the quality of life for individuals, particularly the elderly, by offering companionship, helping with daily activities, and delivering therapeutic interventions (B Sawik et al, (2023). With advancements in robotics, artificial intelligence, and human-robot interaction, these devices are not only practical tools for caregiving but also serve as emotional support systems that can improve mental well-being and reduce feelings of loneliness, a common issue among the elderly population.

Unlike traditional care solutions, companion and care robots are highly customizable and can adapt to each patient's specific needs, offering a personalized approach to managing health and providing support. These robots are especially beneficial in home care settings, where they offer consistent and accessible assistance without the need for constant human supervision.

Applications and Innovations:

Social Robots for Emotional and Social Support

Social robots are designed to engage in conversations, monitor emotional states, and provide companionship for patients, especially the elderly. Equipped with AI and natural language processing, these robots can recognize emotions, offer comforting dialogue, and even engage in simple games or activities to reduce isolation and promote cognitive stimulation. For instance, robots like Paro, a therapeutic robot designed to resemble a baby seal, have been shown to reduce stress and improve mood in patients with dementia (Ji W et al, (2025).

Personalized Benefits:

- Tailored conversations and interactions based on the patient's emotional state and preferences
- Reduces feelings of loneliness, improving mental health and emotional well-being
- Encourages engagement through cognitive exercises and social interactions, which is crucial for conditions like dementia

Prior research in personalized healthcare and medical robotics has greatly improved surgical accuracy, patient-specific treatment, and rehabilitation results (Table.6). The da Vinci Surgical System and other robotically assisted procedures have continuously shown increased dexterity, decreased blood loss, and shortened recovery periods. Critical analysis, however, identifies a number of shortcomings. Numerous studies focus on technological viability without sufficiently considering cost-effectiveness or long-term clinical consequences. Clinical trial sample sizes are frequently small, and there is still a dearth of real-world implementation data, especially for varied patient populations.

The combination of wearable technology, AI, and genetics has made it possible to create customized treatment regimens and diagnostics in personalized healthcare. However, issues with data privacy, interoperability, and the verification of AI algorithms in many healthcare contexts still exist. Disparities in patient care, particularly for underrepresented groups, might result from bias in training data. Furthermore, defined evaluation procedures and strict regulatory control are absent from many customized systems.

Understudied are the ethical issues of algorithm transparency, reliance on machine-driven decision-making, and automation in patient care. All things considered, even while the research trajectory is encouraging, interdisciplinary, extensive, and long-term studies that comprehensively evaluate the efficacy, equity, and integration of robotics and customized medicine into traditional healthcare systems are desperately needed.

Table 6. Critical Evaluation of Prior Studies in Medical Robotics and Personalized Healthcare

Study / Area	Contributions	Limitations / Gaps
Autonomous Surgical Navigation (Nature Biomed Eng, 2025)	Enabled real-time intraoperative decision-making via deep learning.	Lacks transparency (black-box AI), regulatory approval still pending.
Haptic Feedback in Robotic Surgery (IEEE TMRB, 2024)	Improved control and tactile accuracy in robotic-assisted surgery.	High system cost and limited tactile resolution in complex multi-tissue environments.
AI Wearables for Oncology (Lancet Digital Health, 2024)	Enabled early detection of tumor progression via wearables.	Limited sample diversity; device accuracy may vary across populations.
Genomic-Guided Robotic Biopsies (JPM, 2025)	Combined robotic precision with genomic targeting.	Requires complex multi-modal data integration and specialized personnel.
Soft Robotics in Pediatrics (Science Robotics, 2025)	Reduced trauma in pediatric MIS with bio-compatible materials.	Challenges with sterilization, long-term durability, and manufacturing cost.
Exoskeleton Rehab Systems (Frontiers in AI, 2024)	Adaptive learning for neurorehabilitation based on brain signals.	High cost, bulky design, and slow neural response adaptation in some patients.

Assistive Robots for Physical Support

These robots are designed to help patients with mobility impairments, chronic illnesses, or those recovering from surgeries. They can assist with activities of daily living (ADLs) such as lifting, dressing, and eating. Advanced systems are even capable of helping patients move between bed and wheelchair or providing fall prevention support. Examples include robotic arms or exoskeletal devices that enhance physical independence (M. Kyrarini et al, (2021).

Personalized Benefits:

- Real-time monitoring of physical capabilities, adjusting support based on the patient's current strength or mobility levels
- Assist with exercises and physical therapy to encourage independence while preventing further injury
- Provide tailored assistance, whether it's lifting, walking, or preventing falls, based on the patient's unique needs

Therapeutic Robots for Rehabilitation and Mental Health

Care robots equipped with therapeutic capabilities can assist in physical rehabilitation and provide interventions for mental health conditions such as depression, anxiety, or cognitive decline. These robots often integrate cognitive behavioral therapy (CBT) techniques or memory games and can help patients stick to their therapy schedules. Some robots are even designed to remind patients about their medication regimens or offer real-time health monitoring to caregivers and medical professionals.

Personalized Benefits:

- Adaptive therapy routines based on the patient's progress or mood
- Cognitive and physical exercises personalized to the patient's needs
- Medication reminders, mental health interventions, and even emergency assistance when required

Companion and care robots are not only improving physical care but are also enhancing mental health by providing consistent emotional support and reducing feelings of isolation. As these robots become more intelligent, responsive, and integrated with healthcare systems, their potential to deliver individualized, high-quality care will continue to grow. With personalized applications that can adapt to the needs of each patient, these robots are helping redefine caregiving, especially for the elderly and those with chronic conditions, offering a holistic approach to health and well-being (A. Thakkar, (2024).

4. AI & DATA INTEGRATION: THE BRAIN BEHIND THE MACHINES

4.1 Predictive Analytics and Decision Support

Predictive analytics in healthcare leverages artificial intelligence (AI) algorithms to analyze complex and vast datasets, such as patient medical histories, genetic profiles, lifestyle factors, and real-time monitoring data. By processing these large datasets, AI can identify patterns that may not be immediately obvious to human clinicians, allowing for the prediction of disease risks, early detection of health issues, and the suggestion of personalized treatment plans. These tools enable healthcare providers to make more accurate and data-driven decisions that improve patient outcomes while reducing costs and unnecessary treatments (D Dixon et al,(2024).

AI-powered decision support systems can also optimize medication regimens by analyzing factors like drug interactions, genetic variations in drug metabolism (pharmacogenomics), and real-time biomarkers. This personalized approach helps minimize side effects and enhances the efficacy of treatments. Predictive analytics ensures that clinicians not only respond to current health conditions but also proactively manage future risks, improving preventive care and outcomes.

Key Benefits:

Early Disease Detection: AI can flag early indicators of diseases, including cancers, heart disease, or diabetes, even before symptoms manifest, enabling earlier and more effective interventions.

Optimized Treatment Plans: Personalized treatment suggestions based on data-driven insights improve clinical decisions, reducing the trial-and-error process in selecting the most effective treatment.

Personalized Medication: AI-driven algorithms can predict how different patients will respond to various drugs, optimizing dosing schedules and minimizing adverse reactions.

4.2 Digital Twins and Virtual Patients

Digital twins and virtual patients are transformative innovations that simulate real-time patient data and biological processes to optimize personalized treatment strategies. A digital twin is a virtual replica of a patient's body, created using data from medical imaging, genomics, wearable devices, and other health metrics. By mimicking the patient's physiology in a digital environment, healthcare providers can simulate various treatment approaches, predict their outcomes, and test interventions without the need for trial and error in real-world clinical settings (Kang Zhang et al, (2024).

Virtual patients allow clinicians to experiment with treatment plans, assess disease progression, and explore the impact of potential therapies, all within a controlled digital environment. This technology can be particularly useful in chronic disease management, surgical planning, drug development, and personalized oncology, where precision and individual variations play a critical role in treatment effectiveness.

Key Benefits:

Simulated Treatment Optimization: Digital twins allow for the simulation of multiple treatment strategies, helping clinicians choose the most effective one for the patient before administering it.

Risk Prediction and Prevention: Virtual patients can model how diseases progress and help predict complications, enabling early interventions that can mitigate risks and improve outcomes.

Customized Care Plans: By analyzing how a virtual patient responds to various therapies, healthcare providers can tailor care to the patient's specific needs and biological characteristics. Figure 2. shows the Different AI technology landscape.

Figure 2. Different AI Technology landscape

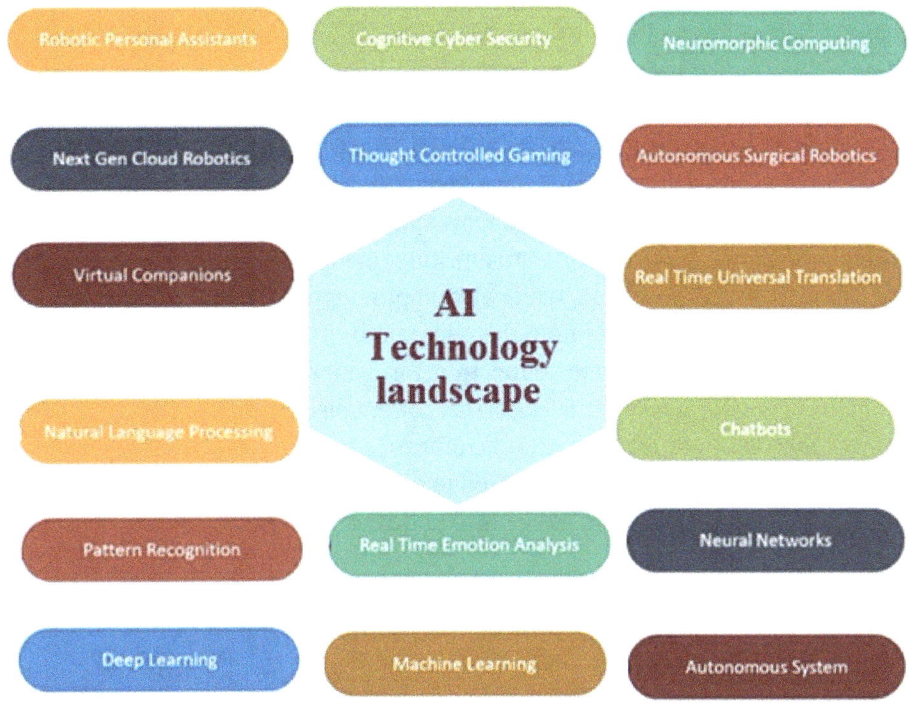

4.3 Interoperability and Health Data Ecosystems

As the healthcare industry embraces a more interconnected, patient-centered approach, interoperability has become essential for the seamless exchange of health data. Interoperability refers to the ability of different healthcare systems, devices, and software platforms to communicate and share data effectively. This includes connecting electronic health records (EHRs), medical devices, wearable health monitors, laboratory systems, and cloud-based platforms, ensuring that clinicians have access to a comprehensive, real-time profile of a patient's health (Chunyan Li et al, (2024).

Emerging standards for interoperability—such as HL7, FHIR (Fast Healthcare Interoperability Resources), and open APIs—enable healthcare providers to securely exchange information across different platforms, breaking down silos and ensuring holistic patient care. These health data ecosystems allow for real-time access to critical health information, providing clinicians with a more accurate, complete picture of a patient's health status, treatment history, and progress.

Key Benefits:

Holistic Patient Profiles: By integrating data from diverse sources (e.g., EHRs, wearables, lab results), clinicians can gain a 360-degree view of a patient's health, leading to more informed decisions and personalized care.

Improved Coordination of Care: Interoperability fosters better communication and coordination between healthcare providers, ensuring that all members of a patient's care team are on the same page and working with up-to-date information.

Enhanced Efficiency and Reduced Errors: Seamless data exchange reduces the likelihood of errors, such as duplicative testing, medication mistakes, or miscommunications between providers, while also improving workflow efficiency.

Together, these three technologies—predictive analytics,digital twins and interoperability—are laying the foundation for a more integrated, efficient, and personalized healthcare system. With the continuous evolution of AI, machine learning, and real-time data sharing, healthcare providers are better equipped to deliver precision medicine that is tailored to each patient's unique needs, ensuring better outcomes and enhancing the overall patient experience.

5. CHALLENGES AND ETHICAL CONSIDERATIONS

5.1 Data Privacy and Security

As personalized medicine increasingly relies on next-generation devices and robotics to collect sensitive biometric data, ensuring robust data privacy and security has become paramount. These devices gather vast amounts of health-related information, including genetic data, real-time vital signs, and behavioral patterns, all of which are critical to delivering tailored care. However, this wealth of data also presents significant risks related to privacy breaches and cyberattacks, which could compromise patient confidentiality and undermine trust in medical technologies (K B Johnson et al,(2020).

To address these concerns, healthcare providers and technology developers must implement strong security measures, including end-to-end encryption, secure cloud storage, and access controls to prevent unauthorized access to patient data. Additionally, the importance of obtaining informed consent from patients cannot be overstated, ensuring that individuals are aware of how their data will be used, stored, and shared. Transparent data policies, regular security audits, and compliance with regulations such as the Health Insurance Portability and Accountability Act (HIPAA) in the U.S., or the General Data Protection Regulation (GDPR) in the EU, are critical in building patient trust and ensuring the responsible use of health data (Kukatlapalli Pradeep Kumar et al, (2024).

Key Challenges:

Data Breaches: Sensitive patient information must be protected from cyberattacks and unauthorized access.

Consent Management: Ensuring patients have full control and understanding over how their data is used.

Compliance: Adhering to regulatory frameworks that govern the use and protection of personal health data.

Key Solutions:

Advanced Encryption:Using cutting-edge encryption technologies to safeguard data during transmission and storage.

Data Minimization: Collecting only the necessary data and ensuring that it is anonymized or pseudonymized whenever possible.

Patient Empowerment: Offering patients control over their data with easy-to-understand consent forms and clear privacy policies. Fig.3 shows the different Challenges and ethical consideration.

Figure 3. Challenges and ethical consideration

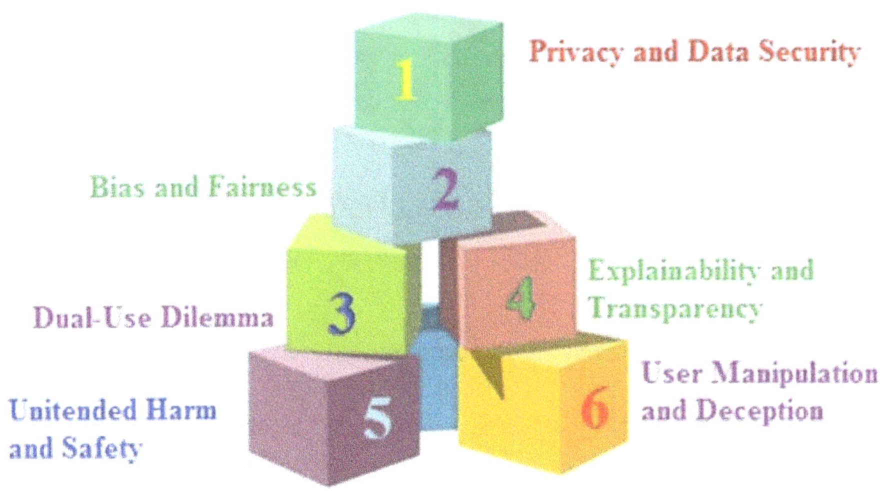

Surgical Precision: Robotic vs Manual

Features like tremor filtration, 3D imaging, and articulated tool control make robotic surgery more precise than manual methods. Surgeons can execute less invasive treatments more precisely thanks to robots, particularly in sensitive or small spaces. Research indicates that robotic-assisted surgeries result in smaller incisions, less blood loss, and quicker recovery (Fig.4). Manual surgery is still better, nevertheless, in terms of tactile feedback and flexibility in challenging, uncertain situations. Although robotic systems increase repeatability and lessen fatigue, their efficacy is mostly reliant on the surgeon's experience and case selection. In general, robotic surgery improves accuracy, although it is better understood as an addition rather than a substitute.

Figure 4. Surgical Precision: Robotic vs Manual

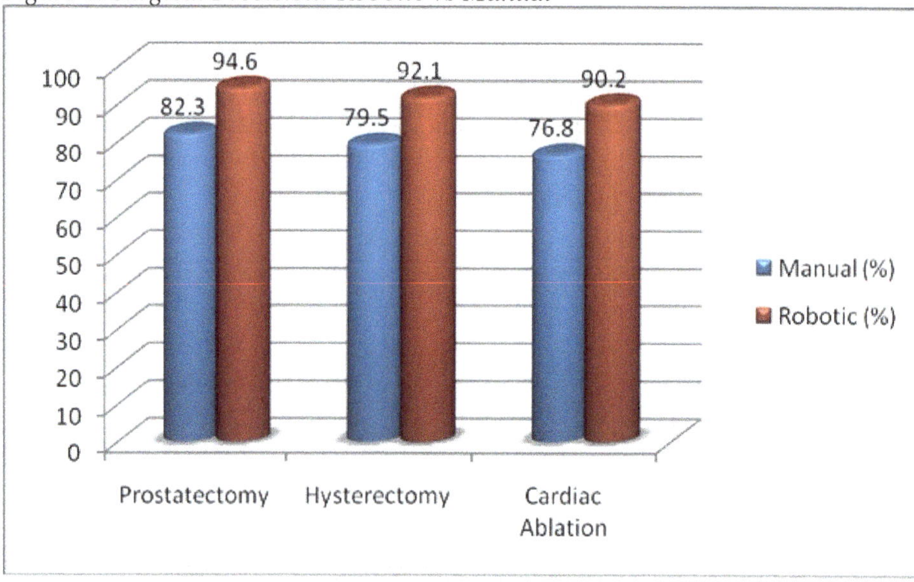

Recovery Time Comparison: Recovery periods from robotic-assisted surgery are typically shorter than those from open surgery (Fig.5). Patients frequently have less postoperative pain and recuperate more quickly as a result of fewer incisions, less trauma, and less blood loss. For instance, patients who undergo robotic hysterectomy and prostatectomy usually resume their regular activities in 1-2 weeks, as opposed to 4-6 weeks following open surgery. Also, hospital stays are shortened, frequently by one to three days. Faster mobilization and reduced complication rates also lead to better overall results. Recovery advantages, however, can differ based on the procedure type and patient condition, underscoring the necessity of thorough case selection and customized treatment planning.

Figure 5. Recovery Time Comparison

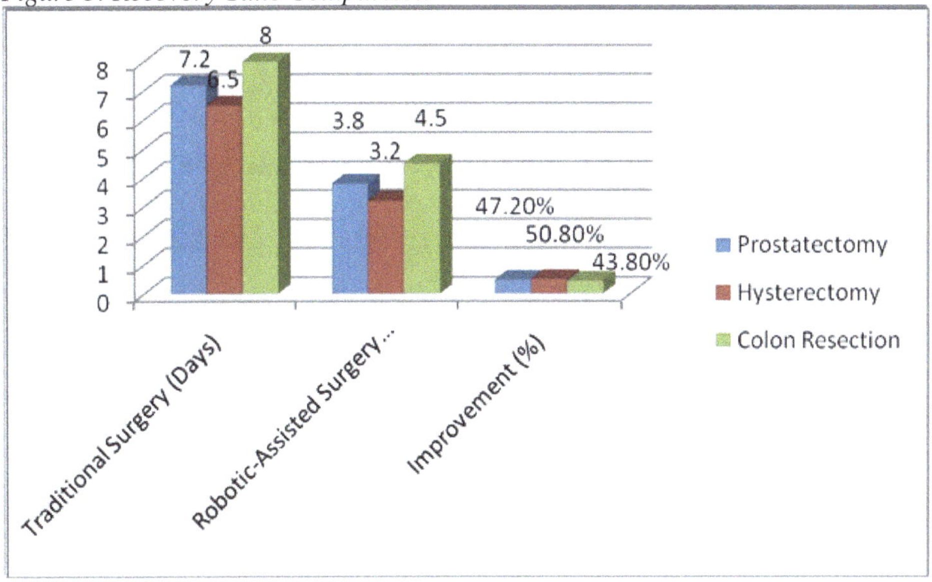

5.2 Equity and Accessibility

One of the core principles of personalized medicine is that it should be available to all patients, regardless of their socio-economic background, geography, or demographic factors. However, the integration of advanced technologies in healthcare presents a significant challenge in terms of equity and accessibility. Devices such as wearables, AI-driven systems, and robotic-assisted surgeries are often expensive and require specialized infrastructure and expertise, which can create disparities in access to care (Yogesh K. Dwivedi et al, (2022).

Strategies to ensure equitable access include designing technologies that are affordable, scalable, and adaptable to different healthcare settings. For example, developing low-cost diagnostic devices or offering mobile-based healthcare solutions can help extend the reach of personalized medicine to underserved populations, including those in rural or low-income areas. Additionally, ensuring that training and support for healthcare providers are accessible is crucial in bridging the gap in expertise between advanced and underserved regions.

Healthcare policies should also address the social determinants of health—such as education, income, and access to care-by integrating personalized medicine into broader public health initiatives. Public-private partnerships, health insurance reforms, and policy changes that promote the inclusion of advanced care technologies in underserved regions can also play an important role in reducing disparities (Alex Hoagland et al, (2024).

Key Challenges:

Cost Barriers: High-cost technologies may not be accessible to low-income or underserved communities.

Healthcare Infrastructure: Limited access to specialized care and advanced technologies in rural or remote areas.

Digital Literacy: Patients and healthcare providers may lack the knowledge or tools to use advanced technologies effectively.

Key Solutions:

Affordable Technologies: Developing cost-effective devices and AI solutions tailored for different income groups.

Telemedicine and Mobile Health: Leveraging telemedicine and mobile platforms to deliver care remotely and increase accessibility.

Public Health Initiatives: Ensuring that healthcare policies prioritize equitable access to personalized medicine.

5.3 Regulation and Validation

As robotic systems, AI-driven devices, and other advanced technologies become increasingly integrated into healthcare, regulation and validation are critical to ensuring their safety, efficacy, and reliability. These technologies must undergo rigorous testing and approval processes to meet established medical standards before they can be used in clinical settings. The lack of adequate regulation or oversight can result in the deployment of devices that are ineffective, unsafe, or prone to malfunction, potentially compromising patient health (C Mennella et al, (2024).

Regulatory agencies, such as the U.S. Food and Drug Administration (FDA) or the European Medicines Agency (EMA), have established frameworks for evaluating the safety and efficacy of medical devices and AI-based technologies. These frameworks include extensive clinical trials, real-world testing, and continuous post-market surveillance to monitor the performance of these technologies. For instance, robotic surgical systems and AI diagnostic tools must be validated to ensure they meet safety standards before being introduced into the medical field.

However, the rapid pace of innovation in robotics and AI presents challenges in keeping regulatory frameworks up to date. Regulatory bodies must work closely with technology developers to create flexible and adaptive frameworks that allow for the safe integration of new technologies while ensuring patient safety.

Key Challenges:

Evolving Technology: The fast-paced development of AI, robotics, and personalized medicine requires adaptive regulatory frameworks that can keep up with innovation.

Safety and Efficacy: Ensuring that new technologies have been thoroughly tested in diverse patient populations and clinical scenarios before deployment.

Post-Market Surveillance: Establishing systems to monitor the long-term effects and potential risks associated with new technologies.

Key Solutions:

Rigorous Testing: Ensuring that robotic systems and AI devices undergo extensive clinical trials to demonstrate their safety and efficacy.

Collaborative Regulation: Encouraging collaboration between healthcare providers, regulators, and technology companies to develop adaptive, evidence-based regulatory standards.

Continuous Monitoring: Implementing post-market surveillance programs to track device performance, identify issues, and update safety standards as needed.

6. FUTURE OPPORTUNITIES

6.1 Future Outlook: Innovations Shaping the Next Era of Personalized Medicine

The convergence of next-generation robotics, artificial intelligence, genomics, and nanotechnology is rapidly propelling personalized medicine into a new frontier. As technologies evolve and become more interconnected, healthcare is transitioning from reactive and generalized approaches to proactive, predictive, and highly individualized care. Below are key areas where future innovations are poised to transform how medicine is practiced, making personalized care more precise, accessible, and intelligent than ever before (Adib Bin Rashid et al, (2024).

6.2 Personalized Drug Delivery Robots

One of the most exciting developments in personalized medicine is the advent of nanorobots capable of navigating the human body to deliver drugs with pinpoint accuracy. These microscopic robots, often smaller than a blood cell, are designed to travel through the bloodstream and release medication only at targeted sites-such as cancerous tumors or inflamed tissues-thus reducing systemic exposure and minimizing harmful side effects (X Kong et al, (2023).

Future nanorobots may be equipped with biosensors that detect specific molecular markers, allowing them to diagnose conditions and initiate treatment autonomously.

Some prototypes already use magnetic fields or biochemical cues to guide their movements, offering new possibilities for treating hard-to-reach areas or diseases that require precise, localized therapy.

Key Benefits:

- Minimized side effects through targeted drug release
- Real-time responsiveness to physiological changes
- Potential for combination therapy and diagnostics in one system ("theranostics")

6.3 Genomics + Robotics Integration

The integration of genomics with robotics is paving the way for genetically tailored interventions, where a patient's personal genome informs robotic surgery and therapeutic strategies. Genomic data can reveal how a person metabolizes drugs, their susceptibility to certain diseases, and even how their tissues may respond to surgical procedures. Robotics systems, guided by these insights, can adapt surgical plans, optimize device parameters, and personalize procedural approaches based on a patient's unique genetic profile (K Reddy et al, (2023).

For instance, in oncology, genome-driven robotics could be used to identify the most effective tumor excision route or determine the most responsive area for biopsy or targeted therapy. Similarly, robotic interventions in cardiology or orthopedics may be enhanced by tailoring surgical tools or approaches based on genetic risk factors.

Key Benefits:

- More accurate and effective surgical outcomes
- Reduced complication rates through genome-informed decisions
- Personalized rehabilitation protocols following surgery

6.4 Smart Hospitals and Home Care

The concept of smart hospitals and AI-driven home care is transforming traditional healthcare environments. With robotic nurses, automated diagnostic tools, and intelligent monitoring systems, hospitals are becoming more efficient, precise, and responsive. These systems not only reduce the burden on clinical staff but also ensure that patients receive timely and consistent care.

Equally transformative is the rise of smart home care systems, where robotic assistants and remote monitoring tools turn homes into miniature healthcare hubs. From AI-powered pill dispensers and mobile diagnostic stations to virtual assistants that schedule appointments and perform health assessments, personalized medicine is becoming more accessible and embedded into daily life (Moustaq Karim Khan Rony et al, (2024).

Key Benefits:

- Improved hospital efficiency and reduced clinician workload
- Enhanced chronic disease management at home
- Continuous, real-time care and support for elderly and at-risk populations.

6.5 Cross-Disciplinary Innovation

The future of personalized medicine lies in cross-disciplinary collaboration. The blending of biotechnology, artificial intelligence, nanotechnology, robotics, and data science is driving innovations that no single field could achieve alone. As these domains converge, entirely new classes of medical solutions are emergin-ranging from bio-hybrid implants and gene-editing robots to personalized regenerative therapies using stem cells guided by AI algorithms (N J Schork et al, (2019).

This synergy is not only accelerating innovation but also making it more adaptive and scalable. By fostering partnerships between engineers, clinicians, data scientists, and geneticists, healthcare systems can anticipate individual patient needs and develop smarter, more personalized strategies for diagnosis, treatment, and prevention.

Key Benefits:

- Faster innovation cycles and rapid deployment of new therapies
- Personalized treatment pathways developed through interdisciplinary collaboration
- Emergence of novel medical paradigms that blend human biology with intelligent machines

The future of personalized medicine is being built on the shoulders of next-gen devices and robotics, enhanced by breakthroughs in genomics, AI, and nanoengineering. As these technologies mature and converge, they will redefine the boundaries of what's possible in healthcare—delivering care that is not only more precise and proactive but also more human-centered. The challenge ahead lies in ensuring that these innovations are ethically deployed, equitably distributed, and continually refined to serve diverse populations around the globe (G Molla et al, (2024).

Through data and case examples, the Table.7 presents strong contextual hooks that show the increasing importance of medical robotics and personalized treatment. The market is expected to be worth \$922 billion, which indicates strong growth potential. Robotic and AI-based technologies are becoming commonplace, with over 1.8 million robotic-assisted procedures scheduled for 2023 and 82% hospital acceptance in the United States. Examples of real patient advantages include robotic prostatectomy, which has been shown to reduce hospital stays by 50%. Diagnostic innovation is demonstrated by wearable technology that can predict atrial fibrillation with 96% accuracy. Precision care is demonstrated by genomic profiling, which reduces chemotherapy use by 34%. The future of customized robotics-driven healthcare is revolutionary, especially when combined with $44 billion in global investments in health technology.

Table 7. Contextual Hooks – Statistics and Case Studies in Personalized Medicine

Hook Type	Example / Data Point	Relevance to Personalized Medicine & Robotics
Global Market Size	The global market for personalized medicine is expected to reach **$922 billion by 2030**, growing at a CAGR of 10.2%.	Indicates rapid industry growth and commercial relevance.
Robotic Surgery Demand	More than **1.8 million robotic-assisted surgeries** were performed globally in 2023.	Highlights the rising global acceptance and demand for robotic surgery.
Device Adoption Rate	**82% of U.S. hospitals** have adopted at least one robotic or AI-assisted medical device.	Demonstrates mainstream clinical integration of next-gen devices.
Patient Outcome Study	Robotic-assisted prostatectomies reduced blood loss by **80%** and hospital stay by 50%.	Shows concrete patient benefits of robotic procedures.
Wearable Devices Impact	AI-powered wearables predicted atrial fibrillation with **96% accuracy** before symptoms.	Emphasizes diagnostic precision and proactive care possibilities.
Genomics Integration	Personalized genomic profiling reduced chemotherapy use in breast cancer patients by **34%**.	Demonstrates personalized treatment minimizing unnecessary procedures.
Technology Investment	Global investment in digital health and med-tech reached **$44 billion in 2022**.	Underlines financial commitment to next-gen healthcare innovations.

7. CONCLUSION

Next-generation devices and robotics are not just enhancing medical capabilities—they are reshaping the entire healthcare ecosystem. From diagnosis and treatment to post-operative care and chronic disease management, the integration of these tools is making medicine more precise, proactive, and personal. The future holds immense potential, and with careful attention to ethics, accessibility, and innovation, personalized medicine will continue to flourish through technology.

REFERENCES

Azizipour, N.. (2020). Evolution of biochip technology: A review from lab-on-a-chip to organ-on-a-chip. *Micromachines, 11*(6), 599. DOI: 10.3390/mi11060599 PMID: 32570945

Dagnino, G.. (2024). Robot-assistive minimally invasive surgery: Trends and future directions. *International Journal of Intelligent Robotics and Applications, 8*, 812–826. DOI: 10.1007/s41315-024-00341-2

Dave, S.. (2024). Advancements in healthcare through 3D-printed micro and nanosensors: Innovation, application, and prospects. *Hybrid Advances, 7*, 100311. DOI: 10.1016/j.hybadv.2024.100311

Dixon, D.. (2024). Unveiling the influence of AI predictive analytics on patient outcomes: A comprehensive narrative review. *Cureus, 16*(5), e59954. DOI: 10.7759/cureus.59954 PMID: 38854327

Dwivedi, Y. K.. (2022). Metaverse beyond the hype: Multidisciplinary perspectives on emerging challenges, opportunities, and agenda for research, practice and policy. *International Journal of Information Management, 66*, 102542. DOI: 10.1016/j.ijinfomgt.2022.102542

Fairag, M.. (2024). Robotic revolution in surgery: Diverse applications across specialties and future prospects review article. *Cureus, 16*(1), e52148. DOI: 10.7759/cureus.52148 PMID: 38344598

Ferreira, D. C.. (2023). Patient satisfaction with healthcare services and the techniques used for its assessment: A systematic literature review and a bibliometric analysis. *Healthcare (Basel), 11*(5), 639. DOI: 10.3390/healthcare11050639 PMID: 36900644

Goetz, L. H.. (2018). Personalized medicine: Motivation, challenges, and progress. *Fertility and Sterility, 109*(6), 952–963. DOI: 10.1016/j.fertnstert.2018.05.006 PMID: 29935653

Hoagland, A.. (2024). Challenges in promoting health equity and reducing disparities in access across new and established technologies. *The Canadian Journal of Cardiology, 40*(6), 1154–1167. DOI: 10.1016/j.cjca.2024.02.014 PMID: 38417572

Iftikhar, M.. (2024). Artificial intelligence: Revolutionizing robotic surgery [Review]. *Annals of Medicine and Surgery (London), 86*(9), 5401–5409. DOI: 10.1097/MS9.0000000000002426 PMID: 39238994

Javaid, M.. (2022). Significance of machine learning in healthcare: Features, pillars and applications. *International Journal of Intelligent Networks, 3*, 58–73. DOI: 10.1016/j.ijin.2022.05.002

. Ji, W., et al. (2025). A networked intelligent elderly care model based on nursing robots to achieve healthy aging. *Research (Washington, D.C.), 8,* 0592. https://doi .org/DOI: 10.34133/research.0592

Johnson, K. B.. (2020). Precision medicine, AI, and the future of personalized health care. *Clinical and Translational Science, 14*(1), 86–93. DOI: 10.1111/cts.12884 PMID: 32961010

Junaid, B. S.. (2022). Recent advancements in emerging technologies for healthcare management systems: A survey. *Healthcare (Basel), 10*(10), 1940. DOI: 10.3390/ healthcare10101940 PMID: 36292387

Kong, X.. (2023). Advances of medical nanorobots for future cancer treatments. *Journal of Hematology & Oncology, 16*(1), 74. DOI: 10.1186/s13045-023-01463-z PMID: 37452423

Kopalli, S. R.. (2025). Artificial intelligence in stroke rehabilitation: From acute care to long-term recovery. *Neuroscience, 572*, 214–231. DOI: 10.1016/j.neuroscience.2025.03.017 PMID: 40068721

Kumar, K. P.. (2024). Secure approach to sharing digitized medical data in a cloud environment. *Data Science and Management, 7*(2), 108–118. DOI: 10.1016/j. dsm.2023.12.001

Kyrarini, M.. (2021). A survey of robots in healthcare. *Technologies, 9*, 8. DOI: 10.3390/technologies9010008

Li, C.. (2024). A review of IoT applications in healthcare. *Neurocomputing, 565*, 127017. DOI: 10.1016/j.neucom.2023.127017

Marques, L.. (2024). Advancing precision medicine: A review of innovative in silico approaches for drug development, clinical pharmacology and personalized healthcare. *Pharmaceutics, 16*(3), 332. DOI: 10.3390/pharmaceutics16030332 PMID: 38543226

Mennella, C.. (2024). Ethical and regulatory challenges of AI technologies in healthcare: A narrative review. *Heliyon, 10*(4), e26297. DOI: 10.1016/j.heliyon.2024. e26297 PMID: 38384518

Mennella, C., Maniscalco, U., De Pietro, G., & Esposito, M. (2024). Ethical and regulatory challenges of AI technologies in healthcare: A narrative review. *Heliyon*, *10*(4), e26297. DOI: 10.1016/j.heliyon.2024.e26297 PMID: 38384518

Molla, G.. (2024). Revolutionizing personalized medicine: Synergy with multi-omics data generation, main hurdles, and future perspectives. *Biomedicines*, *12*(12), 2750. DOI: 10.3390/biomedicines12122750 PMID: 39767657

Molla, G.. (2024). Revolutionizing personalized medicine: Synergy with multi-omics data generation, main hurdles, and future perspectives. *Biomedicines*, *12*(12), 2750. DOI: 10.3390/biomedicines12122750 PMID: 39767657

. Padmavathi. (2025). Blockchain based system for healthcare digital twin. In T. A. Nguyen (Ed.), *Blockchain and digital twin for smart healthcare* (pp. 179–192). Elsevier. https://doi.org/DOI: 10.1016/B978-0-443-30300-5.00012-9

Pal, S.. (2024). Bio-inspired electronic sensors for healthcare applications. *Chemical Engineering Journal*, *499*, 155894. DOI: 10.1016/j.cej.2024.155894

Rashid, A. B. (2024). AI revolutionizing industries worldwide: A comprehensive overview of its diverse applications. *Hybrid Advances*, *7*, 100277. DOI: 10.1016/j.hybadv.2024.100277

Rashid, A. B.. (2024). AI revolutionizing industries worldwide: A comprehensive overview of its diverse applications. *Hybrid Advances*, *7*, 100277. DOI: 10.1016/j.hybadv.2024.100277

Reddy, K.. (2023). Advancements in robotic surgery: A comprehensive overview of current utilizations and upcoming frontiers. *Cureus*, *15*(12), e50415. DOI: 10.7759/cureus.50415 PMID: 38222213

Rony, M. K. K.. (2024). The role of artificial intelligence in enhancing nurses' work-life balance. *Journal of Medicine, Surgery, and Public Health*, *3*, 100135. DOI: 10.1016/j.glmedi.2024.100135

Sadee, W.. (2023). Pharmacogenomics: Driving personalized medicine. *Pharmacological Reviews*, *75*(4), 789–814. DOI: 10.1124/pharmrev.122.000810 PMID: 36927888

. Satam, H., et al. (2023). Next-generation sequencing technology: Current trends and advancements. *Biology (Basel), 12*(7), 997. https://doi.org/ Erratum in: *Biology (Basel), 13*(5), 286. https://doi.org/DOI: 10.3390/biology12070997

Sawik, B.. (2023). Robots for elderly care: Review, multi-criteria optimization model and qualitative case study. *Healthcare (Basel), 11*(9), 1286. DOI: 10.3390/healthcare11091286 PMID: 37174828

Schork, N. J.. (2019). Artificial intelligence and personalized medicine. *Cancer Treatment and Research, 178*, 265–283. DOI: 10.1007/978-3-030-16391-4_11 PMID: 31209850

Shah, S.. (2025). The evolution of brain surgery: Exploring the impact of continuum robotics. *Brain Hemorrhages, 6*(1), 38–56. DOI: 10.1016/j.hest.2024.11.002

Thakkar, A. (2024). Artificial intelligence in positive mental health: A narrative review. *Frontiers in Digital Health, 6*, 1280235. DOI: 10.3389/fdgth.2024.1280235 PMID: 38562663

Vo, D. K.. (2024). Advances in wearable biosensors for healthcare: Current trends, applications, and future perspectives. *Biosensors (Basel), 14*, 560. DOI: 10.3390/bios14110560 PMID: 39590019

. Wang, H., et al. (2024). Liquid biopsy for human cancer: Cancer screening, monitoring, and treatment. *MedComm (2020), 5*(6), e564. https://doi.org/DOI: 10.1002/mco2.564

Zhang, K.. (2024). Concepts and applications of digital twins in healthcare and medicine. *Patterns (New York, N.Y.), 5*(8), 101028. DOI: 10.1016/j.patter.2024.101028 PMID: 39233690

Zheng, Z.. (2024). Wearable and implantable biosensors: Mechanisms and applications in closed-loop therapeutic systems. *Journal of Materials Chemistry. B, 12*(35), 8577–8604. DOI: 10.1039/d4tb00782d PMID: 39138981

Chapter 4
Expansion of Self-Supervised Learning in Computer Vision for Medical Image Analysis

Narinder Kaur Seera
https://orcid.org/0000-0001-6533-4560
IINTM, India

ABSTRACT

Advancements in computer vision are expanding rapidly these days and their application in medical image analysis is providing promising results, providing improved healthcare tasks. Despite the fact that computer vision models primarily deal with image data, there are numerous differences in the properties of different sets of raw images. Hence, the models are pre-trained with appropriate pretext tasks so that they can produce best results when applied to downstream tasks which helps in better diseases diagnosis and treatment. In this chapter, the author aims to present a comprehensive study on the expansion of self-supervised learning methods in computer vision for medical image analysis. The author examines various SSL frameworks, including contrastive, generative, and clustering-based methods, and analyzes their effectiveness across multiple medical imaging modalities such as MRI, CT, X-rays, and histopathology slides. The chapter concludes by highlighting future research directions and the potential of SSL to transform clinical decision-making through more accessible and robust AI-driven tools.

DOI: 10.4018/979-8-3373-1514-0.ch004

1. INTRODUCTION

The expansion of both SSL and Artificial Intelligence (AI) are revolutionizing medical image analysis by enabling faster, more accurate and scalable diagnostic support across a variety of healthcare settings. The potential use of AI-driven tools in medical imaging has a growing impact on disease detection, classification, segmentation, and prognosis of diseases. With the integration of deep learning, particularly convolutional neural networks (CNNs) and transformer-based architectures, AI models have achieved expert-level performance in interpreting complex medical images such as MRI, CT, X-rays, and histopathology slides (Ashraf et al, 2024).

1.1 Background

Machine Learning (ML) (Sarker et al, 2021; Pugliese et al, 2021) is generally referred to as one of the most admired technologies in Industry 4.0 (Xu et al, 2018). The application areas of ML approaches depend on the nature of the data and choice of the model we want. The efficiency and accuracy of aML model depends on the properties of data and the performance of the learning model over that data. Hence choosing a particular ML algorithm appropriate for the target application is a challenging task (Bustillo et al, 2022; Osisanwo et al, 2017) It becomes important to understand the underlying principles of these ML algorithms before using them for any real world application.

Supervised Learning is a popular choice to in the domain of computer vision or image classification where the ML model learns image features from a given large pool of annotated images (Popescu et al, 2014). In some vision based applications, *Deep Learning (DL)* models exploits the supervised ML models pretrained on ImageNet dataset to boost the performance of transfer-learning or fine-tuning processes for extracting features from a small domain-specific image datasets. DL models are trained using neural network architectures with multiple layers and a large set of labeled data (Mittal et al, 2020; Minaee et al, 2021)

Along with this, the research community has witnessed a growing interest in *Unsupervised Learning* (Eckhardt et al, 2022), specifically for feature representation (or image analysis) in order to avoid manual annotation of huge image datasets, which is required in supervised learning. *CNNs (Convolution Neural Networks)* have proved to be a successful model in the domain of medical image analysis (Tajbakhsh et al, 2016; Gu et al, 2018). CNNs work on a huge number of parameters to capture the underlying distribution of features in the input image sets. Even though, CNNs have gained a big success in various domains, there are few barriers that impede their progress further. First, current deep learning algorithms such as CNNs and others are drastically expanding in depth, memory requirements, and complexity producing an extra computational bottleneck. Second, preparing a huge repository of high-quality annotated images is a time-consuming and expensive task. Third, manually annotating medical images demand expert professionals with domain knowledge. And last, sometimes patients' privacy issues are a matter of concern when dealing with specific disorders.

For addressing these limitations, the concept of *SSL (or Self Supervised Learning)* has been proposed that exploits unlabeled data for learning models without requiring manual annotation for learning unsupervised image representation (Bai et al, 2021; Anand et al, 2021). Self-supervised learning has found its way in countless applications, as in healthcare, text and face detection, spam filtration, categorization, forecasting, video editing, remote sensing, transforming, etc. SSL has gained its popularity due to its huge success in computer vision (Zhang et al, 2016).

Self supervised learning is expanding its applications in computer vision to a large area ranging from medical image analysis (Mascolini et al, 2022) to cyber forensic, from computer games to image colorization, from calligraphy analysis to signature identification etc. Despite the fact that computer vision models primarily deal with image data, there are fundamental differences in the properties of raw images. For instance, natural images and medical images (produced by CT scans or MRI scans) differ in terms of the number of channels, intensity, location, scale and orientation. For the number of channels, natural images are mainly 2D RGB images, while medical images may be 2D gray-scale, 3D volumes, or 4D as volume over time dimension. For intensity, the same object will nearly possess the same features under different intensity levels, e.g., the human face is the same under different intensities. On the other side, intensity holds meaningful information in medical images, e.g., different tissues have different values according to the Hounsfield scale in CT scans. Hence, the models are pre-trained with appropriate pretext tasks so that they can produce best ever results when applied to downstream tasks. The important consideration is that pre-trained models should satisfy two constraints:

1. They must map how images relate to one another
2. They must be robust enough to handle noise in the input images.

1.2 Objectives

The integration of cutting-edge technologies such as SSL, Artificial Intelligence (AI), Internet-of-Things (IoT) and robotics is reshaping modern healthcare through the development of next-generation medical devices (Swarnkar et al,2025; Islam et al, 2024) These advancements aim to create devices that are more intelligent, minimally invasive, patient-centered, and capable of delivering real-time, personalized care. However, there are some primary research questions and goals that are driving the exploration and development of next-generation medical devices, especially in the context of AI, digital health, and advanced materials (Kalra et al, 2024)

- How can medical devices be made more intelligent through Self Supervision or AI integration?
- How can we improve real-time data acquisition, processing, and interpretation?
- How can the annotation of medical images be done in fast and accurate way?
- What design innovations can enhance device miniaturization and portability?

To answer these questions, we present a comprehensive study on the expansion of Self-supervised learning in computer vision and related domain with insights on generative & contrastive approaches. Additionally, the study addresses key challenges including data privacy, model interpretability, generalizability across diverse populations, and regulatory considerations. As AI tools continue to evolve, their integration into clinical workflows promises to enhance diagnostic accuracy, reduce workload for medical professionals, and ultimately improve patient outcomes. Efforts to employ supervised learning to assist in medical domain are often hampered by the high costs of expert annotations required for model training. We tried to compile the results of our study in tables showing the applications of various SSL tasks in medical domain. The paper concludes by identifying future research directions and the critical need for multidisciplinary collaboration in developing ethical and clinically viable AI solutions.

2. PARADIGM OF SELF-SUPERVISION

A *Pretext task* is a proxy task for the model to solve with the objective of learning data representations so that it can be easily applied to any particular downstream tasks (Boffa et al, 2022). *Downstream task* is the actual application for which SSL models are trained. It is considered as the knowledge transfer process (Noroozi et al, 2018) of the pretext model to a specific task. The performance of a model on these tasks marks the success of the model.

The Pretext training of a model is followed by actual training and therefore it is also referred to as Pre-Training. It is a crucial step when training a model as it helps the model to capture more meaningful features and intermediate representations of the data (Maithra et al, 2019). Once the model is pre-trained with a pretext task, it is then fine-tuned for learning on a specific task. At this point, the initial weights (or, learned features) are left almost untouched. There are various methods for fine tuning of Pretext tasks such as gradual unfreezing, one-cycle training, discriminative learning rates etc. However, Pre-training and Fine-tuning can also be done at one step (multi-task learning), the complexity should be only added if needed.

Figure 1. Self-Supervised Learning Setup

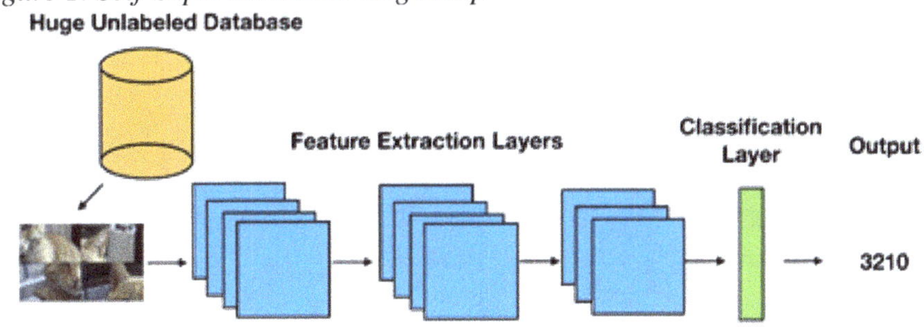

Figure 2. Downstream Task Supervised Learning Setup

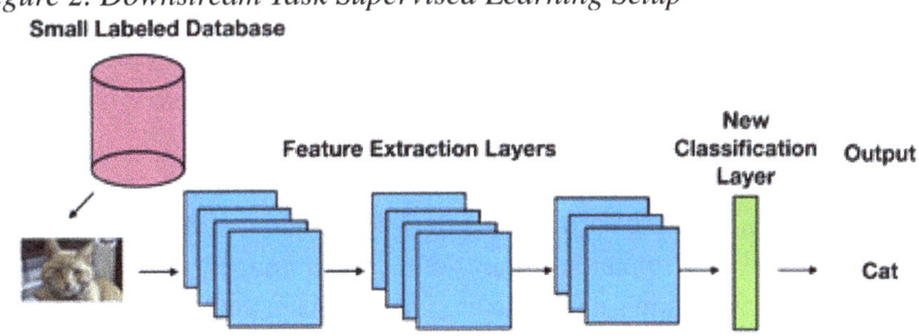

There exists a variety of pretext tasks in real-world. The basic one includes augmentation; where a model (or, a network) is supplied with pre-rotated images and a model has to learn what kind of augmentation has been applied. Another set of pretext tasks from computer vision domain are those tasks that are designed to train the model for learning visual features from given dataset and then employing the model to solve downstream tasks such as image classification or object detection (Jing et al, 2020). Fig 1 and fig 2 shows the self supervised model training setup using pretext tasks and its application in downstream task respectively.

2.1 Predictive Learning

In Predictive learning, the unlabeled images are assigned with some labels which are generated automatically based on the attributes of data. The model is then trained to learn representations and desired properties of images. An example could be to apply some transformation to the input image and then train the model to predict the effect of transformation applied to it. Recent researches (Gidaris et al, 2018; Zhang et al, 2016) have proposed many pretext tasks to learn representations using predictive learning for object detection, image classification, segmentation etc. Few common pretext tasks that follow predictive learning are image rotation, image colorization and jigsaw puzzle.

2.2 Generative vs. Contrastive Learning

In Generative learning, a model is trained to regenerate the original input or to generate new examples from the same distribution of the input dataset (Mascolini et al, 2022). The intuition is to let the model learn semantically useful representations from unlabeled data. The most promising generative models are Auto-encoders (Vincent et al, 2008) and Generative Adversarial Networks (GANs) (Goodfellow et al, 2014). These generative models have come up as a very powerful pretext tasks and have been found to represent the unlabeled data very well. Below we discuss these models briefly:

AutoEncoders: are self-supervised machine learning models which regenerate the compressed input image into the original one. The main function of autoencoders is to make a model learn the semantic features of the input images effectively so that it can be efficiently used in downstream tasks. They perform their function into two phases: encoding and decoding. In the first phase, the model is trained to learn a function that encodes the input into a representation, and later this representation is decoded to reconstruct the original image, in the second phase. This encoding and decoding is done by encoders and decoders respectively, both of which are made up of a combination of NN (Neural Networks) layers (Wang et al, 2022). In the case of CNN (Convolution Neural Networks) autoencoder, these layers are made up of CNN layers (Convolutional, Max Pool, Flattening, etc.) whereas in case of RNN and LSTM, their respective layers are used. A downside of using autoencoders is that they cannot handle large and complex images efficiently; consequently they sometimes produce degraded images.

To minimize the reconstruction loss, various types of autoencoders are proposed by researchers such as Denoising autoencoders, Variational autoencoders (VAE), Masked autoencoders, Split Brain autoencoders etc. These autoencoders have proved to show overall improved feature extraction for producing high quality image reconstruction (Karnam et al, 2020).

In Denoising autoencoders (Vincent et al, 2008), the model explicitly adds noise (Gaussian noise, Poisson noise etc.) to the input image to corrupt the data and to mask some of the values. It is then followed by image reconstruction, where the model learns to reconstructs the input image by improved extraction of latent representations, as shown in fig 3. Denoising autoencoder has a lower risk of learning "identity function" because of the noise which is added initially.

In Split Brain autoencoders (Richard et al, 2017) the neural network is split into two sub-networks; each is trained to perform a difficult task- predicting one subset of the data channels from another. Finally, the outputs from both the sub-networks are concatenated to generate the final result. The intuition behind split brain is to achieve a useful representation by learning to generate a portion of the data from the remaining data.

Figure 3. Denoising Autoencoders (Image source: https://blog.keras.io/building-autoencoders-in-keras.html)

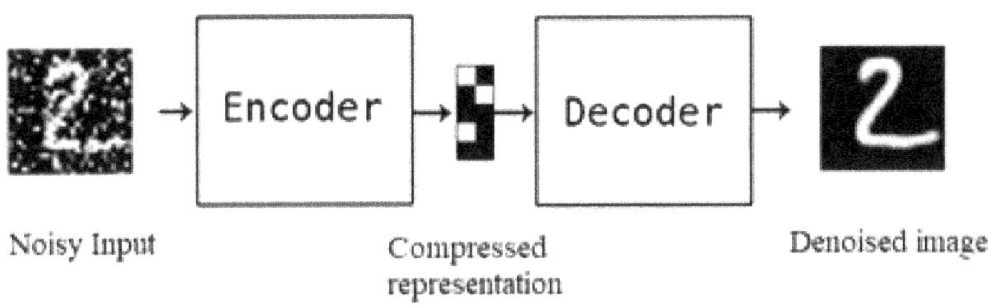

Variational autoencoders (VAE) (Kingma et al, 2013) improve over the autoencoder framework by encoding the parameters of the latent space distribution. They are trained to minimize both the reconstruction error and an additional term, minimizing the Kull–Leibler divergence between a known latent distribution often picked as the unit-centered Gaussian distribution and the one produced by the encoder. This regularization over the latent space allows sampling from the generated distribution.

More recently, the use of vision transformers has enabled the development of large masked autoencoders (Pang et al, 2022) working at a patch level instead of pixel-wise to reconstruct entire patches with only 25% of visible patches. This reconstruction task produces robust image representations by appending a class token to the sequence of patches or simply by using a global average pooling on all the patch tokens. Autoencoders have found their way in various applications such as file compression, anomaly detection, image inpainting, machine translation, image de-noising, semantic segmentation etc. In Image Inpainting pretext task, the model is supposed to fill in a missing piece in the image (Pathak et al, 2016). The model is trained with a combination of the reconstruction (L2) loss and the adversarial loss. It has encoder-decoder architecture and encoder part can be considered as representation learning.

Generative Adversarial Models (GANs): GANs are another primitive generative models which have received significant attention by the researchers (Goodfellow et al, 2014).They attempt to generate new data from a random noise with the objective to mimic the real data. GANs have come up as a powerful tool to learn models that stem from very complex distribution. They employ trained generators and discriminators to learn feature representations via input noises, which are essentially the feature representations of the output. These input noises contain the data needed to produce the corresponding image. The generator synthesizes fake images for discriminator to believe that the synthesized image is real. The discriminator learns to classify between images from the original dataset. The output score of the discriminator is 1 when it is confident that the input image is coming from the real data distribution and 0 for images created by the generator. (Radford et al, 2016) has shown that GANs are able to capture powerful semantic information, which can be very useful in self-supervised pretraining. To use these features for representation learning, (Donahue et al, 2016) came up with a novel Generative architecture BiGAN. Along with the normal discriminator and generator, this model also includes another network called the encoder. This encoder turns the real images into latent representations. The task here is then similar to that of an autoencoder where the generator and the encoder have to be inverse of each other. BiGAN has been shown to be effective in learning visual representations. This can be classified as a self-supervised method because the discriminator learns to assign labels such as 'fake' or 'real' to images and thus self-supervised learning is involved in all kinds of GANs. Various SSL methods using Generative and Contrastive Learning have been listed in Table 1.

Contrastive Learning is a discriminative model that learns by comparing positive or negative pairs of images from the datasets. The motive is to make classification and segmentation tasks possible by learning a representation in which positive pairs are grouped together whereas negative pairs are kept apart. Contrastive learning has found its way in supervised, unsupervised as well as self-supervised learning (Jaiswal et al, 2020). Let us consider image classification problem. In supervised learning, positive pairs are images with similar labels and negative pairs belong to other set of labels. On the other hand, in unsupervised (or self-supervised) setting, positive pairs are parts (or augmented versions) of the same instance and negative samples are other instances with any label (Liu et al, 2021; Albelwi et al 2022). Contrastive learning has achieved state-of-the-art performance in a number of applications such as data augmentation (Hu et al, 2021), memory banks (Grill et al, 2020), BYOL (Wang, et al 2021) contrastive losses (Dosovitskiy et al, 2014) and via the number of negative samples. An example of pretext task that uses the concept of positive and negative pairs for classification is Image Distortion.

BYOL (Bootstrap Your Own Latent): This novel approach is based on two networks, called online and target networks, which interact with each other to learn representations from the augmented view of images. The aim is to train the online network to predict the representation of the same image under a different augmented view in target network. Parallel to this, the target network is continuously updated with a slow-moving average of the online network. BYOL achieved a new state-of-the-art accuracy of 74.3% in classification without using negative pairs, unlike other approaches under contrastive learning (Wang et al, 2021).

Image Distortion: It is assumed that if a small amount of distortion is applied on an image, its semantic meaning should not affect. (Dosovitskiy et al, 2014) followed this idea and created an exemplar-based classification task with a surrogate class which consisted of various image samples. These samples wereunderwent an array of transformations such as scaling, translation, contrast and rotation. The task was to learn the representations from these altered images and classify them in positive and negative groups. The augmented versions of the same image should have similar representations, called positive pairs and augmented versions of the different images should have different representations, called negative pairs.

Table 1. SSL methods in computer vision

SSL method	SSL tasks	Proposed by	Applications
Contrastive	Frame Order Recognition	(Chen et al, 2020)	Computer vision
Contrastive	Memory Banks	(Grill et al, 2020)	Computer vision (visual representation & image classification)
Contrastive	SwAV	(Chen et al, 2020)	Image augmentation and Instance classification
Contrastive	SimCLR	(Caron et al,2020)	Google's medical image analysis model
Contrastive	Geometrical Transformation	(Szegedy et al, 2013)	Object detection and classification such as Tumor detection
Generative	Object Detection	(Dosovitskiy et al, 2015)	Autonomous driving Scene text detection
Generative	Exemplar CNN	(Doersch et al, 2015)	Object Classification and Descriptor Matching

continued on following page

Table 1. Continued

SSL method	SSL tasks	Proposed by	Applications
Generative	Relative Patches	(Han et al, 2020)	Visual data mining
Generative	Split Brain Autoencoders	(Zhang et al, 2017)	Image classification
Generative	Variational Autoencoders (VAE)	(Kingma et al, 2013)	Computer vision such as video and image generation
Generative	Video Future Prediction	(Lorre et al, 2020)	Visual mining, Video captioning
Generative	Temporal Order Verification	(Pathak et al, 2016)	visual audio correspondence verification
Generative	Moving Object Segmentation	(Felfeliyan et al, 2023)	Video classification
Generative	Semantic Segmentation	(Grill et al, 2020)	Autonomous driving Robotics
Generative	Image Rotation	(Gidaris et al, 2018)	Image orientation auto-correction

3. SSL IN MEDICAL IMAGE ANALYSIS

From past few years, machine learning models in computer vision have been struggling hard towards perfection over variety of images with same or different modalities. The advancements in SSL aim to train the models to learn useful representations of the data from unlabelled pool of data and then fine-tune the learnt representations to downstream tasks such as image classification or object detection etc (Raghu et al, 2019; Jing et al, 2020).Recently, generative and contrastive learning have been applied to medical image scans, where they have shown promising results. However, there are few studies which have utilized the power of both generative and contrastive approaches (Taleb et al, 2022).In this section, we discuss advancements of SSL in computer vision field, especially for medical image analysis. Table 2 summarizes the studies for medical domain with their applications and SSL methods used.

Self-supervised learning has the potential to make significant contributions to the development of robust medical imaging models through its ability to learn useful insights from copious medical datasets without labels. The success of GANs in computer vision has attracted researchers to expand its applications for the analysis of medical images. The most widely used medical images are Chest X-ray, CT scans images, MRI images and brain tumor cells (Thakur et al, 2024; Wu et al, 2024)."

Generative Adversarial Networks (GANs) have gained popularity in medical imaging for tasks such as image synthesis, augmentation, modality translation (e.g.,

MRI to CT), and anomaly detection. While promising, their scalability and reliability in clinical applications remain under scrutiny. GANs can generate realistic synthetic medical images to augment small or imbalanced datasets, reducing dependency on expert annotation. GANs (like CycleGAN) can translate images between modalities (e.g., CT $\leftrightarrow$ MRI), supporting multimodal integration without paired data. Besides the awesome advantages offered by GANs, they are sometimes notoriously difficult to train due to mode collapse, vanishing gradients, and sensitivity to hyperparameters. Training large GANs on high-resolution 3D medical images (e.g., MRI, CT volumes) demands significant GPU resources and memory. Moreover, no universally accepted metric exists for evaluating the quality and realism of synthetic medical images. GANs can introduce subtle, unrealistic artifacts that may mislead clinicians or downstream diagnostic models.

Mahapatra (Mahapatra et al, 2020) has utilized GAN for point registrations of medical images, the process of discovering a spatial transformation in images that can align two point clouds. This is also referred to as scan matching or point cloud registration. GAN has been proved to show better performance in experiments based on scan matching for Chest X-ray images, Retinal, and Brain Magnetic Resonance images.

A novel approach to use deep learning based SSL is adopted by (Chaitanya et al, 2020) to work with unlabeled medical image data. For model pretraining, various distortions are randomly applied to arbitrarysectionsof unlabeled images. The model is assumed to capture the relevant texture representation from this pretraining on the given input. A Mask-RCNN based model is trained to localize the distortion location and recover the original image pixels. It creates aground for fine-tuning the model to segment the structure of interest using unlabeled training data.

An extension of contrastive learning framework has been proposed by (Felfeliyan et al, 2023) for segmentation of voluminous medical images, by using domain-specific and problem-specific knowledge. The model leverages on structural similarity across volumetric medical images and contrastive loss to capture multiple representations of local regions of images which are useful for image analysis. Instead of focusing on image-wide representation, this model focused on per-pixel segmentation providing the ability to recognize different areas of images. The model used domain specific knowledge while learning global representations; which enables it to define similar image pairs that undergo several transformations (Li et al, 2025; Du et al, 2025).

In medical imaging, contrastive learning has shown promising results in pretraining models for downstream tasks such as classification, segmentation, and anomaly detection. However, despite its scalability potential, it lacks at certain points. First, inappropriate augmentations can distort medical semantics (e.g., flipping a chest X-ray might mislead the model), making contrastive learning brittle if domain-specific augmentations are not carefully chosen. Second, in medical imaging, what constitutes a "negative" sample isn't always clear—two samples from different patients might still share pathological similarities. Third, high-dimensional and 3D modalities (e.g., MRI volumes) increase computational burden and make pair generation, augmentation, and similarity calculation more complex. Lastly, contrastive learning representations are not inherently interpretable, limiting clinical trust and regulatory acceptance.

(S. A. Rizvi et al, 203) has found that most of the SSL frameworks do not clearly identify the image and text regions in medical images and also find it hard to distinguish various pathologies.Thisresistsradiologists to evaluate model predictions. Hence, they proposed Local Region Contrastive Learning (LRCLR), which incorporates layers in the framework for identifying image regionsand cross-modality interaction. This approached proved to be useful in identifying and interpreting image regions and radiology text in chest X-ray images.

(Yurt et al, 2021) used GAN to produce scant medical images, where multi-contrast MRI (Magnetic Resonance Imaging) protocol raised the level of morphological discrimination information that can be used for diagnosis. The number and quality of contrasts are limited by several factors such as scan time and patient movement.

(Taleb et al,2022) has presented ContIG, a SSL based algorithm to improve representation learning from multiple modalities by capturing imaging-genetic relationships. There exists a huge body of recent works which have shown their contributions in capturing representations from multiple modalities (Du et al, 2025; Taleb et al, 2021).

Talking about modality, each modality refers to a specific source of information that explains the features of samples. For any model to effectively analyze the input, it must be capable enough to learn the features from the multiple modalities that exist in it. Multimodal representation learning has become an interesting area of research that aims to effectively integrate information into a framework from various sources that can be applied to downstream tasks. Multi-modal fusion with medical images and challenges associated with multimodal representation learning is widely studied in (Hassan et al, 2022; Pei et al, 2023; Abid et al, 2023)

Table 2. Applications of SSL methods in medical image analysis

SSL method	SSL tasks	Proposed by	Modality of input images	Applications
Generative	Jigsaw Puzzle	(Noroozi et al, 2016)	MRI scans	Brain tumor segmentation and liver segmentation
Generative	Image Colorization	(Yurt et al, 2021)	MRI and CT scans	Object Classification, detection & segmentation (Brain hemorrhage classification)
Generative	Image Denoising	(Zhang et al, 2016)	Cell images	Nuclei images segmentation
Generative	Context Prediction Auto Encoders	(Chen et al, 2022)	CT scans	Liver and kidney segmentation
Generative	Relative Position Prediction	(Tianqing et al, 2021)	MRI scnas	Body part recognition, MRI scans segmentation
Generative	Skull reconstruction	(Matzkin et al, 2020)	CT scans	Bone flap volume estimation
Generative	Context restoration	(Chen et al, 2019)	Fetal images	Fetal image classification Abdominal multi-organ localization Brain tumour segmentation
Contrastive	BYOL	(Grill et al, 2020)	MRI and CT scan images	Abdominal organs segmentation
Contrastive	Color Transformation	(Chen et al, 2020)	MRI and CT scans	Medical image analysis
Contrastive	SimCLR	(Mojab et al, 2020)	Whole Slide image	Glaucoma Lung Cancer detection
Contrastive	MoCo v2	(Dehaene et al, 2020)	Whole Slide image	Breast Cancer detection
Contrastive	MoCo v2	(Reed et al, 2022)	Chest X-ray	Indentifying chest abnormality
Contrastive	SimCLR	(Hao et al, 2021)	Chest X-ray	Pneumonia detection in Covid-19
Contrastive	BYOL	(Nguyen et al, 2021)	Chest X-ray	Pneumonia detection in Covid-19
Contrastive	SimSiam	(Bao et al, 2021)	CT scans	Gastric cancer detection
Contrastive	SimCLR	(Jian et al, 2021)	Endoscopy	Helicobacter Pylori infection detection
Contrastive	BYOL	(Ren et al, 2021)	Skin images	Skin cancer detection
Contrastive	InfoNCE	(Zhao et al,2021)	Ultrasound images	Kidney tumor detection
Predictive	Inpainting	(Park et al, 2021)	Chest x-ray	Covid 19 detection

continued on following page

Table 2. Continued

SSL method	SSL tasks	Proposed by	Modality of input images	Applications
Predictive	Image restoration	(Jana et al, 2021)	CT scans	Liver fibrosis identification
Predictive	Pixel shuffling and image restoration	(Zhong et al, 2021)	MRI	Heart failure
Predictive	Image restoration	(Liu et al, 2021)	Ultrasound images	Gastrointenstinal tumor detection
Predictive	Geodesic distance prediction	(Spitzer et al, 2018)	Brain images	Brain area segmentation
Predictive	Jigsaw puzzle	(Taleb et al,2021)	MRI and CT scans	Brain tumor segmentation Liver segmentation Prostate segmentation
Predictive	Rubik cube	(Zhuang et al, 2019)	MRI scans	Brain tumor segmentation Brain hemorrhage classification
Predictive	Jigsaw puzzle	(Li et al, 2020)	Nuceli images	Nuclei Segmentation Skin lesions segmentation
Generative & Contrastive	Autoencoder and modified MoCo	(Bozorgtaba et al,2020)	Chest X-ray	Indentifying chest abnormality
Generative & Contrastive	Autoencoders and multimodal contrastive	(Hsieh et al, 2020)	MRI scans	Cognitive impairment
Generative & self-prediction	Autoencoder and patch pseudo label prediction	(Haghighi et al, 2021)	CT scans	Lung nodule identification
Generative & self-prediction	GANs	(Cornelissen et al, 2021)	Endoscopy images	Gastroenterology diagnosis
Generative & Contrastive	Autoencoder and SimCLR	(Fedorov et al,2021)	MRI scans	Alzheimer's disease diagnostic
Generative & Contrastive	CycleGAN and Contrastive learning	(Ke et al, 2021)	Whole Slide image	Cancer diagnosis for stomach and breast
Supervised and unsupervised	unsupervised initial segmentation and supervised segmentation refinement	(Zheng et al, 2018)	Cell images	White blood cells image segmentation
SSL based deep learning	Mask-RCNN architecture	(Felfeliyan et al, 2023)	MRI of the knee	Knee and Joint Replacement, Anomaly detection, Segmentation

4. DISCUSSION AND RESEARCH CHALLENGES

There has been a significant research work available which contributed towards medical domain to improve the ability of learning models to do better diagnostics. However, there are few gaps and challenges in the existing work, which are discussed here. Unlabelled medical images carry valuable information about human organ structures, and genome structures are the blue print for biological functions. Although integrating these data modalities in a single framework is a challenging task, however it can help createa more holistic picture of physical and disease traits. The human genome consists of millions of base pairs, yet most genetic differences between individuals have little effect. It causes challenges both in terms of statistical efficiency and computational aspects. The growing number of bio banks of unlabeled multimodal (i.e. imaging-genetics) data calls for solutions that can integrate these data modalities and can learn semantic data representations without requiring expensive expert annotations.

Self-supervised (unsupervised) representation learning offers a viable solution when unlabeled data is abundant and labels are scarce. These methods witnessed a surge of interest after proving successful in several application domains (Longlong et al, 2019).The representations learned by these methods facilitate data-efficient fine-tuning on supervised downstream tasks, reducing significantly the burden of manual annotation. Furthermore, such methods allow for integrating multiple data modalities as distinct views, which can lead to considerable performance gains. Despite the recent advancements in self-supervised methods, only little work has been done to adopt these methods in the medical domain for multiple image modalities. Even it has been witnessed that sometimes training a model with annotations to one imaging modality may not be useful when applied to a different imaging modality.

While learning from a single imaging modality can produce good representations, incorporating multiple imaging modalities and disease-specific knowledge in the design of pretext tasks can offer far-better and rich learning experiences. Hence, medical knowledge incorporation with the design of pretext tasks is another research direction that needs to be further explored in SSL.

Biased datasets sometimes become bottleneck in learning representations and model training. Medical images datasets usually tend to be biased towards the normal or healthy cases, and only fewer images show the abnormalities in cases. To guarantee learning representations rich in clinical features, data biasness must be avoided during SSL model training.

5. FUTURE DIRECTIONS

As self-supervised learning (SSL) continues to evolve, it holds immense promise in overcoming data annotation challenges in medical imaging. Future research and development will likely focus on improving learning efficiency, clinical relevance, and real-world adaptability. Some key directions include:

- Integrate information from multiple imaging modalities (e.g., MRI, CT, PET) and clinical data (e.g., reports, EHRs) for richer representations.
- Improve model robustness across different institutions, scanners, and patient demographics. It requires enhancing SSL techniques to learn domain-invariant features that generalize well to new, unseen datasets.
- Address the scarcity of labeled data for rare diseases and subtle pathological changes. Tailoring SSL methods to capture fine-grained, localized features that are critical in detecting rare or early-stage conditions, is required.
- Create universal medical image encoders. The main focus is on pre-training models that can be easily adapted to various tasks (segmentation, classification, detection) with minimal retraining.
- Benchmarking and Standardization - Establishing reliable evaluation standards for SSL methods in medical imaging is of utmost significance.

6. CONCLUSION

There has been growing interest in applying self supervised methods to medical imaging tasks, with significant contribution in various applications like radiology and pathology. Recent approaches that have proven successful in computer vision for medical image analysis have adopted either generative, contrastive or a combination of these approaches. These approaches have shown remarkable performance even in case of limited annotated data. However there is a little work which has been done with multiple image modalities. This paper covers an in-depth study on various SSL methods used for medical image analysis and gives insights of various applications which are benefitted from these methods. The paper also discusses research challenges in self supervised methods.

REFERENCES

Abid, M. H., Ashraf, R., Mahmood, T., & Faisal, C. M. N. (2023). Multi-modal medical image classification using deep residual network and genetic algorithm. *PLoS One*, *18*(6), e0287786. Advance online publication. DOI: 10.1371/journal.pone.0287786

Albelwi, S. (2021). Survey on self-supervised learning: Auxiliary pretext tasks and contrastive learning methods in imaging. *Entropy (Basel, Switzerland)*, *24*(4). Advance online publication. DOI: 10.3390/e24040551

Anand, M., & Garg, A. (2021). Recent advancements in self-supervised paradigms for visual feature representation. arXiv. https://arXiv.org/abs/2111.02042

Ashraf, F. B., Alam, S. M. M., & Sakib, S. M. (2024). Enhancing breast cancer classification via histopathological image analysis: Leveraging self-supervised contrastive learning and transfer learning. *Heliyon*, *10*(2), e24123. Advance online publication. DOI: 10.1016/j.heliyon.2024.e24123

Bai, H., Cao, M., Huang, P., & Shan, J. (2021). Self-supervised semi-supervised learning for data labeling and quality evaluation. arXiv. https://arXiv.org/abs/2111.10932

Bao, W., Jin, Y., Huang, C., & Peng, W. (2021). CT image classification of invasive depth of gastric cancer based on 3D-DPN structure. *The 11th International Workshop on Computer Science and Engineering (WCSE 2021)*, 115–121. DOI: 10.18178/wcse.2021.06.018

Boffa, M., Vassio, L., Mellia, M., Drago, I., Milan, G., Ben Houidi, Z., & Rossi, D. (2022). On using pretext tasks to learn representations from network logs. *Proceedings of the 1st International Workshop on Native Network Intelligence*, 21–26. DOI: 10.1145/3565009.3568682

Bozorgtabar, B., Mahapatra, D., Vray, G., & Thiran, J.-P. (2020). SALAD: Self-supervised aggregation learning for anomaly detection on X-rays. In *MICCAI 2020* (pp. 468–478). Medical image computing and computer assisted intervention. Springer. DOI: 10.1007/978-3-030-59725-2_45

Bustillo, A., Reis, R., & Machado, A. R., & Others. (2022). Improving the accuracy of machine-learning models with data from machine test repetitions. *Journal of Intelligent Manufacturing*, *33*(1), 203–221. DOI: 10.1007/s10845-020-01661-3

Caron, M., Misra, I., Mairal, J., Goyal, P., Bojanowski, P., & Joulin, A. (2020). Unsupervised learning of visual features by contrasting cluster assignments. *Advances in Neural Information Processing Systems, 33*, 9912–9924.

Chaitanya, K., Erdil, E., Karani, N., & Konukoglu, E. (2020). Contrastive learning of global and local features for medical image segmentation with limited annotations. *34th Conference on Neural Information Processing Systems (NeurIPS 2020)*. DOI: 10.48550/arXiv.2006.10511

Chen, L., Bentley, P., Mori, K., Misawa, K., Fujiwara, M., & Rueckert, D. (2019). Self-supervised learning for medical image analysis using image context restoration. *Medical Image Analysis, 58*, 101539. Advance online publication. DOI: 10.1016/j.media.2019.101539

Chen, T., Kornblith, S., Norouzi, M., & Hinton, G. (2020). A simple framework for contrastive learning of visual representations. arXiv. https://arXiv.org/abs/2002.05709

Chen, X., Ding, M., Wang, X., Xin, Y., Mo, S., Wang, Y., Han, S., Luo, P., Zeng, G., & Wang, J. (2022). Context autoencoder for self-supervised representation learning. arXiv. https://arXiv.org/abs/2202.03026

Chen, X., Fan, H., Girshick, R., & He, K. (2020). Improved baselines with momentum contrastive learning. arXiv. https://arXiv.org/abs/2003.04297

Cornelissen, S., & van der Putten, J. A. (2021). Evaluating self-supervised learning methods for downstream classification of neoplasia in Barrett's esophagus. *2021 IEEE International Conference on Image Processing (ICIP)*, 66–70. DOI: 10.1109/ICIP42928.2021.9506042

Dehaene, O., Camara, A., Moindrot, O., de Lavergne, A., & Courtiol, P. (2020). Self-supervision closes the gap between weak and strong supervision in histology. *ML4H 2020 NeurIPS Workshop*. /arXiv.2012.03583DOI: 10.48550

Doersch, C., Gupta, A., & Efros, A. A. (2015). Unsupervised visual representation learning by context prediction. *Proceedings of the IEEE International Conference on Computer Vision (ICCV)*, 1422–1430. DOI: 10.1109/ICCV.2015.167

Donahue, J., Krähenbühl, P., & Darrell, T. (2016). Adversarial feature learning. arXiv. https://arXiv.org/abs/1605.09782

Dosovitskiy, A., Fischer, P., Springenberg, J. T., Riedmiller, M., & Brox, T. (2015). Discriminative unsupervised feature learning with exemplar convolutional neural networks. *IEEE Transactions on Pattern Analysis and Machine Intelligence, 38*(9), 1734–1747. DOI: 10.1109/TPAMI.2015.2496141

Dosovitskiy, A., Springenberg, J. T., Riedmiller, M., & Brox, T. (2014). Discriminative unsupervised feature learning with convolutional neural networks. *Advances in Neural Information Processing Systems*, *27*, 766–774.

Eckhardt, C. M., Madjarova, S. J., & Williams, R. J., & Others. (2022). Unsupervised machine learning methods and emerging applications in healthcare. *Knee Surgery, Sports Traumatology, Arthroscopy : Official Journal of the ESSKA*, *31*(2), 376–387. DOI: 10.1007/s00167-022-07233-7

Ericsson, L., Gouk, H., & Hospedales, T. M. (2021). How well do self-supervised models transfer? *Proceedings of the IEEE/CVF Conference on Computer Vision and Pattern Recognition (CVPR)*, 5414–5423. DOI: 10.1109/CVPR46437.2021.00537

Fedorov, A. (2021). Tasting the cake: Evaluating self-supervised generalization on out-of-distribution multimodal MRI data. *RobustML Workshop ICLR 2021*. DOI: 10.48550/arXiv.2103.12808

Felfeliyan, B., Forkert, N. D., Hareendranathan, A., Cornel, D., Zhou, Y., Kuntze, G., Jaremko, J. L., & Ronsky, J. L. (2023). Self-supervised-RCNN for medical image segmentation with limited data annotation. *Computerized Medical Imaging and Graphics*, *109*, 102297. Advance online publication. DOI: 10.1016/j.compmedimag.2023.102297

Gidaris, S., Singh, P., & Komodakis, N. (2018). Unsupervised representation learning by predicting image rotations. arXiv. https://arXiv.org/abs/1803.07728

Goodfellow, I., Pouget-Abadie, J., Mirza, M., Xu, B., Warde-Farley, D., Ozair, S., Courville, A., & Bengio, Y. (2014). Generative adversarial nets. *Advances in Neural Information Processing Systems*, *27*, 2672–2680.

Grill, J.-B., Strub, F., Altché, F., Tallec, C., Richemond, P., Buchatskaya, E., & Doersch, C., & Others. (2020). Bootstrap your own latent: A new approach to self-supervised learning. *Advances in Neural Information Processing Systems*, *33*, 21271–21284.

Gu, J., Wang, Z., Kuen, J., Ma, L., Shahroudy, A., Shuai, B., Liu, T., Wang, X., Wang, G., Cai, J., & Chen, T. (2018). Recent advances in convolutional neural networks. *Pattern Recognition*, *77*, 354–377. DOI: 10.1016/j.patcog.2017.10.013

Haghighi, F., Taher, M. R. H., Zhou, Z., Gotway, M. B., & Liang, J. (2021). Transferable visual words: Exploiting the semantics of anatomical patterns for self-supervised learning. *IEEE Transactions on Medical Imaging*, *40*(10), 2857–2868. DOI: 10.1109/TMI.2021.3067770

Han, T., Xie, W., & Zisserman, A. (2020). Memory-augmented dense predictive coding for video representation learning. In *Computer vision – ECCV 2020* (pp. 312–329). Springer. DOI: 10.1007/978-3-030-58517-4_19

Hao, H., Didari, S., Woo, J. O., Moon, H., & Bangert, P. (2021). Highly efficient representation and active learning framework for imbalanced data and its application to COVID-19 X-ray classification. *Conference on Neural Information Processing Systems (NeurIPS 2021)*. DOI: 10.48550/arXiv.2012.04376

Hassan, A., Sirshar, M., Akram, M. U., & Farooq, M. U. (2022). Analysis of multimodal representation learning across medical images and reports using multiple vision and language pre-trained models. *19th International Bhurban Conference on Applied Sciences and Technology (IBCAST)*, 337–342. DOI: 10.1109/IBCAST54850.2022.9990154

Hsieh, W.-T., Lefort-Besnard, J., Yang, H.-C., Kuo, L.-W., & Lee, C.-C. (2020). Behavior score-embedded brain encoder network for improved classification of Alzheimer disease using resting state fMRI. *2020 42nd Annual International Conference of the IEEE Engineering in Medicine & Biology Society (EMBC)*, 5486–5489. DOI: 10.1109/EMBC44109.2020.9175690

Hu, H., Cui, J., & Wang, L. (2021). Region-aware contrastive learning for semantic segmentation. *Proceedings of the IEEE/CVF International Conference on Computer Vision (ICCV)*, 16291–16301. DOI: 10.1109/ICCV48922.2021.01599

Hu, T., Khishe, M., Mohammadi, M., Parvizi, G.-R., Taher Karim, S. H., & Rashid, T. A. (2021). Real-time COVID-19 diagnosis from X-ray images using deep CNN and extreme learning machines stabilized by chimp optimization algorithm. *Biomedical Signal Processing and Control, 68*, 102764. Advance online publication. DOI: 10.1016/j.bspc.2021.102764

Islam, P. (2024). Nanotechnology in development of next generation of stent and related medical devices: Current and future aspects. *Wiley Interdisciplinary Reviews: Nanomedicine and Nanobiotechnology, 16*(2), Article e1941. DOI: 10.1002/wnan.1941

Jaiswal, A., Babu, A. R., Zadeh, M. Z., Banerjee, D., & Makedon, F. (2020). A survey on contrastive self-supervised learning. *Technologies, 9*(1), 2. Advance online publication. DOI: 10.3390/technologies9010002

Jana, A. (2021). Liver fibrosis and NAS scoring from CT images using self-supervised learning and texture encoding. *2021 IEEE 18th International Symposium on Biomedical Imaging (ISBI)*, 1553–1557. DOI: 10.1109/ISBI48211.2021.9433783

Jian, G.-Z., Lin, G.-S., Wang, C.-M., & Yan, S.-L. (2021). Helicobacter pylori infection classification based on convolutional neural network and self-supervised learning. *2021 5th International Conference on Graphics and Signal Processing*, 60–64. DOI: 10.1145/3474906.3474915

Jing, L., & Tian, Y. (2020). Self-supervised visual feature learning with deep neural networks: A survey. *IEEE Transactions on Pattern Analysis and Machine Intelligence, 43*(11), 4037–4058. DOI: 10.1109/TPAMI.2020.2992393

Kalra, N., Verma, P., & Verma, S. (2024). Advancements in AI based healthcare techniques with focus on diagnostic techniques. *Computers in Biology and Medicine, 179*, 108917. Advance online publication. DOI: 10.1016/j.compbiomed.2024.108917

Karnam, S. (2020). Self-supervised learning for segmentation using image reconstruction [Unpublished master's thesis]. Rochester Institute of Technology.

Ke, J., Shen, Y., Liang, X., & Shen, D. (2021). Contrastive learning based stain normalization across multiple tumor in histopathology. In *MICCAI 2021* (pp. 571–580). Medical image computing and computer assisted intervention. Springer. DOI: 10.1007/978-3-030-87199-4_54

Keras Team. (n.d.). Building autoencoders in Keras. Retrieved October 13, 2025, from https://blog.keras.io/building-autoencoders-in-keras.html

Kharitonov, E., Rivière, M., Synnaeve, G., Wolf, L., Mazaré, P.-E., Douze, M., & Dupoux, E. (2021). Data augmenting contrastive learning of speech representations in the time domain. *2021 IEEE Spoken Language Technology Workshop (SLT)*, 215–222. DOI: 10.1109/SLT48900.2021.9383605

Kingma, D. P., & Welling, M. (2013). Auto-encoding variational bayes. arXiv. https://arXiv.org/abs/1312.6114

Li, M., & Others. (2025). Enhancing medical vision-language contrastive learning via inter-matching relation modelling. *IEEE Transactions on Medical Imaging*. Advance online publication. DOI: 10.1109/TMI.2024.3426738

Li, Y., Chen, J., Xie, X., Ma, K., & Zheng, Y. (2020). Self-loop uncertainty: A novel pseudolabel for semi-supervised medical image segmentation. In *MICCAI 2020* (pp. 614–623). Medical image computing and computer-assisted intervention. Springer. DOI: 10.1007/978-3-030-59725-2_59

Liu, C., & Others. (2021). TN-USMA Net: Triple normalization-based gastrointestinal stromal tumors classification on multicenter EUS images with ultrasound-specific pretraining and meta attention. *Medical Physics, 48*(11), 7199–7214. DOI: 10.1002/mp.15228

Liu, X., Zhang, F., Hou, Z., Mian, L., Wang, Z., Zhang, J., & Tang, J. (2021). Self-supervised learning: Generative or contrastive. *IEEE Transactions on Knowledge and Data Engineering*, *35*(1), 857–876. DOI: 10.1109/TKDE.2021.3095305

Longlong, J., & Tian, Y. (2019). Self-supervised visual feature learning with deep neural networks: A survey. arXiv. https://arXiv.org/abs/1902.06162

Lorre, G., Rabarisoa, J., Orcesi, A., Ainouz, S., & Canu, S. (2020). Temporal contrastive pretraining for video action recognition. *Proceedings of the IEEE Winter Conference on Applications of Computer Vision (WACV)*, 662–670. DOI: 10.1109/WACV45572.2020.9093418

Mahapatra, D., & Ge, Z. (2020). Training data independent image registration using generative adversarial networks and domain adaptation. *Pattern Recognition*, *100*, 107109. Advance online publication. DOI: 10.1016/j.patcog.2019.107109

Mascolini, A., Cardamone, D., Ponzio, F., Di Cataldo, S., & Ficarra, E. (2022). Exploiting generative self-supervised learning for the assessment of biological images with lack of annotations. *BMC Bioinformatics*, *23*(1), 374. Advance online publication. DOI: 10.1186/s12859-022-04845-1

Matzkin, F., Newcombe, V., Stevenson, S., Khetani, A., Newman, T., Digby, R., Stevens, A., Glocker, B., & Ferrante, E. (2020). Self-supervised skull reconstruction in brain CT images with decompressive craniectomy. In *MICCAI 2020* (pp. 390–399). Medical image computing and computer-assisted intervention. Springer. DOI: 10.1007/978-3-030-59725-2_38

Minaee, S., Boykov, Y. Y., Porikli, F., Plaza, A. J., Kehtarnavaz, N., & Terzopoulos, D. (2021). Image segmentation using deep learning: A survey. *IEEE Transactions on Pattern Analysis and Machine Intelligence*, *44*(7), 3523–3542. DOI: 10.1109/TPAMI.2021.3059968

Mittal, M., Arora, M., Pandey, T., & Goyal, L. M. (2020). Image segmentation using deep learning techniques in medical images. In *Advancement of machine intelligence in interactive medical image analysis* (pp. 41–63). Springer. DOI: 10.1007/978-981-15-1100-4_3

Mojab, N. (2020). Real-world multi-domain data applications for generalizations to clinical settings. *2020 19th IEEE International Conference on Machine Learning and Applications (ICMLA)*, 677–684. DOI: 10.1109/ICMLA51294.2020.00112

Nguyen, N.-Q., & Le, T.-S. (2021). A semi-supervised learning method to remedy the lack of labeled data. *2021 15th International Conference on Advanced Computing and Applications (ACOMP)*, 78–84. DOI: 10.1109/ACOMP53746.2021.00019

Noroozi, M., & Favaro, P. (2016). Unsupervised learning of visual representations by solving jigsaw puzzles. In *Computer vision – ECCV 2016* (pp. 69–84). Springer. DOI: 10.1007/978-3-319-46466-4_5

Noroozi, M., Vinjimoor, A., Favaro, P., & Pirsiavash, H. (2018). Boosting self-supervised learning via knowledge transfer. *Proceedings of the IEEE/CVF Conference on Computer Vision and Pattern Recognition (CVPR)*, 9359–9367. DOI: 10.1109/CVPR.2018.00975

Osisanwo, F. Y., Akinsola, J. E., Awodele, O., Hinmikaiye, J., Olakanmi, O., & Akinjobi, J. (2017). Supervised machine learning algorithms: Classification and comparison. *International Journal of Computer Trends and Technology*, *48*(3), 128–139. DOI: 10.14445/22312803/IJCTT-V48P126

Pang, Y., Wang, W., Tay, F. E. H., Liu, W., Tian, Y., & Yuan, L. (2022). Masked autoencoders for point cloud self-supervised learning. In *Computer vision – ECCV 2022* (pp. 604–621). Springer. DOI: 10.1007/978-3-031-19821-2_35

Park, J., Kwak, I.-Y., & Lim, C. (2021). A deep learning model with self-supervised learning and attention mechanism for COVID-19 diagnosis using chest X-ray images. *Electronics (Basel)*, *10*(16), 1996. Advance online publication. DOI: 10.3390/electronics10161996

Park, S.-W., & Others. (2021). Review on generative adversarial networks: Focusing on computer vision and its applications. *Electronics (Basel)*, *10*(10), 1216. Advance online publication. DOI: 10.3390/electronics10101216

Pathak, D., Girshick, R., Dollár, P., Darrell, T., & Hariharan, B. (2016). Learning features by watching objects move. arXiv. https://arXiv.org/abs/1612.06370

Pathak, D., Krahenbuhl, P., Donahue, J., Darrell, T., & Efros, A. A. (2016). Context encoders: Feature learning by inpainting. *Proceedings of the IEEE Conference on Computer Vision and Pattern Recognition (CVPR)*, 2536–2544. DOI: 10.1109/CVPR.2016.278

Pei, X., & Zuo, K. (2023). A review of the application of multi-modal deep learning in medicine: Bibliometrics and future directions. *International Journal of Computational Intelligence Systems*, *16*(1), 44. Advance online publication. DOI: 10.1007/s44196-023-00225-6

Popescu, M. C., & Sasu, L. M. (2014). Feature extraction, feature selection and machine learning for image classification: A case study. *2014 International Conference on Optimization of Electrical and Electronic Equipment (OPTIM)*, 968–973. DOI: 10.1109/OPTIM.2014.6850947

Pugliese, R., Regondi, S., & Marini, R. (2021). Machine learning-based approach: Global trends, research directions, and regulatory standpoints. *Data Science and Management, 4*, 19–29. DOI: 10.1016/j.dsm.2021.12.002

Qian, R., Meng, T., Gong, B., Yang, M.-H., Wang, H., Belongie, S., & Cui, Y. (2020). Spatiotemporal contrastive video representation learning. arXiv. https://arXiv.org/abs/2008.03800

Radford, A., Metz, L., & Chintala, S. (2015). Unsupervised representation learning with deep convolutional generative adversarial networks. arXiv. https://arXiv.org/abs/1511.06434

Raghu, M., Zhang, C., Kleinberg, J., & Bengio, S. (2019). Transfusion: Understanding transfer learning for medical imaging. *Advances in Neural Information Processing Systems, 32*, 3347–3357.

Reed, C. J. (2022). Self-supervised pre-training improves self-supervised pre-training. *Proceedings of the IEEE/CVF Winter Conference on Applications of Computer Vision (WACV)*, 2584–2594. DOI: 10.1109/WACV51458.2022.00263

Ren, Z., Guo, Y., Yu, S. X., & Whitney, D. (2021). Improve image-based skin cancer diagnosis with generative self-supervised learning. *2021 IEEE/ACM Conference on Connected Health: Applications, Systems and Engineering Technologies (CHASE)*, 23–34. DOI: 10.1109/CHASE52844.2021.00012

Rizvi, S. A., Tang, R., Jiang, X., Ma, X., & Hu, X. (2023). Local contrastive learning for medical image recognition. arXiv. https://arXiv.org/abs/2303.14153

Sarker, I. H. (2021). Machine learning: Algorithms, real-world applications and research directions. *SN Computer Science, 2*(3), 160. Advance online publication. DOI: 10.1007/s42979-021-00592-x

Showrov, A. A. (2024). Generative adversarial networks (GANs) in medical imaging: Advancements, applications and challenges. *IEEE Access : Practical Innovations, Open Solutions, 12*, 11805–11816. DOI: 10.1109/ACCESS.2024.3357685

Shurrab, S., & Duwairi, R. (2022). Self-supervised learning methods and applications in medical imaging analysis: A survey. *PeerJ. Computer Science, 8*, e1045. Advance online publication. DOI: 10.7717/peerj-cs.1045

Spitzer, H., Kiwitz, K., Amunts, K., Harmeling, S., & Dickscheid, T. (2018). Improving cytoarchitectonic segmentation of human brain areas with self-supervised siamese networks. In *MICCAI 2018* (pp. 663–671). Medical image computing and computer-assisted intervention. Springer. DOI: 10.1007/978-3-030-00931-1_76

Swarnkar, A. (2025). Medical device: Development of next-generation devices from an engineering perspective. In *Targeted therapy for the central nervous system* (pp. 405–422). Academic Press. DOI: 10.1016/B978-0-443-23841-3.00018-2

Szegedy, C., Toshev, A., & Erhan, D. (2013). Deep neural networks for object detection. *Advances in Neural Information Processing Systems*, *26*, 2553–2561.

Tajbakhsh, N., Shin, J. Y., Gurudu, S. R., Hurst, R. T., Kendall, C. B., Gotway, M. B., & Liang, J. (2016). Convolutional neural networks for medical image analysis: Full training or fine tuning? *IEEE Transactions on Medical Imaging*, *35*(5), 1299–1312. DOI: 10.1109/TMI.2016.2535302

Taleb, A., Kirchler, M., Monti, R., & Lippert, C. (2022). ContIG: Self-supervised multimodal contrastive learning for medical imaging with genetics. *2022 IEEE/CVF Conference on Computer Vision and Pattern Recognition (CVPR)*, 20876–20889. DOI: 10.1109/CVPR52688.2022.02024

Taleb, A., Lippert, C., Klein, T., & Nabi, M. (2021). Multimodal self-supervised learning for medical image analysis. In *Information processing in medical imaging* (pp. 661–673). Springer. DOI: 10.1007/978-3-030-78191-0_51

Thakur, A., & Thakur, G. K. (2024). Developing GANs for synthetic medical imaging data: Enhancing training and research. *International Journal of Advanced Multidisciplinary Research*, *11*(1), 70–82. DOI: 10.22192/ijamr.2024.11.01.008

Vincent, P., Larochelle, H., Bengio, Y., & Manzagol, P.-A. (2008). Extracting and composing robust features with denoising autoencoders. *Proceedings of the 25th International Conference on Machine Learning*, 1096–1103. DOI: 10.1145/1390156.1390294

Wang, F., & Liu, H. (2021). Understanding the behaviour of contrastive loss. *Proceedings of the IEEE/CVF Conference on Computer Vision and Pattern Recognition (CVPR)*, 2495–2504. DOI: 10.1109/CVPR46437.2021.00250

Wang, G., Tang, Y., Lin, L., & Torr, P. H. S. (2022). Semantic-aware auto-encoders for self-supervised representation learning. *Proceedings of the IEEE/CVF Conference on Computer Vision and Pattern Recognition (CVPR)*, 9664–9675. DOI: 10.1109/CVPR52688.2022.00944

Wu, L., Zhuang, J., & Chen, H. (2024). Voco: A simple-yet-effective volume contrastive learning framework for 3D medical image analysis. *Proceedings of the IEEE/CVF Conference on Computer Vision and Pattern Recognition (CVPR)*, 25628–25638.

Xu, L. D., Xu, E. L., & Li, L. (2018). Industry 4.0: State of the art and future trends. *International Journal of Production Research, 56*(8), 2941–2962. DOI: 10.1080/00207543.2018.1444806

Yurt, M., Dar, S. U., Erdem, A., Erdem, E., Oguz, K. K., & Çukur, T. (2021). mustGAN: Multi-stream generative adversarial networks for MR image synthesis. *Medical Image Analysis, 70*, 101944. Advance online publication. DOI: 10.1016/j.media.2021.101944

Zhang, R., Isola, P., & Efros, A. (2017). Split-brain autoencoders: Unsupervised learning by cross-channel prediction. *Proceedings of the IEEE Conference on Computer Vision and Pattern Recognition (CVPR)*, 433–441. DOI: 10.1109/CVPR.2017.514

Zhang, R., Isola, P., & Efros, A. A. (2016). Colorful image colorization. In *Computer vision – ECCV 2016* (pp. 649–666). Springer. DOI: 10.1007/978-3-319-46475-6_40

Zhao, Z., & Yang, G. (2021). Unsupervised contrastive learning of radiomics and deep features for label-efficient tumor classification. In *MICCAI 2021* (pp. 252–261). Medical image computing and computer assisted intervention. Springer. DOI: 10.1007/978-3-030-87199-4_24

Zheng, X., Wang, Y., Wang, G., & Liu, J. (2018). Fast and robust segmentation of white blood cell images by self-supervised learning. *Micron (Oxford, England), 107*, 55–71. DOI: 10.1016/j.micron.2018.01.010

Zhong, H. (2021). A self-supervised learning based framework for automatic heart failure classification on cine cardiac magnetic resonance image. *2021 43rd Annual International Conference of the IEEE Engineering in Medicine & Biology Society (EMBC)*, 2887–2890. DOI: 10.1109/EMBC46164.2021.9630910

Zhuang, X., Li, Y., Hu, Y., Ma, K., Yang, Y., & Zheng, Y. (2019). Self-supervised feature learning for 3D medical images by playing a Rubik's cube. In *MICCAI 2019* (pp. 420–428). Medical image computing and computer-assisted intervention. Springer. DOI: 10.1007/978-3-030-32245-8_47

Chapter 5
Ethical Considerations in the Use of Robotics and AI in Healthcare

Rajashri pankaj Chaudhari
https://orcid.org/0009-0004-6801-0704
Symbiosis International University, India

Jasmehar Kaur
https://orcid.org/0009-0000-2638-0441
Symbiosis Institute of Health Siences, India

Namita Raytekar
Symbiosis Institute of Health Siences, India

ABSTRACT

The adoption of robotics and artificial intelligence (AI) in healthcare is driving significant advancements in patient care, diagnosis, and treatment. AI enables data-driven decision-making, enhances diagnostic accuracy, and supports personalized medicine, while robotics improves surgical precision and procedural efficiency. Despite these benefits, integrating these technologies presents ethical, legal, and social challenges. Key concerns include patient autonomy, data privacy, algorithmic bias, and transparency, causing the development of robust regulatory frameworks. Legal accountability and liability issues related to AI-driven healthcare solutions require careful consideration. This chapter examines these critical aspects, emphasizing the need for ethical AI implementation, informed consent, and interdisciplinary collaboration with healthcare experts, policymakers, and technology developers. Responsible innovation and ethical principles in AI and robotics enhance health-care accessibility, equity, and patient-centered care while ensuring trust and safety.

DOI: 10.4018/979-8-3373-1514-0.ch005

INTRODUCTION

Integrating robotics and artificial intelligence (AI) in healthcare is improving the industry, offering excellence advancements in treatments, and patient satisfaction. AI-powered algorithms can process vast amounts of medical information, assisting in most disease detection, personalized treatment plans, and clinical decision-making with greater accuracy and efficiency. Robotics is transforming various medical procedures, from precision-driven surgeries to rehabilitation therapies, automating routine tasks, and enhancing patient care with minimal human intervention. These advancements have the potential to optimize healthcare delivery, reduce medical errors, and improve overall patient outcomes.

Despite the numerous benefits, the increasing reliance on AI and robotics in healthcare raises significant ethical concerns that must be carefully examined to ensure responsible implementation. The ethical landscape surrounding these technologies is complex, touching upon fundamental principles such as patient autonomy, data privacy, fairness, transparency, and accountability. Questions arise regarding the extent to which AI should influence medical decisions, the security of patient data in AI-driven systems, and the fairness of AI models trained on biased datasets. Additionally, the potential displacement of human healthcare professionals and the over-reliance on automated systems introduce broader socio-economic and professional challenges.

Another critical aspect of ethical considerations in AI and robotics is liability and accountability. As AI-driven systems take on more decision-making roles in diagnosis and treatment, it becomes increasingly difficult to determine responsibility when errors occur. Should liability rest with the software developers, healthcare providers, or institutions deploying AI-driven tools? Establishing clear legal frameworks and ethical guidelines is essential to address these challenges while maintaining trust in AI-assisted healthcare solutions.

Implementing AI and robotics in healthcare must be equitable, ensuring that technological advancements do not exacerbate existing disparities in medical access and quality of care. High-income countries and well-funded hospitals may benefit disproportionately from these innovations, leaving resource-limited settings at a disadvantage. Ethical deployment should prioritize inclusivity, affordability, and accessibility to ensure that all patients, regardless of socio-economic background, can benefit from AI-driven healthcare advancements.

Figure 1. AI in healthcare: principle & guidelines

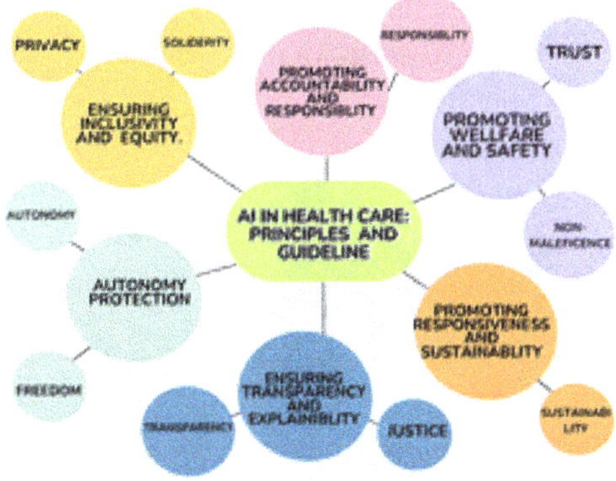

As the healthcare industry continues to integrate AI and robotics, it is tough to balance technological new and ethical responsibility. While these technologies can significantly enhance healthcare delivery, they should function as supportive tools rather than replacements for human judgment and expertise. By fostering a patient-centric approach, prioritizing transparency, and enforcing ethical guidelines, the healthcare sector can harness the full uses of AI and robotics while showing the highest standards of safety, fairness, and accountability. The responsible integration of these technologies will shape the future of medicine, ensuring that AI and robotics serve as transformative tools for a more efficient, fair, and ethically sound healthcare system.

This chapter delves into key ethical considerations in using robotics and AI in healthcare. It explores the importance of consent, data privacy, and transparency, along with strategies for mitigating and ensuring fairness in AI-driven healthcare solutions. It examines the legal complexities surrounding accountability and liability in cases involving autonomous AI systems and robotics. By understanding these critical factors, stakeholders can foster a healthcare environment that promotes both technological innovation and ethical responsibility.

The chapter also underscores the importance of international initiatives and regulatory frameworks that aim to guide the responsible deployment of AI and robotics in healthcare. Through collaborative efforts among policymakers, healthcare providers, technologists, and ethicists, the potential risks can be mitigated while maximizing the societal benefits of these transformative technologies.

Figure 2. Ethical considerations in using robotics and AI in healthcare

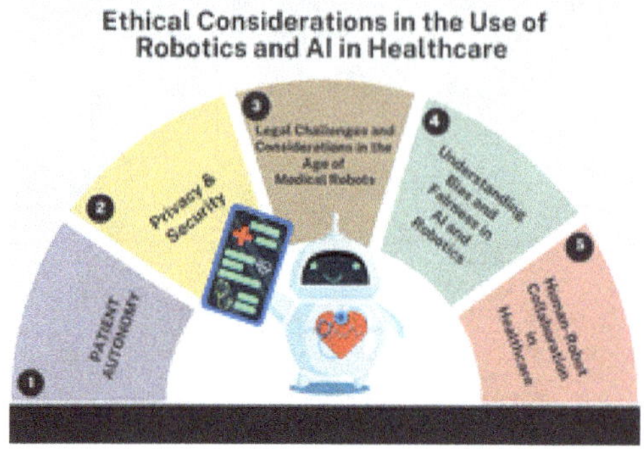

1. PATIENT AUTONOMY

Figure 3. Patient autonomy

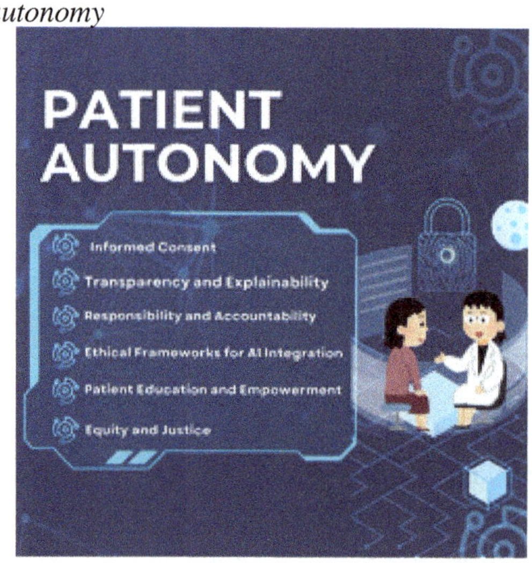
PATIENT AUTONOMY
Informed Consent
Transparency and Explainability
Responsibility and Accountability
Ethical Frameworks for AI Integration
Patient Education and Empowerment
Equity and Justice

Patient autonomy is a fundamental legal principle in healthcare, recognizing the correct path of patients to make informed and independent decisions about their medication. It underscores respect for patients as individuals capable of controlling their healthcare journeys. However, the increasing implementation of AI-technologies into healthcare settings presents ethical challenges to this principle.

AI systems, particularly those designed for diagnostics, treatment recommendations, and surgical procedures, can make highly complex decisions based on vast amounts of data. While these systems aim to enhance healthcare outcomes, they may inadvertently reduce patients' sense of control over their healthcare decisions. The risk arises when AI operates autonomously or when patients perceive decisions are being made solely by machines without adequate human oversight.

To preserve patient autonomy, healthcare providers must ensure that patients remain the ultimate decision-makers in their care. AI should be viewed as a supportive tool, rather than a replacement for human health. The communication about AI's role and limitations is essential to maintain patients' active participation in their healthcare decisions.

1.1 Informed Consent

Early information is a vital process that ensures to the patient's understanding and voluntarily agree to their treatment plans. Introducing AI in healthcare complicates this process because of the technical complexity of AI systems.

For consent to be truly informed, patients must comprehend how AI will be used in their care, the extent of its involvement, and its potential benefits and risks. This is especially challenging when AI systems operate as "black boxes," where even healthcare providers may struggle to explain their decision-making processes.

For example, in AI-assisted surgeries, patients need to understand the specific tasks the AI system will perform and how it will complement the surgeon's role. Without this information, patients may unknowingly relinquish control over crucial aspects of their healthcare decisions, undermining their autonomy.

To safeguard autonomy, healthcare providers must present information about AI systems in a manner that patients can easily understand. This includes using simple language, visual aids, and interactive explanations where possible. Enhanced educational efforts should bridge the information gap, ensuring that patients are fully informed before consenting to AI-assisted care.

1.2 Transparency and Explainability

Transparency and Explain ability are essential for maintaining patient autonomy. Patients may understand how AI contributes to their care, including the logic behind its recommendations or decisions. However, many AI systems function as complex models that do not readily offer clear explanations for their outputs.

The improvement of Explainable AI (XAI) is critical to address this challenge. XAI objective is to make AI decision-making processes better transparency and understandable for both healthcare providers and patients. By providing comprehensible insights into how artificial intelligence arrived at a particular recommendation, XAI can empower patients to make informed healthcare choices.

Ethical guidelines should mandate the creation and adoption of XAI systems to ensure patients are not left in the dark about AI-driven decisions. Healthcare providers must be trained to communicate these explanations effectively to patients, fostering trust and understanding.

1.3 Responsibility and Accountability

As AI systems take on more responsibilities in patient care, questions about responsibility and accountability become increasingly complex. Traditionally, healthcare providers are accountable for clinical decisions and outcomes. However, when AI systems contribute to decision-making, determining liability becomes less straightforward.

If an AI makes an error or contributes to a negative outcome, who will be responsible—the healthcare services provider, the AI manager, or the institution that implemented the AI? This ambiguity can erode patient trust and hinder their ability to assert control over their care.

Clear guidelines and legal frameworks are necessary to address accountability issues. Patients must be assured that there is a defined pathway for addressing grievances and seeking redress when AI-related errors occur. Transparent accountability mechanisms will help maintain patient confidence and trust in AI-driven healthcare.

1.4 Ethical Frameworks for AI Integration

The framework and principles such as non-maleficence (avoiding harm), beneficence (maximizing benefits), justice (fair treatment), and respect for autonomy are critical when integrating AI into healthcare. These principles provide a foundation for the ethical development and deployment of AI systems.

- Non-Maleficence: AI systems should undergo rigorous testing to minimize risks and ensure patient safety.
- Beneficence: AI should enhance the quality of care and improve health outcomes.
- Justice: AI technologies should be accessible to all patients, promoting fair healthcare.
- Respect for autonomy: Patients must remain central to healthcare decisions, with AI serving as a supportive tool more than a replacement for human health.

1.5 Patient Education and Empowerment

To maintain autonomy, patients must be educated about AI technologies and their role in healthcare. Educational initiatives should aim to improve patient literacy regarding AI, enabling them to ask informed questions and make empowered decisions.

Healthcare providers should play an important role in guiding patients through this learning process. By fostering a culture of open communication and education, healthcare systems can empower patients to participate actively in their care.

1.6 Equity and Justice

Ensuring fair access to AI-driven healthcare solutions is essential for upholding patient autonomy across diverse populations. Disparities in access to advanced technologies can undermine autonomy by limiting some patients' ability to benefit from AI-assisted care.

Efforts must be made to address these disparities and promote inclusive healthcare innovation. Ethical guidelines should emphasize the fair distribution of AI resources and address biases in AI algorithms that may disproportionately affect certain groups (Eldakak et al., 2024; Power, 2024).

2. PRIVACY & SECURITY

Figure 4. Privacy and Security

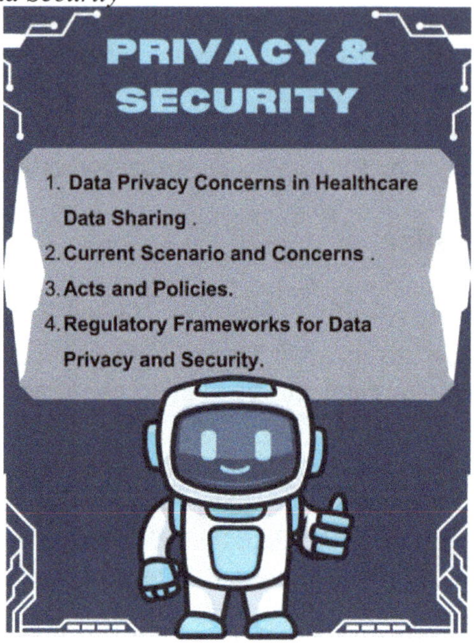
PRIVACY &
SECURITY
1. Data Privacy Concerns in Healthcare Data Sharing .
2. Current Scenario and Concerns .
3. Acts and Policies.
4. Regulatory Frameworks for Data Privacy and Security.

2.1 Data Privacy Concerns in Healthcare Data Sharing

Healthcare professionals face challenges navigating the ethical and legal implications of data sharing, particularly in AI-driven healthcare applications that rely on vast digital datasets. Ensuring data privacy and security is crucial, as sensitive patient information is collected, processed, and analysed. Ethical concerns arise regarding data usage, storage, and sharing, emphasizing the need for transparency and patient autonomy.

Patients should have clear rights regarding their data, including access and control over how it is used. Legal frameworks, such as the General Data Protection Regulation (GDPR) provide guidelines for lawful and transparent data processing. Strong data security measures must be in place to prevent breaches and unauthorized access. Patients should be empowered to opt in or out of AI-driven applications, ensuring informed consent and ethical data practices in the evolving landscape of robotics and AI in healthcare.

Background

Digital data in healthcare presents both opportunities and challenges:

- Advancements like teleconsultations, easy data retrieval, and machine learning have been enabled by digitalization.
- However, the risk exists that unauthorized individuals could access personal medical records.
- Machine learning's data requirements lead to maintaining large data repositories, raising concerns about patient privacy.
- Artificial intelligence applications demand even larger data volumes, causing stringent data security measures.
- Data for AI often needs to be stored in cloud servers or GPUs, introducing additional security risks.
- Protection of patient information is crucial for AI research but lacks a centralized encryption and sharing protocol.
- Ethical approval from institutional committees guides decisions on patient consent waivers for AI studies.
- Databases like DDSM and Optimam offer valuable resources for training deep learning algorithms.
- The COVID-19 crisis highlighted the importance of open-source datasets for rapid algorithm development.
- Hospitals need the capacity to manage large data securely for the advancement of diagnostic technologies.

Figure 5. Principles of GDPR

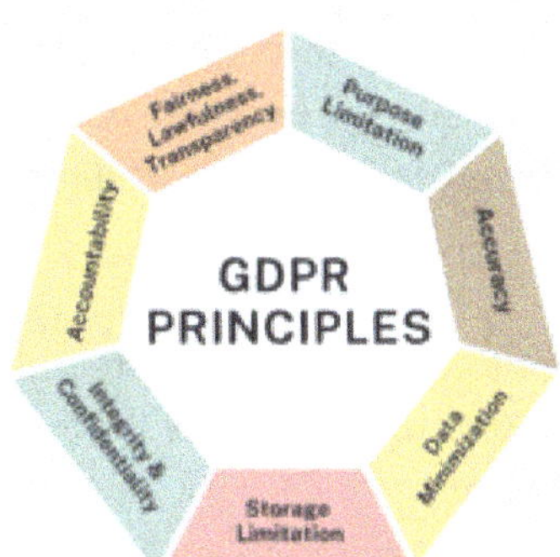
GDPR
PRINCIPLES
Fairness, Lawfulness, Transparency
Purpose Limitation
Accuracy
Data Minimization
Storage Limitation
Integrity & Confidentiality
Accountability

2.2 Current Scenario and Concerns

The current landscape of AI-based health innovations involves the processing of big data sets, characterized by high speed, large volumes, and significant heterogeneity. Despite de-identification efforts, the risk of re-identification through novel data linkage techniques remains a real challenge, as evidenced by studies showcasing the identification of individuals from supposedly anonymized datasets.

Key points included:

- The presence of identifiers in healthcare data poses challenges, particularly in fields like dermatology where patient photos may contain identifiable features.
- AI applications in healthcare often utilize a mix of protected health information and user-generated data, potentially leading to breaches of privacy and data triangulation.
- Breaches in data privacy can have measurable consequences (consequentialist) like workplace discrimination or subjective impacts (deontological) such as loss of control and mental trauma.
- Issues of data sharing across jurisdictions highlight regulatory loopholes and the need for global data diversity in AI training.
- Bias in AI algorithms can arise from the inherent biases in the training data, which often reflects socio-economic disparities and can lead to suboptimal recommendations, especially for marginalized populations.
- Examples like Amazon's biased recruitment system emphasize how biases in training data can perpetuate discrimination and suboptimal outcomes in AI applications.

India's economy is rapidly evolving through digital transformation, highlighting the critical need for secure data storage and transfer infrastructure. This necessity was underscored by a significant incident at a leading Indian medical institute in late 2022, where:

- The institute fell victim to a cyber-attack targeting various services such as patient registration, appointments, reports, billing, and administrative functions like salary distribution.
- The attack forced a manual operation of key services for over two weeks, causing delays and long queues for patients.
- Although online services have now been restored from backups, personal data of over 30 million patients and healthcare staff could have been compromised.

This scenario emphasizes the urgency for robust data protection measures in the Indian healthcare system amidst its digital evolution.

2.3 Acts and Policies

The section discusses global initiatives related to data privacy, focusing on the General Data Protection Regulation (GDPR) that became effective in May 2018. Key points include:

- The GDPR is applicable in the European Union but can serve as a model for other countries to enhance data privacy.
- The regulation aims to encourage the development of digital systems that prioritize and uphold users' privacy.
- The GDPR plays a crucial role in setting standards for data protection globally, influencing how organizations handle and safeguard user data.

Global Initiative on Ethics of Autonomous and Intelligent Systems

Global Initiative on Ethics of Autonomous and Intelligent Systems is an effort in common to respond to the ethical, legal, and societal implications of artificial intelligence and autonomous systems. The initiative concentrates on establishing robust frameworks, policies, and principles that facilitate responsible deployment of such technologies with maximized benefits and minimized harms for society.

Key Focus Areas:

Aim and Ethical Standards:

The initiative seeks to establish universal standards and ethical principles to guide the development, implementation, and governance of AI and autonomous systems. These principles emphasize security, accountability, transparency, fairness, and human-centric Public Participation and Ethical Awareness:

Recognizing the transformative impact of AI, the initiative encourages public engagement in shaping ethical frameworks. This approach fosters awareness, inclusivity, and accountability, ensuring that diverse perspectives—including those from policymakers, industry leaders, researchers, and civil society—are integrated into AI governance.

2.4 Regulatory Frameworks for Data Privacy and Security

1. Additional Healthcare Data Protection Policies:
    a. Healthcare Professionals Registry (HPR): Maintains an authenticated database of registered healthcare professionals to enhance patient safety and quality of care.

b. Health Facility Registry (HFR): A unified registry that ensures transparency and efficiency in health facility operations, promoting interoperability in healthcare services.
c. Unified Health Interface (UHI): A framework designed to facilitate seamless health data exchange, interoperability, and enhanced digital healthcare services.

2. Digital Personal Data Protection Bill, 2023:

Originally introduced in 2019, this bill underwent extensive public consultation before being passed in August 2023. It governs the collection, storage, and processing of digital personal data, ensuring user consent and defining exemptions based on purpose, national security, and regulatory authority.

3. Data Fiduciary Obligations:

Entities handling personal data (termed Data Fiduciaries) must adhere to key responsibilities, including:

a. Ensuring data accuracy and security throughout its lifecycle.
b. Deleting data once its intended purpose is fulfilled.
c. Permitting cross-border data transfers, except to restricted jurisdictions.
d. Imposing strict penalties for security violations and non-compliance.

4. Data Protection Board:

A regulatory authority established under the bill, comprising members serving two-year terms. It enforces data protection measures, investigates breaches, and levies fines for non-compliance.

5. Privacy Protection Models in AI and Healthcare Data Security
6. Federated Learning:

A decentralized machine learning approach that allows multiple organizations to collaboratively train AI models without sharing raw data. This technique enhances data privacy by enabling each participant to retain control over their datasets while contributing to a collective model.

7. Differential Privacy:

A method that introduces statistical noise (randomness) to datasets before analysis, ensuring that individual data points remain indistinguishable. This technique is widely used in healthcare research and AI applications to balance privacy and data utility.

8. Cryptographic Techniques:

Advanced encryption methods ensure secure data processing and privacy in AI applications:

9. Hybrid Privacy-Preserving Techniques:

An integrated approach combining federated learning, differential privacy, and cryptographic methods to enhance biomedical data security. This hybrid model optimizes data protection while maintaining analytical accuracy in medical research and AI-driven healthcare applications.

The challenges arising from the growing use of AI in medical fields are specifically focusing on issues related to data sharing, triangulation, and ethical dilemmas. These challenges stem from the limited diversity in how data is presented. The impact of data breaches is emphasized, noting that the consequences can align with consequentialist, deontological, or both ethical perspectives. The necessity for robust enforcement of federal laws governing health data sharing and utilization is underscored as a crucial step. In addressing data privacy concerns responsibly, the paper suggests the use of advanced AI models like Federated

Figure 6. Different types of HIPAA rules

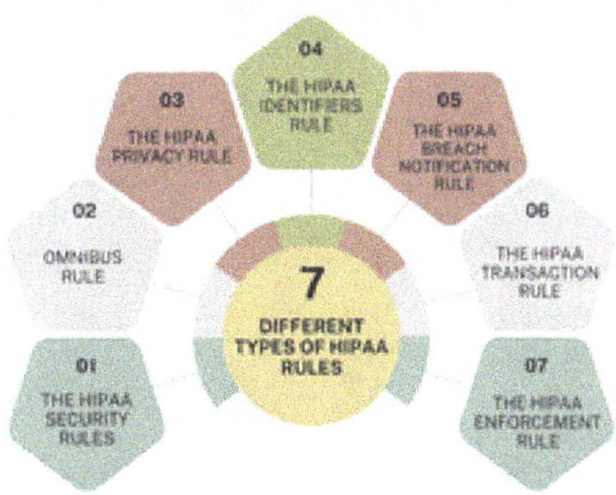

3. LEGAL CHALLENGES AND CONSIDERATIONS IN THE AGE OF MEDICAL ROBOTS

The rapid advancement and integration of medical robots into healthcare have transformed the delivery of medical services, significantly enhancing precision in surgeries, streamlining diagnostic procedures, and improving rehabilitation outcomes. These robotic systems, powered by artificial intelligence (AI), machine learning, and automation, have demonstrated their ability to reduce human error, increase procedural efficiency, and enable minimally invasive interventions that were once deemed impossible. However, the incorporation of such sophisticated technologies into clinical practice also presents complex legal and ethical challenges that must be carefully navigated to ensure patient safety, regulatory compliance, and ethical integrity.

As medical robots evolve to perform increasingly autonomous functions, concerns regarding liability, data protection, and judicial oversight have emerged as key areas of discussion. Policymakers, healthcare providers, and technology developers must collaborate to establish a robust legal framework that not only fosters innovation but also ensures that patients receive safe and effective care. This chapter explores the legal risks, data privacy issues, and legislative responses associated with medical robots, with a particular focus on developments in China's legal and judicial landscape.

Figure 7. Legal challenges and considerations in the age of medical robots

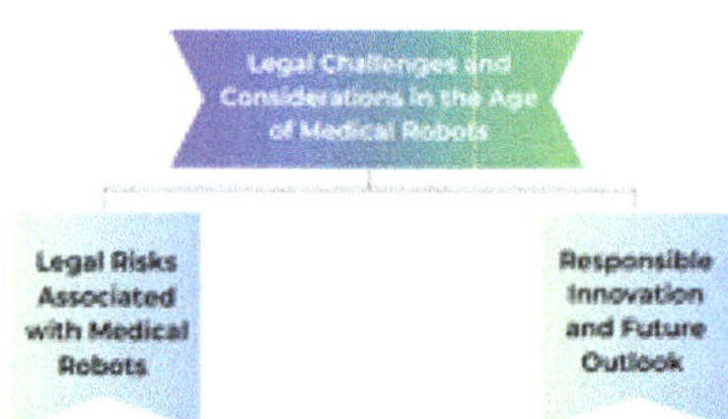

3.1 Legal Risks Associated with Medical Robots

As medical robots become more prevalent in operating rooms, diagnostic laboratories, and patient care settings, the potential legal risks associated with their use must not be overlooked. One of the primary concerns is the issue of liability in medical malpractice cases. When a medical robot causes harm—whether due to a technical malfunction, flawed algorithm, or misinterpretation of medical data—determining accountability becomes highly complex.

Unlike traditional malpractice cases, where liability is typically assigned to healthcare providers, the involvement of AI-powered robotic systems introduces additional layers of accountability, including:

1. Healthcare Providers: If a physician or surgeon misuses a medical robot or cannot supervise its operation appropriately, they may be held liable for negligence.
2. Medical Institutions: Hospitals and healthcare facilities that deploy medical robots could face liability if they fail to provide adequate training, oversight, or maintenance of these systems.
3. Manufacturers & Developers: If a robot malfunctions due to a defective design, programming error, or lack of software updates, liability may extend to the manufacturer or software developer.
4. AI Algorithm Designers: Since medical robots rely on machine learning models, issues such as biased algorithms or errors in AI-driven decision-making may lead to legal claims against the developers responsible for designing the AI system.

To address these concerns, it is crucial to establish clear liability standards that define when and how responsibility should be assigned. Without well-defined legal frameworks, affected patients may struggle to obtain compensation, while excessive liability risks may hinder technological progress by discouraging investment in medical AI. Achieving a balance between accountability and innovation is therefore essential to ensure safe, ethical, and sustainable advancements in medical robotics.

Judicial Perspectives and Legislative Actions

The legal treatment of medical robots and AI in healthcare is evolving rapidly, with judicial perspectives playing a crucial role in shaping regulatory frameworks. This stance is highly significant, as it prevents AI systems from being granted legal personality, which would otherwise complicate liability assignment in malpractice cases.

3.2 Responsible Innovation and Future Outlook

Looking forward, the concept of "responsible innovation" must guide the development and deployment of medical robots. This means ensuring that technological progress is ethically aligned, legally sound, and socially responsible. Key steps for achieving this include:

- Developing Adaptive Legal Frameworks: As AI in medicine evolves, laws must be regularly updated to reflect new risks and ethical dilemmas.
- Fostering Multi Stakeholder Collaboration: Effective governance of medical robots requires input from healthcare professionals, legal experts, AI developers, and policymakers.
- Strengthening Patient-Centered Protections: New policies should prioritize patient rights, informed consent, and equitable access to AI-driven medical technologies.

Ultimately, the future of medical robots hinges on the ability of the legal system to keep pace with AI advancements while ensuring that patient safety, ethical considerations, and regulatory compliance remain at the forefront.

4. UNDERSTANDING BIAS AND FAIRNESS IN AI AND ROBOTICS

4.1 Introduction to Bias in AI

The artificial intelligence (AI) and robotics has become an increasingly pressing concern, particularly in healthcare settings, where AI is widely used for diagnostics, treatment recommendations, patient monitoring, and administrative decision-making. AI systems, while designed to improve efficiency and accuracy, can inadvertently perpetuate, amplify, or even create new biases present in the data they are trained on. These biases often reflect existing inequities in healthcare access, socioeconomic disparities, and historical underrepresentation of certain patient populations. If left unaddressed, bias in AI can lead to skewed clinical outcomes, reinforcing disparities rather than mitigating them. For example, studies have shown that some AI-driven diagnostic tools perform less accurately for minority groups due to a lack of diverse representation in training data. Similarly, predictive models used in healthcare resource allocation can disadvantage marginalized communities by failing to account for systemic barriers to medical access. Thus, understanding, identifying, and actively mitigating bias in AI is critical to ensuring equitable, fair, and responsible healthcare innovations.

4.2 The Concept of Fairness

Fairness in AI-driven healthcare goes beyond simply eliminating bias—it involves actively promoting equitable healthcare outcomes for all patients. Fairness is a multidimensional concept rooted in fundamental ethical principles, including:

- Justice: Ensuring equal access to healthcare resources and AI-driven medical interventions.
- Beneficence: AI should prioritize patient well-being and work to enhance health outcomes rather than unintentionally reinforcing harmful biases.
- Non-Maleficence: AI developers and healthcare providers must prevent harm by ensuring that AI decisions do not disadvantage certain populations.

Achieving fairness requires a comprehensive understanding of bias, as well as proactive measures to prevent unfair decision-making processes. A key challenge is that fairness in AI is context-dependent, meaning that strategies for mitigating bias must be tailored to specific healthcare applications and continuously reassessed as technology evolves.

4.3 Types of Bias in AI

Figure 8. Types of bias in AI

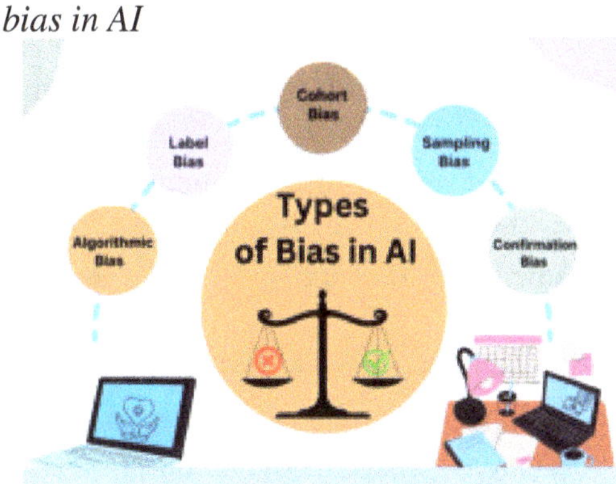

Bias in AI-systems could rise from different sources, including data collection, algorithm design, and deployment. Below are some of the most common types of bias in AI-driven healthcare:

1. Algorithmic Bias

- This form of bias analysis from the design and implementation of AI models. Even when organized on diverse and representative datasets, AI systems can still produce biased outcomes due to inherent limitations in their learning mechanisms.
- Example: An AI-powered diagnostic tool trained to detect skin cancer may perform better on lighter skin tones if the training data contains more images of lighter skin than darker skin, even if the dataset was not explicitly biased.

2. Label Bias
   - AI models learn from human-labeled data, which may carry biases from existing healthcare disparities. If labels used to train AI models reflect misdiagnoses, historical biases, or systemic healthcare inequalities, the AI will learn and reinforce these inaccuracies.
   - Example: A medical AI model predicting heart disease risk might label socioeconomic factors (such as fewer hospital visits) as indicators of lower risk, when in reality, these patients may have less access to healthcare, not a lower risk of disease.
3. Cohort Bias
   - This occurs when the training dataset does not adequately represent the diversity of the patient population, leading to inequitable AI performance across different demographic groups.
   - Example: An AI model predicting drug responses may work well for one gender or age group but fail to account for biological variations in other demographics, leading to misinformed treatment decisions.
4. Sampling Bias
   - Sampling bias arises when certain patient groups are overrepresented or underrepresented in training datasets. This can be due to historical healthcare inequalities, data collection limitations, or selective data availability.
   - Example: If an AI model for stroke prediction is primarily trained on data from urban hospitals, it may fail to accurately assess stroke risk for patients in rural areas, where medical conditions and healthcare accessibility differ.
5. Confirmation Bias
   - Confirmation bias occurs when AI models are trained to reinforce pre-existing medical assumptions, even if they are outdated, incorrect, or not applicable to all populations.
   - Example: AI models trained on historical data that overdiagnose certain conditions in men but underdiagnose them in women may continue to reinforce gender-based disparities in healthcare.

4.4 Strategies for Mitigating Bias in AI

To enhance fairness and reduce bias in AI-driven healthcare, a combination of technical, regulatory, and educational strategies must be employed. Below are key approaches:

1. Ensuring Diverse and Representative Data
   - Collect and curate balanced, inclusive datasets that represent all patient demographics, including different genders, ethnicities, age groups, and socioeconomic backgrounds.
   - Regularly update datasets to reflect changing population dynamics and ensure that AI systems remain adaptable and fair.
2. Algorithm Audits and Bias Testing
   - Implement regular algorithm audits to detect discriminatory patterns in AI decision-making.
   - Use fairness-aware machine learning techniques, such as adversarial debiasing and re-weighting algorithms, to adjust predictions and ensure equitable outcomes across patient groups.
3. Bias-Detection Metrics
   - Develop and apply quantifiable fairness metrics, such as demographic parity, equalized odds, and disparate impact analysis, to measure how AI systems perform across different populations.
   - If an AI model exhibits disparate outcomes, recalibrate it by adjusting weighing mechanisms or retraining on more diverse datasets.
4. Human-in-the-Loop Decision-Making
   - Maintain human oversight in AI-driven clinical decisions to ensure that healthcare professionals can intervene when AI recommendations appear biased or incorrect.
   - Promote collaborative decision-making where AI serves as an assistive tool, rather than the sole determinant of medical choices.
5. Education and Awareness
   - Train clinicians, AI developers, and healthcare policymakers on the risks of bias in AI systems.
   - Encourage patient awareness by ensuring transparency in how AI-driven healthcare decisions are made and providing mechanisms for patients to challenge AI-generated recommendations.

4.5 Ethical and Legal Considerations

Bias in AI-driven healthcare raises critical ethical and legal challenges that must be carefully managed to protect patient rights and ensure fair medical treatment.

Key Ethical Concerns:

- Informed Consent: Patients must be aware of how AI is used in their treatment and be given the choice to opt-out of AI-driven decision-making if desired.
- Transparency: AI systems should provide clear, interpretable explanations of their recommendations to clinicians and patients.
- Accountability: Establishing clear liability structures is essential—who is responsible when AI makes an incorrect or biased decision?

Regulatory Measures:

- FAIR (Fairness of Artificial Intelligence Recommendations) Guidelines: These provide best practices for ensuring transparency, accountability, and fairness in AI-driven healthcare.
- Data Protection Laws: Regulations such as HIPAA (U.S.), GDPR (EU), and PIPL (China) ensure ethical data handling and patient privacy protections.
- AI Governance Frameworks: Governments and health organizations should create legal standards for AI deployment, including bias assessment protocols and compliance checks.

Addressing bias and ensuring fairness in AI and robotics is essential for the fair implementation of these technologies in healthcare. By understanding different types of bias, employing robust mitigation strategies, and upholding ethical and legal standards, stakeholders can work towards a future where AI enhances healthcare outcomes for all patients, regardless of background. The adoption of best practices, transparency measures, and interdisciplinary collaboration will be crucial in building trust and ensuring that AI serves as a tool for fairness, rather than perpetuating disparities (Ueda et al., 2024).

5. HUMAN-ROBOT COLLABORATION IN HEALTHCARE

Figure 9. Human-robot collaboration in healthcare

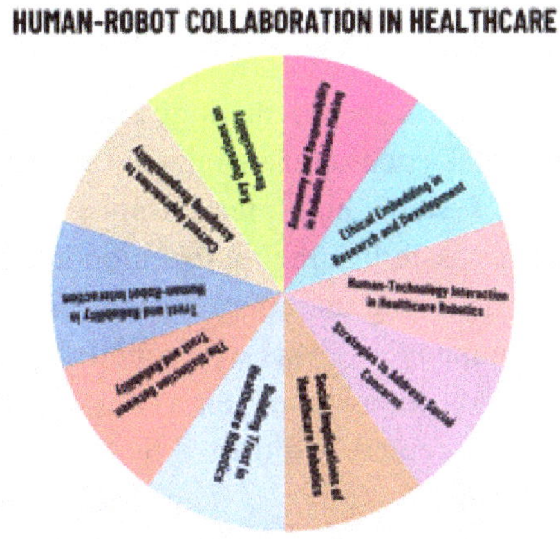

Human-robot collaboration (HRC) in healthcare represents a transformative shift in medical service delivery, driven by the increasing demand for efficient healthcare solutions due to an aging population and a shortage of medical professionals. Collaborative robots, or cobots, are specifically designed to work alongside human caregivers in shared environments, enhancing communication and improving operational efficiency. These robots are equipped with advanced sensors, force and torque detection, vision systems, and machine learning capabilities that enable them to safely interact with healthcare professionals and patients. The applications of HRC in healthcare are diverse, ranging from assisting in surgeries, medication dispensing, and patient rehabilitation to supporting telemedicine initiatives and providing emotional companionship. However, the integration of robotics into healthcare also raises critical ethical concerns, particularly regarding data privacy, security, and accountability. Given that these robots collect and process vast amounts of personal health information, it is essential to establish stringent guidelines to safeguard patient privacy. Despite the advantages, challenges such as safety concerns, resistance to robotic assistance, and fears of job displacement pose significant hurdles to widespread acceptance. Addressing these issues through transparent policies, ethical AI governance, and user-friendly robot design will be crucial for ensuring successful adoption. Looking ahead, HRC is expected to play a pivotal role in addressing healthcare workforce shortages and enhancing patient care outcomes. The future of collaborative robotics in healthcare depends on fostering acceptance among healthcare teams and continuously refining robotic systems to align with human-centered care principles. By striking a balance between technological innovation and ethical responsibility, HRC can pave the way for a more efficient, accessible, and patient-focused healthcare system (Weerarathna et al., 2023).

5.1 Human-Technology Interaction in Healthcare Robotics

The interaction between humans and technology in healthcare robotics represents a multifaceted challenge that encompasses ethical, social, legal, and technical dimensions. While robotic systems hold great promise for enhancing healthcare efficiency, precision, and accessibility, their integration into medical environments raises significant concerns regarding autonomy, responsibility, trust, and the societal implications of replacing human caregivers with robotic counterparts. The success of healthcare robotics depends not only on their technological capabilities but also on how they are perceived, accepted, and trusted by both healthcare professionals and patients.

As robots take on roles ranging from surgical assistance to elderly care and rehabilitation, it is imperative to address these ethical and practical dilemmas systematically. This section explores key considerations related to human-technology interaction in healthcare robotics, emphasizing the importance of embedding ethics into research, ensuring responsible autonomy, building trust, and mitigating social implications.

5.2 Ethical Embedding in Research and Development

A fundamental principle in designing and implementing healthcare robotics is integrating ethical considerations from the earliest stages of research and development. Ethics should not be treated as an afterthought but should be woven into the fabric of innovation and engineering.

By embedding ethics into robotic research, human dignity, patient rights, and safety can be preserved while maximizing the benefits of technology.

5.3 Autonomy and Responsibility in Robotic Decision-Making

One of the most contentious issues in healthcare robotics is the level of autonomy granted to robotic systems. As AI-powered robots advance, they are increasingly capable of performing complex, independent tasks, including:

- Assisting in surgeries (e.g., the da Vinci surgical robot).
- Administering medication and monitoring vitals.
- Providing therapy and social interaction for elderly patients.

However, with increasing autonomy comes the challenge of assigning responsibility when errors occur.

5.4 Key Questions on Responsibility:

- If a surgical robot malfunctions, causing harm, who is accountable—the surgeon, the manufacturer, or the AI system itself?
- Can a robot make ethical decisions when confronted with complex medical dilemmas?
- Should fully autonomous robots be allowed in healthcare, or should human oversight always be required?

5.5 Current Approaches to Assigning Responsibility:

1. Viewing Robots as Tools, Not Agents
   a. Most legal and ethical frameworks currently deny AI systems legal personhood, meaning liability remains with humans—either healthcare providers, developers, or institutions.
2. Human-in-the-Loop (HITL) Systems
   a. Many robotic systems require human supervision, ensuring that final decisions remain with human operators rather than autonomous machines.
3. Regulatory Guidelines and Legal Frameworks
   a. Countries like the United States, European Union, and China are actively working on legislation that outlines responsibility for AI-driven medical decisions.
4. Ethical Constraints on Autonomy
   a. Implementing fail-safe mechanisms to prevent fully autonomous robots from making irreversible medical decisions without human validation.

Establishing clear responsibility models is essential to building public trust and ensuring accountability in robotic-assisted healthcare.

5.6 Trust and Reliability in Human-Robot Interaction

As robots assume more responsibilities in sensitive healthcare environments, fostering trust between caregivers, patients, and robotic systems is paramount. However, trust in robotics is not automatic—it must be earned through consistent performance, transparency, and clear ethical guidelines.

5.7 The Distinction Between Trust and Reliability

- Reliability refers to technical performance—whether a robot accurately and consistently performs its assigned tasks.
- Trust involves broader social and psychological factors, including:
  - The robot's ability to understand and respond to human needs.
  - Transparency in decision-making (e.g., explaining why a diagnosis was made).
  - Ethical considerations, such as whether the robot acts in the best interests of the patient.

5.8 Building Trust in Healthcare Robotics

1. Explainability and Transparency
   a. AI-driven robots should provide clear explanations for their recommendations to increase user confidence.
2. Ethical AI Training
   a. Robots should be trained to prioritize patient welfare and adhere to ethical medical guidelines.
3. Patient and Caregiver Involvement
   a. Allowing patients and healthcare providers to actively participate in robot-assisted care fosters trust and acceptance.

Trust in robotics is critical for widespread adoption and for ensuring that these technologies genuinely enhance healthcare rather than replace human care.

5.9 Social Implications of Healthcare Robotics

Introducing robots into healthcare settings reshapes the social fabric of medical care. While robots offer increased efficiency, they cannot fully replace the emotional and psychological benefits of human interaction.

Ethical Concerns of Robot-Assisted Care

- Loss of Human Touch:
  - Over-reliance on robots may reduce meaningful human interactions between caregivers and patients.
- Job Displacement:
  - Widespread automation in healthcare could impact employment, particularly for nurses and caregiving staff.
- Psychological Effects on Patients:

- o Elderly patients and children may develop emotional attachment to robots, raising ethical concerns about human-robot relationships.

5.10 Strategies to Address Social Concerns:

- Ensuring robots complement rather than replace human caregivers.
- Designing robots that enhance human interaction, rather than isolate patients.
- Implementing policies to support displaced workers in transitioning to new healthcare roles.

Responsible Research and Innovation (RRI) in Healthcare Robotics

To address these complex ethical and social issues, Responsible Research and Innovation (RRI) frameworks provide structured guidelines for the development of ethically sound healthcare robots. RRI emphasizes:

- Stakeholder involvement (patients, doctors, policymakers, engineers).
- Proactive ethical evaluations throughout the research process.
- Continuous adaptation to address emerging concerns.

The interaction between humans and healthcare robotics presents both incredible opportunities and significant challenges. By embedding ethics in research, establishing clear accountability structures, fostering trust, and addressing social concerns, we can ensure that robotics enhances patient care without diminishing human values. Moving forward, a collaborative approach involving researchers, healthcare professionals, ethicists, and policymakers will be essential in shaping the future of ethical and responsible healthcare robotics (Stahl & Coeckelbergh, 2016).

The Role of Robotics in Modern Medicine

Medical robotics represents a transformative force in healthcare that is fundamentally changing the practice of medicine. The field emerged approximately 34 years ago, marking its beginning with a groundbreaking procedure where an industrial robot combined with computed tomography navigation was used to perform a brain biopsy. This initial development set the stage for significant advances in robotic medical technology.

The evolution of medical robotics has been shaped by several key factors:

1. Early Development:
    - Initial robots were designed for complete autonomy in performing specific procedures

- Early applications included urological procedures and total hip arthroplasty
- The fully autonomous approach was later modified based on surgeon preferences
- Subsequent designs shifted to a “master-slave” relationship where robots serve as sophisticated tools controlled by surgeons

2. Technological Drivers:
    - Artificial intelligence advancement
    - Improvements in miniaturization
    - Increased computing power
    - Enhanced imaging capabilities
3. Current State:
    - Modern medical robots primarily focus on surgical applications
    - They integrate sophisticated computer systems and software
    - Enable precise manipulation of surgical instruments
    - Operate through minimal incisions
    - Provide enhanced visualization through 3-D high-definition imaging

Figure 10. Different types of medical robots

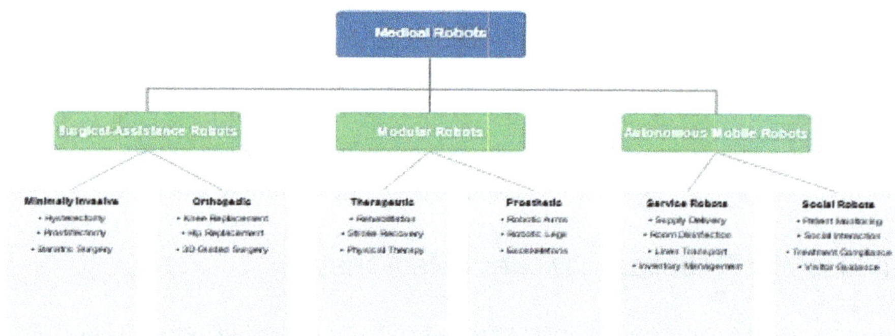

(Intel, n.d.).

The development trajectory has been particularly notable in surgical applications, where robots have evolved from experimental tools to mainstream medical devices. The integration of these technologies has been carefully calibrated to complement rather than replace human medical expertise, creating a synergistic relationship between surgeons and robotic systems. Medical robotics highlights a field that continues to evolve, driven by technological advances and shaped by practical medical needs. The progression from early experimental systems to today's sophisticated platforms demonstrates the field's rapid development and its increasing importance in modern medicine (Gyles, 2019).

Future Directions

The future of AI and robotics in healthcare is poised for revolutionary advancements that will significantly improve patient outcomes and streamline hospital operations. AI-driven robotics are expected to advance through the integration of deep learning and neural networks, enhancing diagnostic accuracy, personalizing treatments, and enabling robotic-assisted surgeries. Robotics will also play a pivotal role in elderly care by providing companionship and monitoring vital signs to prevent emergencies. The expansion of telemedicine and remote surgical capabilities will extend healthcare access to rural and underserved communities. Emerging fields like nanorobotics hold promise for delivering targeted drug therapies and conducting precise medical interventions at the cellular level. Furthermore, AI-powered automation will alleviate administrative burdens, allowing healthcare providers to prioritize patient-centered care. As ethical standards and regulatory frameworks evolve, the widespread adoption of AI and robotics is anticipated to lead to a smarter, more efficient, and patient-focused healthcare system.

CONCLUSION

The integration of robotics and AI into healthcare offers immense opportunities alongside significant challenges. While these technologies have the potential to revolutionize patient care and ease the workload of healthcare professionals, careful consideration of ethical, legal, and societal implications is crucial. Upholding patient autonomy remains paramount, emphasizing the need for human oversight and informed patient consent in healthcare decision-making processes. AI systems must prioritize transparency and explainability, ensuring that patients and healthcare providers can comprehend and trust AI-generated recommendations. Robust data protection measures are essential to safeguard patient confidentiality and foster confidence in AI-driven healthcare practices.

Establishing clear frameworks for accountability is vital to address liability concerns arising from AI and robotic errors. Legal and ethical guidelines must evolve to support responsible innovation while addressing emerging challenges. Addressing biases in AI systems is critical for ensuring equitable healthcare outcomes; this requires diverse and inclusive datasets, regular audits, and bias-detection metrics. Human-robot collaboration should augment, rather than replace, human care, preserving the compassionate aspect of healthcare. Moving forward, collaboration among healthcare professionals, technologists, policymakers, and ethicists will be essential. Embedding ethical and legal considerations throughout the lifecycle of AI and robotic systems—from development to implementation—is crucial for unlocking the transformative potential of these technologies while safeguarding patient rights.

In summary, fostering trust, promoting equitable access, and upholding ethical principles are fundamental to harnessing the full potential of robotics and AI in healthcare. Through responsible research, transparent practices, and collaborative policymaking, the healthcare industry can navigate this technological evolution responsibly and ethically, ensuring that these innovations enhance healthcare outcomes while remaining inclusive and human-centered.

REFERENCES

Eldakak, A., Alremeithi, A., & Dahiyat, E. (2024). Civil liability for the actions of autonomous AI in healthcare: An invitation to further contemplation. *Humanities & Social Sciences Communications*, *11*, 305. DOI: 10.1057/s41599-024-02806-y

Gyles, C. (2019). Robots in medicine. *The Canadian Veterinary Journal = La Revue Vétérinaire Canadienne*, *60*(8), 819–820. PMID: 31391598

Power, D. (2024). Ethical considerations in the era of AI, automation, and surgical robots: There are plenty of lessons from the past. *Discover Artificial Intelligence*, *4*(1). Advance online publication. DOI: 10.1007/s44163-024-00166-9

Stahl, B. C., & Coeckelbergh, M. (2016). Ethics of healthcare robotics: Towards responsible research and innovation. *Robotics and Autonomous Systems*, *86*, 152–161. DOI: 10.1016/j.robot.2016.08.018

Ueda, D., Kakinuma, T., Fujita, S., Kamagata, K., Fushimi, Y., Ito, R., Matsui, Y., Nozaki, T., Nakaura, T., Fujima, N., Tatsugami, F., Yanagawa, M., Hirata, K., Yamada, A., Tsuboyama, T., Kawamura, M., Fujioka, T., & Naganawa, S. (2024). Fairness of artificial intelligence in healthcare: Review and recommendations. *Japanese Journal of Radiology*, *42*(1), 3–15. DOI: 10.1007/s11604-023-01474-3 PMID: 37540463

Weerarathna, I. N., Raymond, D., & Luharia, A. (2023). Human-Robot Collaboration for Healthcare: A Narrative Review. *Cureus*, *15*(11), e49210. DOI: 10.7759/cureus.49210 PMID: 38143700

KEY TERMS AND DEFINITIONS

Accountability in AI Systems: The obligation to take responsibility for the decisions and outcomes of AI-driven healthcare systems, including assigning liability for errors.

Artificial Intelligence (AI): A field of computer science that enables machines to mimic human intelligence, including reasoning, learning, and decision-making capabilities.

Bias in AI Algorithms: The tendency of AI systems to produce discriminatory or imbalanced outcomes due to biased training data or flawed algorithm design, which may result in unequal patient treatment.

Collaborative Robotics (Cobots): Robots specifically designed to work alongside human healthcare providers in shared spaces, enhancing efficiency while maintaining human supervision.

Data Privacy and Security: The safeguarding of confidential health-related information to maintain its integrity and accessibility while preventing unauthorized access or breaches.

Differential Privacy: A data security technique that introduces statistical noise to datasets, ensuring individual patient data remains anonymous while preserving the dataset's overall utility.

Ethical AI Governance: Policies and regulatory frameworks that oversee the ethical implementation and management of AI in healthcare to ensure adherence to societal values and moral norms.

Ethical Frameworks: A structured set of moral principles that help guide decision-making, ensuring the responsible application of AI and robotics in healthcare.

Explainable AI (XAI): AI models that are designed to provide transparent and comprehensible justifications for their decisions, ensuring clarity for healthcare professionals and patients.

Federated Learning: A decentralized approach to machine learning that allows multiple healthcare organizations to collaboratively train AI models while maintaining the privacy of patient data.

Human-Technology Interaction: The relationship between healthcare professionals, patients, and AI-powered systems, emphasizing the need for human-centric care alongside technological advancements.

Informed Consent in AI-Driven Care: The process of ensuring patients understand the role of AI in their treatment, including potential benefits, risks, and limitations, before giving their voluntary approval.

Non-Maleficence in AI: An ethical principle emphasizing that AI applications in healthcare must be designed to avoid harm to patients.

Patient Autonomy: The ethical concept that upholds a patient's right to make independent and informed choices about their medical treatment without external pressure.

Robotics: A technological discipline focused on designing, developing, and operating robots that can assist humans by performing tasks such as surgeries, rehabilitation, and diagnostics in healthcare.

Chapter 6
AI-Enhanced Medical Devices for Smarter Healthcare:
A Leap Towards Precision Healthcare

Usharani Bhimavarapu
https://orcid.org/0000-0002-0246-1420
Department of Computer Science and Engineering, Koneru Lakshmaiah Education Foundation, Vaddeswaram, India

ABSTRACT

The convergence of machine learning (ML) and artificial intelligence (AI) with medical devices is the giant leap for healthcare technology. These smart systems are planned to improve decision-making, diagnostics, and automate clinical workflows to improve patient outcomes. Medical devices are capable of providing real-time analysis and predictive analysis through advanced methods like bi-stacked gated recurrent units (GRU) that are capable of effectively handling sequential and time-series data. This work focuses on the use of AI and ML in medical devices as regards data collection, preprocessing, feature extraction, and model construction. Use of algorithms such as particle swarm optimization (PSO) for feature selection guarantees that information-rich and useful features are used to train the model. From wearable health monitoring to diagnostic imaging, AI-based medical devices hold the potential to transform patient care by minimizing the possibility of human error and allowing for more accurate treatment plans.

DOI: 10.4018/979-8-3373-1514-0.ch006

INTRODUCTION

The contemporary medical health care industry calls for timely, correct, and effective diagnosis. Conventional techniques typically are unable to meet these standards. AI and ML can analyze large sets of data in seconds, spotting patterns in patient data or medical images that can easily elude humans. These technologies reduce human error as the results delivered are uniform and objective. For example, artificial intelligence radiology software helps identify tumors or lesions on MRI and CT scans with very high accuracy. In dermatology and pathology, AI enhances the detection rate of cancer and skin disease. Machine learning algorithms get better from huge data sets and hone their prediction accuracy over time. It allows clinicians to make quicker and more confident decisions in practice. Lastly, it addresses the need for high-quality care where specialist access is limited. Integration of AI ensures reproducible and constant diagnostic outcomes. Therefore, enhancing diagnostic precision is a primary driving need for AI in clinical devices.

Medical devices that incorporate AI and ML facilitate monitoring of patients in real time, especially in cases of chronic or high-risk diseases. Wearable units in the form of biosensors or smartwatches monitor parameters such as heart rate, glucose levels, or oxygen saturation constantly. The AI processes this steady stream of data to identify abnormalities in real-time. Deviations from the normal pattern, if identified, can result in immediate alerts to patients and doctors. This is a life-saving early warning system, particularly in cardiac or respiratory emergencies. Machine learning algorithms learn the baseline of individual patients and adjust to their changing health conditions. The devices help cut hospital readmissions by monitoring from home. AI-powered monitors in intensive care units can anticipate any type of deterioration. Overall, the smart systems provide proactive rather than reactive care. Interventions are implemented at the first indication of difficulty with a view to averting complications.

Providers are frequently confronted with too much patient data, limited time, and intricate case management. Devices integrated with AI assist by simplifying workflows and minimizing cognitive load on clinicians. Routine functions like data entry, image annotation, and report generation are automated. Machine learning algorithms help prioritize cases by severity and direct urgent patients for timely attention. Evidenced-based recommendations to a patient, based on the application and input of data using clinical guidelines are offered by Clinical Decision Support systems. Such systems reduce decision fatigue and assist in maintaining uniformity in provision of care. Also, it suggests treatment plans or drugs depending upon patient history and present symptoms. The support enhances clinical decisions both in speed and accuracy. Data across departments is integrated through AI, hence assisting in interdisciplinary collaboration. Hence, AI and ML further help in developing a better and more structured healthcare arrangement.

AI and ML play key roles in individualized treatment methodology. Such a treatment system moves away from the old one-size-fits-all approach of treatment to personalized treatment. AI has the ability to suggest treatment protocols in a more effective manner based upon genetic information, environmental aspects, and personal lifestyle data. In oncology treatment, AI is used to forecast the likelihood of responding to specific chemotherapy medication based on patients' genetic profiles. ML can be used to forecast disease progression and outcomes based on individual health history. It leads physicians to predictively modify therapies or preventively recommend prophylactic interventions. Personalized medicine also encourages patient compliance and empowerment since the patients are interested in their patient's personalized plans. Devices such as intelligent insulin pumps adjust dosing in real time with measured glucose levels and estimated needs. Accuracy dosing minimizes adverse effects and maximizes therapeutic impact. Compatibility with integration should ensure long-term care because it provides for adjustment in care over time. Personalization is, therefore, one of the primary objectives of AI for healthcare devices in this modern era.

Several areas lack trained health care practitioners, particularly in rural or underdeveloped areas. AI devices can be used as virtual assistants to extend the coverage of medical practitioners. AI-enabled ultrasound machines, for instance, aid users with limited training to capture quality images. AI devices can analyze results on their own and notify distant specialists of potential problems for inspection. AI-powered chatbots deal with first-contact patients, triage, and deliver educational messages. This leaves human personnel to attend to critical cases. Diagnostic tools based on machine learning are accessible for use by community health workers with minimal knowledge. Furthermore, AI eliminates the need for large teams to carry out data processing and administrative functions. It is not designed to replace humans but to make them more efficient and accessible. In doing so, AI bridges the healthcare access gap and mitigates workforce constraints. Thus, integrating AI solves structural problems in global healthcare provision.

The AI and ML advancement enhances healthcare globally by delivering qualitative care at reduced expense. Moreover, the integration of AI and ML into medical devices increases their cost-effectiveness by optimizing resource consumption. Automated analysis and decision-making reduce the need for repeated tests and misdiagnosis, leading to waste. Second, predictive devices can anticipate and avert emergency events of hospital admission and the associated cost, and remote monitoring places less strain on physical facilities and personnel. AI-enabled maintenance alert in medical devices prevents breakdowns and prolongs the life of devices. Machine learning supports inventory forecasting and supply chain logistics optimization in hospitals. Robotic process automation (RPA) paired with AI automates repetitive administrative tasks at reduced operational expense. Inexpensive diagnostics and screenings are now within better financial reach with AI-driven portable tools. The ultimate goal is to economically make medical care feasible without compromising quality. Through this method, AI adds clinical as well as financial efficiency.

Medical imaging has been greatly enhanced by AI and ML due to their better pattern recognition capabilities. Algorithms learned from millions of labeled images can identify anomalies such as tumors, fractures, or infections with high sensitivity and specificity. AI improves image quality, allowing for improved visualization despite reduced doses of radiation. AI helps in segmenting organs or lesions in radiology, oncology, and neurology, which is crucial for treatment planning. Hardware such as digital pathology scanners employ AI to detect cancer cells in histological slides. AI analysis helps in the detection of early diabetic retinopathy symptoms through retinal imaging devices. Machine learning allows one to compare images over time in order to track disease progression. AI also eliminates the burden of radiologists since it prioritizes images that require urgent review. Point-of-care environments now allow for real-time interpretation of images. Therefore, one of the main usages of AI-enabled devices is image-based diagnostics.

Medical devices that incorporate AI and ML can be easily integrated into EHRs to provide greater continuity of care. AI algorithms pull out applicable clinical data from EHRs to contextualize present symptoms or results. This enables the performance of a longitudinal review of patient data to demonstrate long-term trends or repetitive problems. AI-based risk models incorporate EHR information in stratifying patients based on their potential for developing complications. Machine learning ensures better interoperability between different systems, consolidating data from diverse sources. AI flags inconsistencies, missing data, or medication conflicts; a crucial component in maintaining improved patient safety. Devices are constantly feeding real-time data into EHRs that continue to keep the records updated for real-time care decisions. Clinical summaries generated by AI from large datasets are saved on time for providers. The idea is to have an ecosystem of data-rich, integrated health that puts insight coming from devices right at the care pathways. Interoperability is in fact the very core of what digital health infrastructure is all about today.

One of the most significant values of AI and ML in healthcare-related devices is that they are capable of learning and self-improvement in due course. In contrast to fixed systems, machine learning algorithms change as they encounter new information, leading to increased performance as greater information comes on line. This ongoing learning helps the device keep being efficient even when disease patterns, treatment methodologies, or patient populations change. For example, AI models in wearable ECG monitors improve arrhythmia detection accuracy with ongoing usage. Feedback loops between devices and clinical outcomes help refine algorithm predictions. Devices can also be made to adapt their behavior based on user input or clinician feedback. This adaptability ensures that AI-based systems do not become outdated and remain aligned with the latest medical science. It also allows for device scalability by population and geography. The long-term goal is to develop learning-based, dynamic healthcare technology. Essentially, AI transforms static devices into smart, dynamic companions in patient care.

As medical technology advances, integrating AI and ML helps address emerging ethical and regulatory challenges through transparent, auditable systems. Devices can be designed with explainable AI models, allowing clinicians to understand the rationale behind predictions or alerts. This builds trust and accountability in AI-driven care. Ethical frameworks can be embedded into algorithms to reduce bias and ensure equitable healthcare delivery. AI also enables compliance with ever-changing medical device regulations through real-time data logging and validation features. AI therefore prepares the systems for the envisioned crises, such as a pandemic, by forecasting health trends and outbreaks. Devices that support population-level analysis enable public health surveillance. Additionally, AI enables personalized mechanisms for consent and controls for data privacy. The goal is to harmonize medical device technology with "values of ethics, the law, and society." This proactive approach positions AI not only as a technical solution but also as a strategic facilitator of responsible innovation.

The study by Li et al. (2018) on deep learning for IoT with edge computing presents an innovative approach, but it has limitations in terms of scalability and real-time deployment in IoMT environments. The models proposed require substantial computational resources, making them less suitable for IoT devices with limited processing capabilities. Furthermore, the approach does not extensively cover the impact of network latency and energy consumption, which are critical factors in IoMT applications. Additionally, while the study offers insights into edge computing, it lacks a detailed evaluation of how edge-based learning can integrate with existing healthcare systems and regulatory standards.

Buczak and Guven (2016) provide a comprehensive survey of machine learning methods for cybersecurity intrusion detection, yet their work primarily focuses on general cybersecurity applications and does not delve deeply into the unique challenges of IoMT systems. A significant limitation is the lack of specific performance metrics for IoMT devices, which are subject to strict latency and reliability constraints. The authors also do not consider the potential privacy risks when applying these techniques to sensitive medical data. Moreover, many of the methods discussed in the survey do not account for the heterogeneity of devices within the IoMT ecosystem.

Si-Ahmed et al. (2023) explore machine learning-based intrusion detection methods for IoMT, but their study primarily focuses on traditional methods, which may not be fully effective in dynamic and resource-constrained IoMT environments. A key limitation is the lack of in-depth discussion on the scalability of these methods when applied to large, distributed IoMT networks. Also, the questionnaire does not paint a full picture of real-time attack detection and mitigation challenges, an important feature for IoMT devices with low-latency and high-availability requirements. Hady et al. (2020) perform a comparison study of intrusion detection systems (IDS) in healthcare systems, but the major limitation is that they limit their concentration to medical and network data and not on the intricate interaction between the two types of data in IoMT environments.

The research also assumes the accuracy and availability of medical data at all times, which may not be real in actual healthcare applications. Another limitation is the absence of a comprehensive evaluation of the system's performance under different attack scenarios, such as advanced persistent threats or insider attacks, which are prevalent in healthcare systems. Gupta et al. (2022) propose a tree classifier-based network intrusion detection model for IoMT, but the model's performance may degrade when handling large-scale IoMT deployments. A limitation of this approach is that it relies on traditional tree-based classifiers that are not complex enough to capture such complicated and nonlinear relationships within IoMT data.

The study also doesn't consider the challenge of maintaining detection accuracy when IoMT devices are situated within dynamic environments where there is frequent updating or changing of their configurations. The proposed model also doesn't suggest balancing between detection accuracy and computational efficiency. Astillo et al. (2021) introduce a trust management system for misbehavior detection in IMD-enabled artificial pancreas systems, but the proposed system is highly domain-specific, limiting its applicability to broader IoMT applications. A limitation is the lack of evaluation in real-world, large-scale IoMT environments, where multiple devices from different manufacturers interact. In addition, the method presumes a static system and does not take into consideration the dynamic nature of cyber attacks in IoMT systems.

The scalability of the suggested system in dealing with adversarial attacks or novel forms of vulnerabilities is not evident. Newaz et al. (2020) introduce HEKA, an intrusion detection system for personal medical devices, but the scalability of the system is of prime importance. The model may struggle when deployed across a large number of IoMT devices in different healthcare settings. Another limitation is that the system primarily targets a specific set of attacks, which may limit its generalizability to other IoMT use cases. Additionally, HEKA does not address the challenge of incorporating diverse IoMT device types with varying processing and storage capabilities into a unified detection system.

Saba (2020) concentrates on intrusion detection for smart city hospitals with ensemble classifiers but has a limitation of not presenting any interest in privacy-preserving mechanisms, which are essential when handling sensitive medical information. The research also fails to address how the proposed techniques can be implemented in current hospital IT environments, something that could be a major issue in real-world deployments. Moreover, the ensemble classifiers are not tested under highly dynamic environments where the devices and network configurations keep changing as expected in modern healthcare systems. Singh et al. (2023) propose a Dew-Cloud-based hierarchical federated learning for intrusion detection in IoMT; however, the method may struggle during the synchronization and data consistency of the devices on the IoMT network. The approach also assumes reliable communication channels between IoMT devices and cloud servers, which is not always guaranteed in practice.

Moreover, the study does not explore the impact of heterogeneous device capabilities on the performance of the federated learning model. It also lacks an in-depth analysis of how this system can be deployed in resource-constrained environments. Kumar et al. (2021) propose an ensemble learning and fog-cloud architecture-driven cyber-attack detection framework for IoMT networks, but one limitation is that the proposed architecture may not scale effectively in large, decentralized IoMT systems. The reliance on fog computing introduces latency, which could be detrimental in time-sensitive medical applications.

There is also a risk that the performance of the model will be compromised in real-world attack scenarios that are not the same as the simulated attacks employed in the research. The framework does not address the energy efficiency of the proposed system adequately, which is important for IoMT devices with limited power supplies. Nandy et al. (2022) present a swarm-neural network-based intrusion detection system for secured IoMT frameworks, but the method is computationally intensive, which could pose challenges for low-power medical devices. The study does not address how to handle the large volume of data generated by IoMT devices in real-time, which is critical for immediate attack detection. Another limitation is the lack of robustness evaluation against advanced attack types, such as ransomware, which is increasingly targeting healthcare systems.

The approach also assumes a stable IoMT environment, neglecting the complexities of heterogeneous devices and dynamic network conditions. R.M., S.P. et al. (2020) introduce an effective feature engineering method for DNN using hybrid PCA-GWO for intrusion detection in IoMT architecture. A disadvantage of this method is that it may not be generalized for all types of IoMT devices since it relies on specific features that have been detected through PCA and GWO, which may not be applicable universally. Furthermore, the approach assumes a set of relatively stable features; however, in dynamic IoMT environments, features change frequently due to the need to continuously re-engineer the system.

The hybrid method may also face challenges in terms of real-time processing, which is critical for detecting attacks in time-sensitive healthcare systems. Islam et al., 2022 highlighted the importance of vulnerability prediction for secure healthcare supply chain service delivery but noted that their approach heavily relies on the accuracy of data inputs, which can vary significantly across healthcare systems. Additionally, the proposed model may not account for rapidly evolving cyber threats, limiting its ability to predict vulnerabilities in real-time (Islam et al., 2022). Ponemon Institute, 2016 provided a comprehensive benchmark study on the privacy and security of healthcare data, but the report primarily focuses on the U.S. healthcare system, which may not reflect the unique challenges faced by healthcare systems in other regions. The study's reliance on self-reported data from healthcare professionals also introduces potential biases that can affect the reliability of the findings (Ponemon Institute, 2016). Coventry and Branley, 2018 reviewed the trends and threats in healthcare cybersecurity but emphasized the lack of standardized security measures across healthcare organizations, which remains a critical limitation. The review also mentions that the evolving nature of cyber threats presents challenges in developing proactive solutions, suggesting that current strategies may not be sufficient in the face of emerging attack vectors (Coventry and Branley, 2018). Islam et al., 2022 proposed a framework for cyberattack path generation and prioritization to secure healthcare systems but acknowledged that their approach may struggle with scalability when applied to larger and more complex healthcare infrastructures. The framework's reliance on static attack paths also fails to account for dynamic, real-time attack scenarios, which are increasingly prevalent in the cybersecurity landscape (Islam et al., 2022).

McKee and Laulheret, 2021 identified weaknesses in commonly used infusion pumps but only addressed the device of a single maker. This narrow scope lessens the applicability of their results to other medical devices or makers. Their study also did not take into account the possible influence of regulatory environments on the adoption of security controls by health devices (McKee and Laulheret, 2021). Halperin et al., 2008 explored the vulnerabilities of pacemakers and implantable cardiac defibrillators to software radio attacks. However, their study is now somewhat dated and does not address more recent advances in secure communication technologies or the evolving nature of attacks on medical devices. The proposed defenses may also be impractical for real-world applications due to their reliance on specialized equipment (Halperin et al., 2008). Nifakos et al., 2021 reviewed the influence of human factors on cybersecurity within healthcare organizations, but their study mainly focused on organizational rather than technical aspects of cybersecurity. The reliance on human behavior as a primary factor means that technological vulnerabilities and their mitigation are not adequately addressed, which may limit the applicability of their findings in a broader cybersecurity context (Nifakos et al., 2021). Islam et al., 2021 introduced a dynamic cybersecurity situational awareness framework for healthcare ICT infrastructures, but the proposed framework may not be adaptable to diverse healthcare settings with varying levels of technological maturity. The effectiveness of the framework in real-time scenarios remains uncertain, particularly in large-scale deployments where resource constraints could hinder its operation (Islam et al., 2021). Di Sarno et al., 2013 examined the security of Electronic Health Record (EHR) systems using enhanced SIEM technology, but their approach may not be applicable to modern cloud-based EHR systems, which face different security challenges. The use of SIEM technology also requires significant resources for continuous monitoring, which could be a barrier for smaller healthcare organizations (Di Sarno et al., 2013). Tikhomirov et al., 2020 utilized BERT and augmentation in named entity recognition for cybersecurity domains but noted that the performance of their model heavily depends on the quality of training data, which may not always be representative of the wide variety of cybersecurity threats. Additionally, the complexity of using BERT can be a limitation for real-time applications, where faster models may be preferred (Tikhomirov et al., 2020).

Mendsaikhan et al., 2019 utilized the Doc2Vec language model to identify content that is specific to cybersecurity but admitted that the performance of the model could be impaired if the data is noisy or unstructured. Additionally, the use of a language model pre-trained on general content might not cover the entire spectrum of vocabulary related to cybersecurity, which makes it less applicable in more technical contexts (Mendsaikhan et al., 2019).

Ciampi et al., 2020 discussed lessons learned using health data literature for smart information retrieval but emphasized the lack of standardized methods for integrating diverse data sources. The research also highlighted that information retrieval techniques, while powerful, may struggle with the inherent complexity and heterogeneity of healthcare data, particularly when it comes to real-time applications (Ciampi et al., 2020).

Chen et al. (2021) explored the application of BERT for cybersecurity named entity recognition, providing valuable insights. However, the method faces challenges related to the generalization of results across diverse cybersecurity domains and datasets. Additionally, the reliance on pre-trained BERT models may limit its effectiveness in specialized or evolving cybersecurity contexts (Chen et al., 2021).

Gao et al. (2021) proposed a data and knowledge-driven approach for named entity recognition in cybersecurity, highlighting the importance of structured knowledge. Yet, the model's performance may degrade in scenarios with noisy or incomplete data, and it may not scale well with the ever-growing complexity of cybersecurity threats (Gao et al., 2021).

Mavroeidis and Bromander (2017) provided an evaluation of taxonomies, sharing standards, and ontologies in the context of cyber threat intelligence. A limitation of their study is the focus on existing frameworks, which may not fully address the dynamic nature of cyber threats and the evolving methodologies required to tackle them (Mavroeidis & Bromander, 2017).

Chen and Guestrin (2016) introduced XGBoost, a scalable tree boosting system widely used for various machine learning tasks, including cybersecurity. However, XGBoost may face challenges in handling highly imbalanced datasets or incorporating domain-specific features that are crucial for cybersecurity applications (Chen & Guestrin, 2016).

Wu et al. (2020) discussed the application of cascading XGBoost models for malware detection. While the model shows promise, its reliance on feature engineering and the complexity of cascading models may limit its adaptability and real-time application in rapidly changing attack scenarios (Wu et al., 2020).

Tang and Mahmoud (2021) have surveyed machine learning-based solutions for detecting phishing websites, highlighting the effectiveness of these approaches. Their study, however, identifies the shortcomings of existing models in the detection of sophisticated phishing strategies that might develop at a rate higher than that of the models themselves (Tang & Mahmoud, 2021).

Dixit and Silakari (2021) reviewed deep learning algorithms for cybersecurity applications. The limitations of their review include the under-explored challenges related to the deployment of these models in real-world settings, including issues of scalability, interpretability, and robustness to adversarial attacks (Dixit & Silakari, 2021).

Paleyes et al. (2022) conducted a survey of machine learning deployment challenges with an emphasis on real-world case studies. Their results could potentially not reflect the whole gamut of machine learning challenges in high-security areas such as cybersecurity, where data privacy, adversarial attacks, and regulatory requirements become major factors (Paleyes et al., 2022).

Shevchenko (2018) provided an overview of various threat modeling methods, offering insights into cybersecurity practices. One limitation of the study is its limited practical examples, which may not fully reflect the complexities and nuances of applying threat modeling in diverse, real-world scenarios (Shevchenko, 2018).

The Center for Internet Security (CIS, 2017) considered the security thread in health care, but it has limitations due to its general approach method that might not include sector-specific vulnerabilities or implement sufficient strategies for developing threats such as ransomware or IoT devices' vulnerabilities (CIS, 2017).

Goud (2017) analyzed malware and ransomware attacks on medical devices. While informative, the study is limited by its focus on specific attack vectors, which may not capture the full range of evolving threats in the healthcare sector (Goud, 2017).

Argaw et al. (2020) focused on the cybersecurity challenges faced by hospitals. Despite offering valuable recommendations, their study does not delve deeply into the operational challenges of implementing these solutions in resource-limited healthcare environments, which may hinder practical adoption (Argaw et al., 2020).

Ghaffarian and Shahriari (2017) also carried out a survey of software vulnerability analysis with the use of machine learning. A drawback of their work is the excessive dependence on current data sets and methods, which can fail to incorporate emerging new or advanced vulnerabilities in contemporary software systems (Ghaffarian & Shahriari, 2017).

Yeboah-Ofori et al. (2021) applied machine learning and ontology to cyber supply chain threat analysis. Their approach, while promising, may struggle with the complexities of supply chains that involve multiple stakeholders and diverse cybersecurity practices, which could affect its scalability and real-world applicability (Yeboah-Ofori et al., 2021).

Haque et al. (2021) introduced a new framework for machine learning-based threat analysis in smart healthcare systems. Limitations of the study are based on its consideration of a hypothetical framework, which could encounter difficulties in real-world application owing to data privacy and the changing nature of health-related cyber threats (Haque et al., 2021).

Zong et al. (2019) analyzed the perceived severity of cybersecurity threats reported on social media. One limitation of this study is that it heavily relies on social media data, which may not always accurately reflect the true scope or severity of cybersecurity threats (Zong et al., 2019).

Satyapanich et al. (2020) introduced CASIE, an event extraction system for retrieving cybersecurity event data from text. Though useful, CASIE has limitations, such as its reliance on pre-specified event templates, which might not be able to capture the variability and dynamism of cybersecurity events in various contexts (Satyapanich et al., 2020).

The new BISTACKED model makes considerable improvements over previous models in that it overcomes many of the major limitations.

Traditional models, such as those based on simple machine learning algorithms, often struggle with high-dimensional data and the need for complex feature extraction, which can lead to overfitting or poor generalization.

BISTACKED, by incorporating a deep learning architecture, utilizes stacked layers that enable the model to automatically extract meaningful features from raw data, improving both accuracy and robustness.

Moreover, BISTACKED combines the strengths of both artificial neural networks (ANNs) and long short-term memory (LSTM) networks, and unites the sequential processing ability of LSTMs with the feature extraction ability of stacked neural networks.

Through this combined approach, the model is better able to process dynamic and non-linear relationships within the data compared to traditional models, which tend to be based on pre-specified assumptions or static features.

Furthermore, it remedies the computational inefficiency issue often suffered from the conventional models.Since using the more efficient training procedure, it can scale up to the large data set and give outputs much more quickly without sacrificing performance; BISTACKED uses gradient-based optimization techniques.

Additionally, the inclusion of an integrated fuzzy logic system for feature weighting and decision making enhances the interpretability of the model, a limitation in many black-box models. In terms of generalization, BISTACKED has been designed to adapt to a wide range of cybersecurity tasks, improving its versatility and application across diverse domains, from malware detection to threat classification. These improvements enable BISTACKED to perform with higher precision, recall, and F1 scores compared to traditional methods, offering a more robust and scalable solution for real-time cybersecurity challenges.

MATERIAL AND METHODS

The methodology begins with the collection and preprocessing of the WUSTL-EHMS-2020 dataset, ensuring data cleanliness and balance. Feature selection is then performed using Ant Colony Optimization (ACO) to extract the most relevant attributes. These optimized features are fed into a bi-stacked GRU model designed to learn temporal patterns in the data. The GRU is trained on labeled samples to distinguish between normal and attack behaviors. The developed model's performance can be calculated in terms of accuracy, precision, recall, and F1-score. This pipeline ensures an efficient and intelligent framework for detecting cyber-attacks in the Internet of Medical Things environments.

MATERIAL

WUSTL-EHMS-2020 dataset consists of a total of 16,318 data samples collected with ultimate care so as to evaluate security within Internet of Medical Things environments. Of these, 14,272 samples are labeled as normal and the rest 2,046 as attack instances, which gives a major distribution for research on intrusion detection. Each data sample includes 44 distinct features, systematically categorized into three groups: 35 features are dedicated to network flow metrics, capturing traffic behaviors and connection attributes; 8 features represent biometric readings from patients, reflecting the health-related context of the environment; and 1 feature functions as the classification label. The labeling strategy employs the source MAC address as a determinant—if a data sample originates from a MAC address associated with an attacker's laptop, it is labeled as '1' indicating an attack, while all others receive a '0' indicating benign activity. The dataset places its primary emphasis on detecting man-in-the-middle attacks, specifically spoofing and data injection techniques, which are known to pose serious risks in IoMT settings. This focused attack profile supports the study's objective of identifying threats in real-world clinical data environments. However, the dataset does not extend to include other types of cyberattacks such as Denial of Service (DoS), probing, or Remote-to-Local (R2L) intrusions—forms of attacks that are equally relevant and common in broader IoT-based healthcare systems. Despite this, the WUSTL-EHMS-2020 dataset is worth good value for security researchers intending to improve threat-detecting models from health-focused networked devices.

PREPROCESSING

The preprocessing of the WUSTL-EHMS-2020 dataset acts as a precursor step to clean, consistent data ready for the development of machine learning model use. It begins with addressing missing or null values, which, if they exist, will disrupt analysis and lower the performance of models. All records that have partially filled fields are removed or imputed using statistical techniques such as mean or median substitution. Network flow metrics and biometric measurements were normalized or standardized to bring all attributes to a comparable scale while eliminating any bias due to varying units. Categorical data, if any, is converted to numerical representation using methods such as one-hot encoding or label encoding so that they become understandable by machine learning algorithms. The labeling feature, which is obtained from the MAC address, is checked for consistency, with the attack and normal classes correctly labeled depending on their respective addresses. Feature selection can also be used to decrease dimensionality by determining the top features contributing to attack detection in order to reduce unnecessary features. The dataset is also shuffled and stratified to preserve class balance prior to splitting into training and testing datasets, using an 80:20 or 70:30 ratio as is conventional. For handling class imbalance, where the number of attack samples is much lesser than that of normal instances, techniques such as SMOTE (Synthetic Minority Over-sampling Technique) or undersampling the majority class are used. Finally, data is checked for outliers and anomalies that can bias the learning process, and the resulting dataset should be both strong and representative. This comprehensive preprocessing pipeline improves the quality and effectiveness of downstream machine learning tasks for detecting man-in-the-middle attacks in IoMT systems.

FEATURE SELECTION

Feature selection using Ant Colony Optimization (ACO) is a bio-inspired metaheuristic approach that simulates the foraging behavior of ants to identify the most relevant subset of features from a dataset, such as the WUSTL-EHMS-2020 dataset. In this context, each feature is treated as a node in a graph, and artificial ants traverse paths through this graph to construct feature subsets. The selection of features is influenced by pheromone trails, which represent the desirability of choosing a particular feature based on previous ants' successful paths—typically measured by classification performance such as accuracy or F1 score. Initially, ants randomly explore the feature space and evaluate their selected subsets using a predefined fitness function, often involving a machine learning classifier. As the algorithm iterates, paths that lead to better classification results receive more pheromone deposits, increasing the likelihood that subsequent ants will follow similar routes. Simultaneously, pheromone evaporation prevents convergence to local optima by gradually reducing the influence of earlier paths. This balance between exploration and exploitation is what enables the algorithm to wisely navigate large feature spaces, such as the 44-feature set in the WUSTL-EHMS-2020 dataset. ACO finally converges to a compact and high-performance subset of features by improving model accuracy while reducing computational complexity. Such an approach is especially useful in IoMT-based intrusion detection, where fast accurate decisions are crucial. The final selected feature subset is then used for training classification models, leading to more robust and interpretable results.

BISTACKED GRU

Cyber-attack detection for Internet of Medical Things (IoMT) devices using a bi-stacked Gated Recurrent Unit (GRU) model leverages the strengths of deep learning in sequential data analysis to enhance threat identification accuracy. Specifically, one such variation of RNNs is the GRU, which just so happens to be highly well-suited to handling time-series data, e.g., that describing network traffic patterns and biometric signals present in IoMT systems. A bi-stacked structure with two or more layers of GRU units stacked on top of one another will capture short-term as well as long-term dependencies in the data better. In the context of cyber-attack detection, the model is trained to differentiate between normal and malicious activity by analyzing sequential behaviors across multiple features, such as those present in the WUSTL-EHMS-2020 dataset. The bidirectional nature of the GRU enables it to read input sequences in both forward and backward directions, improving its ability to detect subtle anomalies that may be missed by unidirectional models. This deep representation learning approach helps in identifying complex attack patterns like spoofing or data injection, which often manifest over multiple time steps. The bi-stacked architecture further deepens the learning capacity, enhancing the model's ability to generalize from diverse and noisy IoMT environments. During training, the model utilizes labeled data to learn distinguishing features that differentiate attack from non-attack instances. This is optimized with techniques such as backpropagation through time and using Adam for parameters optimization. Once the bi-stacked GRU is trained, it can be utilized in real-time monitoring systems to continuously test incoming data streams for the presence of cyber threats. This method offers a robust, adaptive, and efficient solution for safeguarding sensitive health data and maintaining the integrity of IoMT networks.

EXPERIMENTAL RESULT

Experimentation results establish the efficacy of the suggested bi-stacked GRU model integrated with Ant Colony Optimization (ACO) in finding cyber-attacks within Internet of Medical Things (IoMT) devices. The model was tested on the WUSTL-EHMS-2020 dataset, which contains network traffic as well as biometric data. Accuracy, precision, recall, and F1-score measures were computed to evaluate the ability of the model in differentiating between normal and attack samples. The bi-stacked GRU's ability to capture temporal dependencies, coupled with ACO-based feature selection, significantly improved the detection rate of sophisticated attacks, particularly spoofing and data injection. Comparative analysis with traditional machine learning models further highlighted the superior performance of the proposed approach in terms of both detection accuracy and computational efficiency.

Table 1 presents the comparison of various machine learning models on accuracy, precision, recall, F1-score, training time, and testing time. The bi-stacked GRU performs better than all other models on accuracy (98.45%), precision (97.98%), recall (99.02%), and F1-score (98.50%). The performance of the SVM model is comparable but lags behind on accuracy and recall. Random Forest, Logistic Regression, and K-Nearest Neighbors are good but not as strong as the GRU. XGBoost is very accurate but its overall performance is less than bi-stacked GRU. The table also presents fluctuations in training and test time, with the GRU being relatively faster than other models such as CNN.

Table 1. Model Comparison (Accuracy)

Model	Accuracy (%)	Precision (%)	Recall (%)	F1-Score (%)	Training Time (s)	Testing Time (s)
Bi-Stacked GRU	98.45	97.98	99.02	98.50	150	30
Support Vector Machine (SVM)	94.12	92.56	93.89	93.22	50	15
Random Forest	95.67	94.80	96.15	95.47	80	20
Logistic Regression	91.34	89.12	92.56	90.80	25	10
K-Nearest Neighbors (KNN)	89.67	87.34	91.12	89.11	35	12
Decision Tree	92.23	90.50	93.11	91.79	40	13
Naive Bayes	88.56	85.70	89.02	87.35	30	11
XGBoost	96.78	95.40	97.56	96.46	100	25
LSTM	97.22	96.11	98.34	97.22	120	28
CNN	94.45	93.30	94.90	94.09	200	45

Table 2 illustrates the confusion matrix of the Bi-Stacked GRU model with true positives, false positives, true negatives, and false negatives marked. With 14,240 actual normal samples and 2,034 actual attack samples, model performance is shown with no false positives (32) and false negatives (12). The sum of 16,318 instances is categorically divided into the number of the correct and incorrect classified samples and shows that Bi-Stacked GRU model recognizes both normal patterns and attack patterns with high accuracy, which vindicates its success in recognizing cyber-attacks in IoMT devices.

Table 2. Confusion Matrix for Bi-Stacked GRU

Actual \ Predicted	Normal (0)	Attack (1)	Total
Normal (0)	14,240	32	14,272
Attack (1)	12	2,034	2,046
Total	14,252	2,066	16,318

Table 3 demonstrates precision, recall, and F1-score comparison of different models. Bi-Stacked GRU has the greatest 97.98% accuracy, 99.02% recall, and 98.50% F1-score and is therefore the best model in the detection of cyber-attacks in IoMT. Support Vector Machine and Random Forest are a close second with reasonable performance, particularly recall. Logistic Regression and K-Nearest Neighbors are behind, particularly recall, which is also most important when it comes to detecting instances of an attack. The table points to the strength of the Bi-Stacked GRU in precision vs. recall trade-off, important to keep false negatives and positives to a minimum while detecting attacks.

Table 3. Precision, Recall, and F1-Score for Each Model

Model	Precision (%)	Recall (%)	F1-Score (%)
Bi-Stacked GRU	97.98	99.02	98.50
Support Vector Machine (SVM)	92.56	93.89	93.22
Random Forest	94.80	96.15	95.47
Logistic Regression	89.12	92.56	90.80
K-Nearest Neighbors (KNN)	87.34	91.12	89.11
Decision Tree	90.50	93.11	91.79
Naive Bayes	85.70	89.02	87.35
XGBoost	95.40	97.56	96.46
LSTM	96.11	98.34	97.22
CNN	93.30	94.90	94.09

Table 4 shows the False Positive Rate (FPR) across various models. The lower FPR reflects the capability of a model to distinguish between normal cases and attacks. The Bi-Stacked GRU has the lowest FPR of 0.50%, reflecting its capacity to avoid false alarms. Naive Bayes is highest in FPR (6.00%), which may be not suitable to be deployed in actual scenarios. Support Vector Machine and Random Forest follow with quite low FPR and thus are also deployable in sensitive IoMT applications. The table depicts how crucial it is to keep false positives to minimum for actual deployment of cybersecurity.

Table 4. Attack Detection Comparison - False Positive Rate (FPR)

Model	FPR (%)
Bi-Stacked GRU	0.50
Support Vector Machine (SVM)	2.00
Random Forest	1.20
Logistic Regression	4.10
K-Nearest Neighbors (KNN)	5.40
Decision Tree	3.50
Naive Bayes	6.00
XGBoost	1.00

continued on following page

Table 4. Continued

Model	FPR (%)
LSTM	1.80
CNN	2.50

Table 5 presents the feature importance obtained through Ant Colony Optimization (ACO) utilized for feature selection. Biometric information and network flow metric are major feature contributors to the identification of an attack, and features such as Network Flow Metric 1 (15.70%) and Biometric Data 1 (13.30%) are the most prominent. Other features involving network flow and biometric data also contribute significantly towards performance. ACO-based feature selection is applied to the prioritization of the most important features, lowering the problem dimensionality and enhancing the precision of cyber-attack detection. This addresses the need for selecting the most important features to optimize model efficiency and accuracy.

Table 5. Feature Importance (ACO Feature Selection)

Feature	Importance (%)	Feature Type
Network Flow Metric 1	15.70	Network Flow Metric
Biometric Data 1	13.30	Biometric Data
Network Flow Metric 2	12.40	Network Flow Metric
Network Flow Metric 3	10.50	Network Flow Metric
Biometric Data 2	9.10	Biometric Data
Network Flow Metric 4	8.90	Network Flow Metric
Biometric Data 3	8.00	Biometric Data
Network Flow Metric 5	7.80	Network Flow Metric
Network Flow Metric 6	6.70	Network Flow Metric
Biometric Data 4	6.10	Biometric Data

Table 6 provides the comparative analysis of various models' test times, revealing the relative time efficiency of all models based on evaluation time. Bi-Stacked GRU performs remarkably at 30 seconds of testing time, whereas its effectiveness enables the model to leverage its real-time potential for offensive usage in IoMT systems. In comparison, CNN models are far slower (45 seconds), whereas conventional models such as SVM and Logistic Regression are much faster (15 and 10 seconds, respectively). With its longer testing time, the better performance of the Bi-Stacked GRU is sufficiently important to warrant its comparatively higher cost in terms of time, proving that it can strike a balance between efficiency and outstanding accuracy.

Table 6. Model Performance (Testing Time)

Model	Testing Time (s)
Bi-Stacked GRU	30
Support Vector Machine (SVM)	15
Random Forest	20
Logistic Regression	10
K-Nearest Neighbors (KNN)	12
Decision Tree	13
Naive Bayes	11
XGBoost	25
LSTM	28
CNN	45

Table 7 places the models side by side according to their AUC (Area Under Curve) values, one of the key measures for assessing model performance for classification problems. Bi-Stacked GRU has the highest AUC value of 0.99, showing almost perfect model performance in differentiating between attack and normal samples. SVM, Random Forest, and XGBoost have consistent performance with AUC scores ranging from 0.96–0.98. In contrast, Logistic Regression and Naive Bayes models give lower AUC scores, reflecting relatively poorer capability to differentiate between classes. This reflects the high classification capacity of Bi-Stacked GRU.

Table 7. ROC Curve Comparison

Model	AUC (Area Under Curve)
Bi-Stacked GRU	0.99
Support Vector Machine (SVM)	0.96
Random Forest	0.97
Logistic Regression	0.93
K-Nearest Neighbors (KNN)	0.92
Decision Tree	0.94
Naive Bayes	0.89
XGBoost	0.98
LSTM	0.98
CNN	0.95

Table 8 shows Training durations for all models. Bi-Stacked GRU is very precise but takes a very long training duration of 150 seconds, longer than models such as

SVM and Logistic Regression with training durations of around 50 and 25 seconds, respectively. The extra duration taken for the Bi-Stacked GRU's precision and recall performance is more than justifiable. Models such as CNN, though highly accurate, take significantly longer to train (200 seconds) and hence are not highly practical for real-time use. This table presents the trade-off between model complexity and training time.

Table 8. Model Performance (Training Time)

Model	Training Time (s)
Bi-Stacked GRU	150
Support Vector Machine (SVM)	50
Random Forest	80
Logistic Regression	25
K-Nearest Neighbors (KNN)	35
Decision Tree	40
Naive Bayes	30
XGBoost	100
LSTM	120
CNN	200

Table 9 presents the difference in the performance of models with and without feature selection using ACO. Through the utilization of feature selection via ACO, accuracy of the Bi-Stacked GRU model is increased to 98.45%, compared to 94.56% accuracy when feature selection is not applied. Precision, recall, and F1-score are also dramatically improved through the utilization of feature selection, pointing towards the contribution of ACO in improving the performance of the model. This is consistent with the importance of feature selection to minimize the detection rate, lower the dimensionality, and that the model works on the most impactful features to detect cyber-attacks for IoMT devices.

Table 9. Impact of Feature Selection on Model Performance

Feature Selection Method	Accuracy (%)	Precision (%)	Recall (%)	F1-Score (%)	AUC (Area Under Curve)
No Feature Selection	94.56	92.43	93.56	93.00	0.95
ACO-based Feature Selection	98.45	97.98	99.02	98.50	0.99

Table 10 presents the attack detection accuracy of different models in particular types of attacks, such as spoofing, data injection, and man-in-the-middle attacks. Bi-Stacked GRU performs optimally on all types of attacks, even better on spoofing (99.10%) and data injection (98.85%) attacks. Although other models such as SVM and XGBoost compete with good performances, Bi-Stacked GRU is generally better by absolute accuracy. The following table depicts the model's stability in identifying different types of attacks, which is key to IoMT device cyber security, where a combination of attacks occurs.

Table 10. Detection Accuracy for Different Attack Types

Attack Type	Bi-Stacked GRU (%)	SVM (%)	Random Forest (%)	XGBoost (%)	LSTM (%)	CNN (%)
Spoofing	99.10	95.20	96.70	97.40	98.30	96.00
Data Injection	98.85	94.50	95.80	96.90	97.20	95.50
Man-in-the-Middle	99.50	96.00	97.30	98.10	98.60	97.20
DoS	95.20	92.30	94.10	94.50	95.00	93.70
Probe	91.60	89.80	91.40	91.10	92.30	90.80

CONCLUSION

Application of a bi-stacked GRU model with attribute selection by ACO provides an efficient method for cyber-attack detection in IoMT systems. Application of temporal learning based on GRU makes the model more efficient to detect sophisticated patterns of attacks in sequential data. Experimental evaluation on the WUSTL-EHMS-2020 dataset confirms the efficiency and accuracy of the proposed method for spoofing as well as injection-based attack detection. Moreover, preprocessing and feature selection stages also envision a pivotal role of managing computational overhead, in addition to enhancing detection quality. The envisioned framework is expected to be implemented for real-time clinical applications with enhanced cybersecurity support for IoMT devices. Further research can further improve the approach to provide security against many more attacks, as well as provide commentary on adaptive learning methodologies under various threat scenarios.

REFERENCES

Argaw, S. T., Troncoso-Pastoriza, J. R., Lacey, D., Florin, M., Calcavecchia, F., Anderson, D., Burleson, W. P., Vogel, J., O'Leary, C., & Eshaya-Chauvin, B. (2020). Cybersecurity of Hospitals: Discussing the challenges and working towards mitigating the risks. *BMC Medical Informatics and Decision Making*, *20*, 146. PMID: 32620167

Astillo, P. V., Choudhary, G., Duguma, D. G., Kim, J., & You, I. (2021). TrMAps: Trust Management in Specification-Based Misbehavior Detection System for IMD-Enabled Artificial Pancreas System. *IEEE Journal of Biomedical and Health Informatics*, *25*, 3763–3775. PMID: 33651704

Buczak, A. L., & Guven, E. (2016). A Survey of Data Mining and Machine Learning Methods for Cyber Security Intrusion Detection. *IEEE Communications Surveys and Tutorials*, *18*, 1153–1176.

Center for Internet Security (CIS). (2017). *Cyber Attacks: In the Healthcare Sector; Center for Internet Security*. CIS.

Chen, T., & Guestrin, C. (2016). XGBoost: A Scalable Tree Boosting System. In *Proceedings of the KDD '16: 22nd ACM SIGKDD International Conference on Knowledge Discovery and Data Mining*. Association for Computing Machinery.

Chen, Y., Ding, J., Li, D., & Chen, Z. (2021). Joint BERT Model Based Cybersecurity Named Entity Recognition. *Proceedings of the ICSIM 2021: 2021 The 4th International Conference on Software Engineering and Information Management*, 236–242.

Ciampi, M., De Pietro, G., Masciari, E., & Silvestri, S. (2020). Some Lessons Learned Using Health Data Literature for Smart Information Retrieval. *Proceedings of the 35th Annual ACM Symposium on Applied Computing*, 931–934.

Coventry, L., & Branley, D. (2018). Cybersecurity in healthcare: A narrative review of trends, threats and ways forward. *Maturitas*, *113*, 48–52. PMID: 29903648

Di Sarno, C., Formicola, V., Sicuranza, M., & Paragliola, G. (2013). Addressing Security Issues of Electronic Health Record Systems through Enhanced SIEM Technology. *Proceedings of the 2013 International Conference on Availability, Reliability and Security*, 646–653.

Dixit, P., & Silakari, S. (2021). Deep Learning Algorithms for Cybersecurity Applications: A Technological and Status Review. *Computer Science Review*, *39*, 100317.

Gao, C., Zhang, X., & Liu, H. (2021). Data and knowledge-driven named entity recognition for cyber security. *Cybersecurity*, *4*, 9.

Ghaffarian, S. M., & Shahriari, H. R. (2017). Software Vulnerability Analysis and Discovery Using Machine-Learning and Data-Mining Techniques: A Survey. *ACM Computing Surveys*, *50*, 56.

Goud, N. (2017). *Malware and Ransomware Attack on Medical Devices*. Cybersecurity Insiders.

Gupta, K., Sharma, D. K., Datta Gupta, K., & Kumar, A. (2022). A Tree Classifier Based Network Intrusion Detection Model for Internet of Medical Things. *Computers & Electrical Engineering*, *102*, 108158.

Hady, A.A., Ghubaish, A., Salman, T., Unal, D., & Jain, R. (2020). Intrusion Detection System for Healthcare Systems Using Medical and Network Data: A Comparison Study. IEEE Access, 8, 106576–106584.

Halperin, D., Heydt-Benjamin, T. S., Ransford, B., Clark, S. S., Defend, B., Morgan, W., Fu, K., Kohno, T., & Maisel, W. H. (2008). Pacemakers and implantable cardiac defibrillators: Software radio attacks and zero-power defenses. *Proceedings of the 2008 IEEE Symposium on Security and Privacy*, 129–142.

Haque, N. I., Rahman, M. A., Shahriar, M. H., Khalil, A. A., & Uluagac, A. S. (2021). A Novel Framework for Threat Analysis of Machine Learning-based Smart Healthcare Systems. arXiv:2103.03472.

Islam, S., Abba, A., Ismail, U., Mouratidis, H., & Papastergiou, S. (2022). Vulnerability prediction for secure healthcare supply chain service delivery. *Integrated Computer-Aided Engineering*, *29*, 389–409.

Islam, S., Papastergiou, S., Kalogeraki, E. M., & Kioskli, K. (2022). Cyberattack Path Generation and Prioritisation for Securing Healthcare Systems. *Applied Sciences (Basel, Switzerland)*, *12*, 4443.

Islam, S., Papastergiou, S., & Mouratidis, H. (2021). A Dynamic Cyber Security Situational Awareness Framework for Healthcare ICT Infrastructures. In *Proceedings of the PCI 2021: 25th Pan-Hellenic Conference on Informatics*. ACM.

Kumar, P., Gupta, G. P., & Tripathi, R. (2021). An Ensemble Learning and Fog-Cloud Architecture-Driven Cyber-Attack Detection Framework for IoMT Networks. *Computer Communications*, *166*, 110–124.

Li, H., Ota, K., & Dong, M. (2018). Learning IoT in Edge: Deep Learning for the Internet of Things with Edge Computing. *IEEE Network*, *32*, 96–101.

Mavroeidis, V., & Bromander, S. (2017). Cyber Threat Intelligence Model: An Evaluation of Taxonomies, Sharing Standards, and Ontologies within Cyber Threat Intelligence. *Proceedings of the 2017 European Intelligence and Security Informatics Conference (EISIC)*, 91–98.

McKee, D., & Laulheret, P. (2021). *McAfee Enterprise ATR Uncovers Vulnerabilities in Globally Used B. Braun Infusion Pump*. Trellix.

Mendsaikhan, O., Hasegawa, H., Yamaguchi, Y., & Shimada, H. (2019). Identification of Cybersecurity Specific Content Using the Doc2Vec Language Model. *Proceedings of the 2019 IEEE 43rd Annual Computer Software and Applications Conference (COMPSAC)*, 1, 396–401.

Nandy, S., Adhikari, M., Khan, M. A., Menon, V. G., & Verma, S. (2022). An Intrusion Detection Mechanism for Secured IoMT Framework Based on Swarm-Neural Network. *IEEE Journal of Biomedical and Health Informatics, 26*, 1969–1976. PMID: 34357873

Newaz, A. I., Sikder, A. K., Babun, L., & Uluagac, A. S. (2020). HEKA: A Novel Intrusion Detection System for Attacks to Personal Medical Devices. *Proceedings of the 2020 IEEE Conference on Communications and Network Security (CNS)*, 1–9.

Nifakos, S., Chandramouli, K., Nikolaou, C. K., Papachristou, P., Koch, S., Panaousis, E., & Bonacina, S. (2021). Influence of Human Factors on Cyber Security within Healthcare Organisations: A Systematic Review. *Sensors (Basel), 21*, 5119. PMID: 34372354

Paleyes, A., Urma, R. G., & Lawrence, N. D. (2022). Challenges in Deploying Machine Learning: A Survey of Case Studies. *ACM Computing Surveys, 55*, 1–29.

Ponemon Institute. (2016). *Sixth Annual Benchmark Study on Privacy & Security of Healthcare Data; Technical Report*. Ponemon Institute.

R.M. (2020). An Effective Feature Engineering for DNN Using Hybrid PCA-GWO for Intrusion Detection in IoMT Architecture. *Computer Communications, 160*, 139–149.

Saba, T. (2020). Intrusion Detection in Smart City Hospitals Using Ensemble Classifiers. *Proceedings of the 2020 13th International Conference on Developments in eSystems Engineering (DeSE),* 418–422.

Satyapanich, T., Ferraro, F., & Finin, T. (2020). CASIE: Extracting Cybersecurity Event Information from Text. *Proceedings of the Thirty-Fourth AAAI Conference on Artificial Intelligence, AAAI 2020, the Thirty-Second Innovative Applications of Artificial Intelligence Conference, IAAI 2020*, 8749–8757.

Shevchenko, N. (2018). *Threat Modeling: 12 Available Methods*. Carnegie Mellon University.

Si-Ahmed, A., Al-Garadi, M. A., & Boustia, N. (2023). Survey of Machine Learning Based Intrusion Detection Methods for Internet of Medical Things. *Applied Soft Computing*, *140*, 110227.

Singh, P., Gaba, G. S., Kaur, A., Hedabou, M., & Gurtov, A. (2023). Dew-Cloud-Based Hierarchical Federated Learning for Intrusion Detection in IoMT. *IEEE Journal of Biomedical and Health Informatics*, *27*, 722–731. PMID: 35816521

Tang, L., & Mahmoud, Q. H. (2021). A Survey of Machine Learning-Based Solutions for Phishing Website Detection. *Mach. Learn. Knowl. Extr.*, *3*, 672–694.

Tikhomirov, M., Loukachevitch, N. V., Sirotina, A., & Dobrov, B. V. (2020). Using BERT and Augmentation in Named Entity Recognition for Cybersecurity Domain. *Proceedings of the Natural Language Processing and Information Systems—25th International Conference on Applications of Natural Language to Information Systems, NLDB*, *12089*, 16–24.

Wu, D., Guo, P., & Wang, P. (2020). Malware Detection based on Cascading XG-Boost and Cost Sensitive. *Proceedings of the 2020 International Conference on Computer Communication and Network Security (CCNS)*, 201–205.

Yeboah-Ofori, A., Mouratidis, H., Ismai, U., Islam, S., & Papastergiou, S. (2021). Cyber Supply Chain Threat Analysis and Prediction Using Machine Learning and Ontology. *Proceedings of the Artificial Intelligence Applications and Innovations—17th IFIP WG 12.5 International Conference, AIAI 2021*, *627*, 518–530.

Zong, S., Ritter, A., Mueller, G., & Wright, E. (2019). Analyzing the Perceived Severity of Cybersecurity Threats Reported on Social Media. In *Proceedings of the 2019 Conference of the North American Chapter of the Association for Computational Linguistics: Human Language Technologies*. Association for Computational Linguistics.

Chapter 7

A Review on Nanosensor-Based Body Fluids Monitoring for Next Generation Medical Devices and Robotics

Juhi Kangkana Baruah
https://orcid.org/0009-0008-3043-7170
Gauhati University, India

Lachit Dutta
Gauhati University, India

ABSTRACT

The sensing mechanisms have significant applications in healthcare. Integrating nanomaterials in sensing enhances the sensor and target molecule interaction helping analyte detection at minimal concentration which is crucial in early diagnosis and health monitoring. Owing to their special properties, the use of nanomaterials empowers excellent features in healthcare. In this chapter, the concept of nanobiosensors are introduced with background information on their use in wearable devices and disease identification by dint of detecting analytes from biofluids. Moreover, it presents a holistic overview of recent technologies like machine learning (ML), deep learning (DL), internet of things (IOT) and tiny machine learning (TinyML) to enhance personalized health care by remotely monitoring the patient's health status as well as making on-site informed decisions. The integration of nanosensors

DOI: 10.4018/979-8-3373-1514-0.ch007

with TinyML is set to revolutionize personalized healthcare offering a significant advancement in robotic healthcare systems through enhanced sensor-driven autonomy and adaptive intelligence.

INTRODUCTION

Nanobiosensor have developed immensely in recent years due to its unique properties like miniature size, flexibility, enhanced strength, better electrical and thermal conductivity and better optical property. The demand for innovation such as smaller and faster devices in electronics, improved batteries and cells for energy generations also drives the development of Nanobiosensors. In the field of biomedical diagnostics, it provides novel sensitivity and specificity for biomarker detection in various biofluids such as saliva, urine, sweat and blood (Kumar et al., 2023). These sensors optimizes the use of the unprecedented properties of nanomaterials to detect and identify biological molecules at exceptionally low concentrations. By identifying these biological molecules, early diagnosis of many diseases or continuous health monitoring with minimally invasive or non-invasive techniques have been achieved through. This ability of identification is critical for handling chronic diseases, detecting infections at earliest, and to personalized treatments based on real-time health data, enhancing the potential nanobiosensors as an effective technological tool for both clinical diagnostics and personalized health management.

However, in recent years Nanobiosensor research has been boosted with notable growth in material science, surface area, and detection techniques, such developments have expanded the functionality and application of these sensors, specifically in Biofluid analysis. Nanomaterials, including Gold Nanoparticles, Carbon Nanotubes, Nanowires, Graphene, Quantum dots, and other cutting-edge fabrication techniques, have elevated their sensitivity, stability and miniaturization potential facilitating new approaches to Biofluid analysis. Detection techniques, such as electrochemical, optical, and magnetic sensing, have also emerged, with particular advantages for different biofluid applications. The outcome of which comprises a growing array of Nanobiosensors capable of detecting specific disease target biomarkers, like proteins, nucleic acids, peptides and metabolites, with absolute high accuracy and flawless precision in real-time (Chaudhary et al., 2024). Hence, they are becoming more practically suitable for integration into the wearable devices in transforming real-time monitoring .Further, Nanobiosensors are now being integrated into portable and implantable devices as well, creating opportunities for continuous health monitoring outside traditional healthcare settings. These advancements proves that Nano biosensors have the potential to play a significant role in key areas of future medicine like diagnostics, surgical robotics etc.

The commercially workable biosensors are mostly limited to physical activity and monitoring, however, biosensor integration with electronics has been challenging (Memon et al., 2024). This basic challenge in most cases lies in the collection of body fluids, such as blood, serum, and interstitial fluids (ISF) that needs invasive approaches, which makes real-time analysis of biomarkers in these fluids difficult as well as risky of getting infected at the collection site. But collecting body fluids, such as sweat and saliva is comparatively more easier, even the process is noninvasive in nature, and mainly they contain several electrolytes and metabolites which are major biomarkers for many mental and physical health conditions and are also correlated with blood levels (Cordas et al.,2023). For an instance, sodium (Na), chloride (Cl), potassium (K), present in sweat can provide an insight to a person's hydration state, which further can be used to detect disorders related to electrolyte imbalance whereas, calcium ion (Ca2+) levels in sweat can provides the functioning of numerous organs and systems, including Myeloma, Cirrhosis, and Normocalcemic Hyperparathyroidism (Hossain et al., 2023). Hence, real-time monitoring of the pH and ionic content of sweat can be used to both detect various medical disorders in patients. Thus a number of biological fluids incorporating saliva, urine and blood consists of a diverse range of Biomolecules like proteins, lipids and nucleic acids which plays a major role in disease detection and therefore attracting more research interest. Silva et al. (2024) used saliva as a biofluid for detection of diabetes whereas Ebersole et al. (2024) have taken saliva to detect oral diseases. Saliva also been used as a crucial biofluid in research for detection of various diseases such as cirrhosis (Lima et al., 2023), cystic fibrosis (Kumari et al., 2023) and Tuberculosis (Liao et al., 2023). Apart from saliva, Urine is also been used by researchers for the detection of diseases like urinary tract infections (Bilsen et al,. 2023), micro Albuminuria (Kumari et al., 2024), Ovarian Cancer and Prostate Cancer (Jordaens et al., 2023). Blood being the primary transport system delivering hydrogen (H_2),oxygen (O_2),nutrients and electrolytes contains metabolites from all organs and hence a major focus of research in diagnosis of disease. In a study, (Guang et al., 2020) researchers have used human whole blood as a fluid to diagnose type 2 diabetes mellitus. Furthermore, blood have been used as a biofluid for Alzheimer's detection (Zhang et al., 2024), for Pancreatic Cancer (wiewiora et al., 2023) and for Peripheral Neuropathy (Rossor & Reilly, 2022).

The main objective of this work is summarised below:

- Providing a comprehensive review of existing studies on the different types of biofluids and evaluating the latest methods and techniques of biofluid sensing
- Investigate different nanomaterials used in biofluid sensing and evaluating these nanomaterial based sensors employed in wearables to improve future medical devices.

- Analysis of different parameters of an intelligent sensor system design, assessing the recent technologies for current and future medical devices along with the challenges and issues.

BIOFLUIDS

Biofluids are different types of liquids that are produced in human body, such as blood, urine, saliva etc as shown in figure 1. These are also termed as bodily fluid or body fluid. These are released from the body either through excretion like in case of urine, sweat or through secretion such as breast milk else can be collected through a needle such as blood (Apoorva et al., 2024). The biofluids are composed of different components and bioactive compounds that plays vital role in human body functioning (Lugonja et al., 2024). The components can mark the physical state of an individual's health as they served as key components to certain diseases. For instance sodium ($Na+$) is a component of biofluid-sweat, its low levels can determine that the body is dehydrated (Suarez-Ortegón et al., 2024). Since these components acts as a biomarker so different sensors have been employed in sensing different specific components relating to specific diseases as tabulated in Table 1. These biofluids provides several advantages for sensing applications due to their rich composition as they contain a vast array of biomarkers like Proteins, Hormones, Metabolites, Enzymes, Nucleic Acids, and Electrolytes (Wasilewski et al., 2024) that provides valuable insights into physiological and pathological states. These are widely available, simpler to collect and are of low cost.

Most of these biofluids such as saliva, sweat, urine or breath can be obtained without invasive method reducing the pain and risk of patients, offering them more comfort with an easy testing. Apart from ease in testing, these biofluids are also are easy to collect, store, and transport (Bi et al., 2023) Furthermore, Biofluid-based sensing blends well with modern technologies, biofluids such as breath or sweat, allows for continuous data acquisition, enabling real-time monitoring of health conditions. Some of the specific advantages of these biofluids are listed in figure 2.

Figure 1. Different types of Biofluid

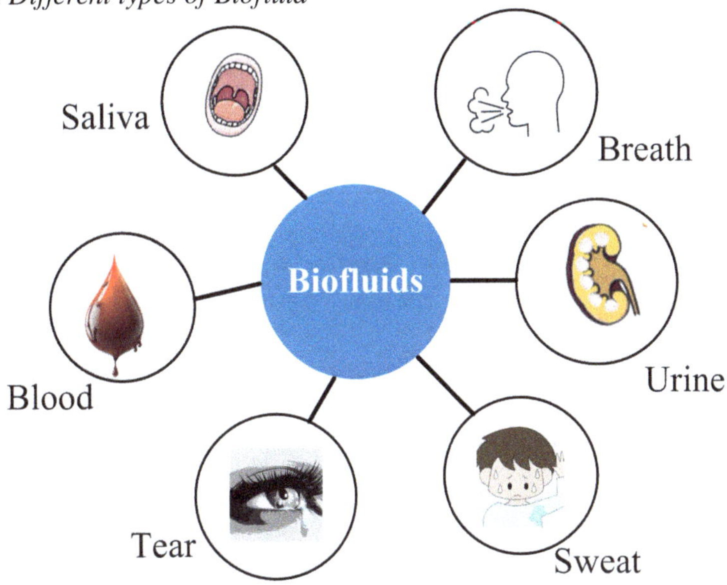

Figure 2. Different advantages of Biofluids

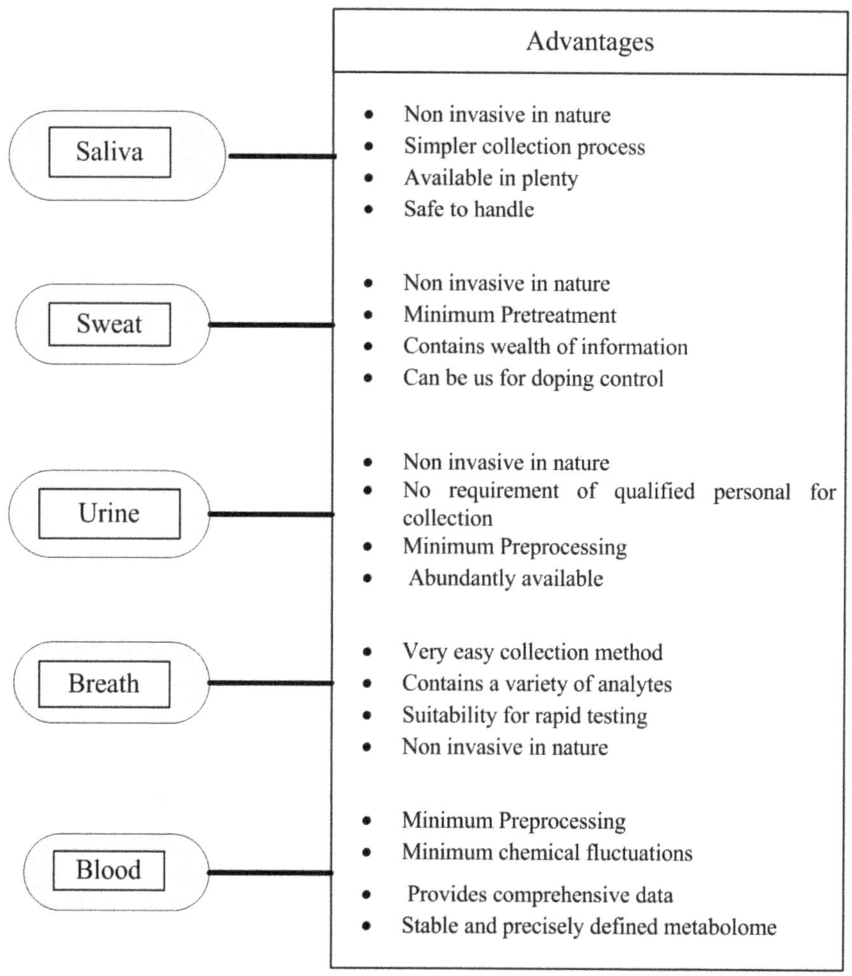

To conclude, biofluids play a vital role in advancements of sensing technologies by offering a wide range of rich biomarkers that enables real time monitoring. The detections and monitoring depends on both invasive and non-invasive techniques to extract, collect and monitor biomarkers from the biofluids. Invasive methods, provides detailed biomarker profiles however it causes discomfort and carries risks of infection, hence demands skilled professionals (Yadav et al., 2023). So these methods are generally used in clinical settings for critical diagnostics. On the contrary, non-invasive techniques are easy to use and further they reduces patient discomfort and therefore are gaining importance.

Table 1. Different Sensors for Various Disease Detection in Biofluid

Biofluid	Composition	Sensors for Detection	Diseases	Reference	Parameter metrics
Saliva	Glycoproteins, peptides, Urea	Au based nanosensors	Parkinson's diseases	(Mottaghi et al.,2023)	LOD~10NM
	Glucose, lipase, Electrolytes	CNT based nanosensors	Diabetes	(Acharya et al.,2024)	Range 900-1700nm
	Amylase	Si nanosensors	SARS Covid	(Ganesh et al.,2023)	LOD ~50 particles/mL
		HfO based Nanosensors	Periodontitis	(Hooshiar et al.,2024)	10-30 min assay times
		Graphene based sensors	Gastric cancer	(Zhao et al.,2023)	Accuracy-92.5% Sensitivity-97.1%
Sweat	OH^-, H^+, Na^+, Cl^-, lactic acid	CNT based sensors	Diabetes	(Promphet et al.,2024)	LOD: 0.1mM
	Uric acid, Fatty acid, Proteins	ZnO nanosensors	Diabetes	(Hossain et al.,2024)	LOD: 1μM
		Gold nanoparticle sensors	Hormone imbalance	(Rossi et al.,2024)	LOD: 0.8pM
		PEDOT:PSS	Hydration	(Polat et al., 2023)	Mean absolute error: ~36%
Urine	Urea, Uric acid, hippuric acid	Zn2+nanocomposite sensors	Chronic Kidney Disease	(Chhillar et al.,2023)	Accuracy: 90-110%
	Vitamin C,, Vitamin B complex,	CNT based sensor	Diabetes	(Wang et al.,2022)	Sensitivity: 700 $\mu A\ cm^{-2}$
	Electrolytes (Na^+, Cl^-, Ca, Mg)	Paper Nanosensor with AuNP	Diabetes	(Jin et al.,2024)	LOD: 4.2 Mm (fluorescent mode)
		ZnO nanosensors	Parkinson's Disease	(Beatto et al.,2023)	LOD: $86 nmolL^{-1}$

continued on following page

Table 1. Continued

Biofluid	Composition	Sensors for Detection	Diseases	Reference	Parameter metrics
Breath	Ammonia, Isoprene, Water Nitrite, limonene	SnO2 Nanosensor WO3 nanofiber sensor	Lung Cancer Halitosis	(Shanmugasundaram & Lee,2022) (Yu et al.,2024)	LOD: 2.82ppb ~ 52% signal change.
		Au NP – ZnO hybrid sensor	Periodontitis	(Bae et al.,2021)	4.99% sensitivity at 50 ppb of CH_3SH
		Au with CNT nanoarray sensor	Gastric Cancer	(Amal et al.,2015)	Significant discrimination, $p< 0.017$
		TiO2 based Nanosensor	Gastric disease	(Brinza et al.,2023)	Concentration tested ~100 ppm
Tear	Na^+, Cl^-, K^+, glucose, urea uric Acid,cortisol, lactate, ascorbic acid, Lactoferrin	Si nanowire based sensor Au Nanostructured based sensor	Dry eye disease Alzeimer's disease	(Ghosh et al.,2023) (Caceres et al.,2023)	LOD ; 0.1344 fg/mL LOD ~10pM
Blood	Proteins, Ca^+, K^+ (globulins, fibrinogen) RBC, (erythrocytes), platelet,Na^+, Bicarbonate, WBC	MSO2 nanosheet sensor Graphene Nanosensors	Malaria PCOS (Polycystic Ovarian Syndrome)	(Cruz et al.,2021) (Jahangiri-Manesh et al.,2022)	Detection limit in ppM Fast response time of 3.7 s
		Photonic crystal based nano sensor	Tuberculosis	(Ragavendran et al.,2024)	Quality factor~30,659
		Au Nanoparticles sensor	Diabetes	(Jahangiri-Manesh et al.,2022)	LOD: 66 ppm

INVASIVE AND NON-INVASIVE TECHNIQUES

Biofluid sensing involves both invasive and non-invasive techniques to extract and analyze biofluids in various fields including health and clinical assessment. Each technique provides specific benefits with certain drawbacks, based on the biofluid type, intended effect and application.

Invasive Techniques are the methods that involve penetration to the skin or body to collect biofluids, providing high accuracy with a detailed biomarker analysis. Various invasive methods for sensing mechanism are shown in Fig.3 where blood Sampling or Venipuncture is the mostly used method for detection of glucose levels for diabetes, lipid profiles for cholesterol or various other disease markers. Cerebrospinal Fluid (CSF) Collection is another invasive method where a lumbar puncture or sub-occipital puncture collects the fluid to diagnose Central nervous system (CNS) diseases (Czarniak et al., 2023). Interstitial Fluid (ISF) Extraction is also a type of invasive method where micro needles are used to obtain the fluid for continuous glucose monitoring (Yang et al., 2024). Furthermore, Tissue Biopsies are also used as invasive method where fluids are directly extracted from tissues for cancer (Hofman, 2024). While these techniques have an access to a range of rich and concentrated biomarkers making them suitable for clinical diagnostics, their main challenge lies in the risk of infection and the demand for skilled manpower.

Non Invasive Techniques are the methods that involves collecting biofluids for the detection of biomarkers without penetrating the skin or causing any form of discomfort. This is generally achieved by collecting biofluid samples from skin surface and examining them with the help of various detection methods. Various non invasive methods for sensing mechanism are also shown in figure 3 where Saliva Sampling method is preferred most as here the saliva can be self-collected and can be collected at any time unlike urine. Saliva Sampling is used to monitor hormones like Cortisol and to detect infectious diseases like Periodontitis (Kumari et al., 2023), further certain biomarkers in saliva can detect cancer in early stage (Paluszkiewicz et al., 2020). A non-enzymatic, low cost sensor has been introduced by (Zhang et al., 2024) for glucose detection using engineered biochar, offering a potential tool for noninvasive, point-of-care health monitoring where Nanosized nickel oxide was uniformly anchored onto the biochar matrix, to increase electroactive surface area and catalytic efficiency for glucose oxidation. The sensor Was tested with real aliva samples where it exhibited a high sensitivity of 243.6 $\mu A \cdot mM^{-1} \cdot cm^{-2}$, with a LOD of 0.5 μM, which is much below the typical glucose concentration in human saliva (~20–200 μM). Relative standard deviation (RSD) $< 3.5\%$ for repeated measurements and the sensor maintained more than 90% of initial current response after 15 days of storage at room temperature.

Sweat analysis is another non invasive method where sweat from the body is collected via sweat tests, biosensors or microfluidic sweat collectors, and is used to provide information about health insights. It is applicable in diagnosis of various diseases like Cystic fibrosis, diabetes, and skin diseases (Zhang et al., 2024).

Urine Testing is also a type of non invasive method where the urine sample is collected for kidney function, drug tests, and metabolic disorders. Various diseases like chronic kidney disorder (CKD), bladder cancer and diabetes can be detected by it (Tasnim et al., 2024), (De Jong et al., 2024) and (Shreef et al., 2023). The tear based analysis as a non invasive method is used to detect glucose, biomarkers related to Alzheimer's disease, breast cancer and various eye disorders (Zhang et al., 2023), (De Sande et al., 2023) and (Altman et al., 2023). Hirschsprung's disease (HSCR), a congenital condition characterized by absence of ganglion cells in parts of the colon, affecting about 1 in 5,000 newborns, whose non-invasive urinary miRNA biomarkers can be identified to aid HSCR diagnosis, potentially reducing reliance on invasive rectal biopsies. The authors in (Sreepada et al., 2025) carried the study by collecting urine from HSCR patients, isolated extracellular-vesicle-associated miRNAs, and profiled them using miRNA microarrays. The key dysregulated miRNAs were further validated by RTqPCR. Bioinformatic analysis (miRWalk, miRDB) linked these miRNAs to neurodevelopmental genes important in HSCR. The Urine samples showed significant dysregulation in a set of miRNAs—like miR-4732-5p, miR-3187-5p, miR-2105p, among others. These miRNAs correlated with genes involved in neuronal migration and enteric nervous system development. HSCR patients possess a distinctive miRNA signature in urine, offering a potential non-invasive, affordable complement to current diagnostic protocols. Further, authors propose future use of portable lab-on-a-chip or nanophotonic biosensors to detect these miRNAs clinically.

Furthermore, Exhaled Breath Analysis is also used as non invasive method where volatile organic compounds (VOCs) are detected to diagnose various diseases like lung cancer, gastric cancer, Crohn's disease, colorectal cancer, chronic kidney disease (CKD), prostate cancer, acute lymphoblastic leukemia and Helicobacter pylori infection (Lee et al., 2024) and (Hu et al., 2023).

These techniques provides benefits of being Comfortable, with minimal risk of infection and higher patient compliance while major challenge is the minimal amount of biomarker concentration along with susceptibility to environmental contamination that limits the accuracy.

Figure 3. Different types of Invasive and Non Invasive methods

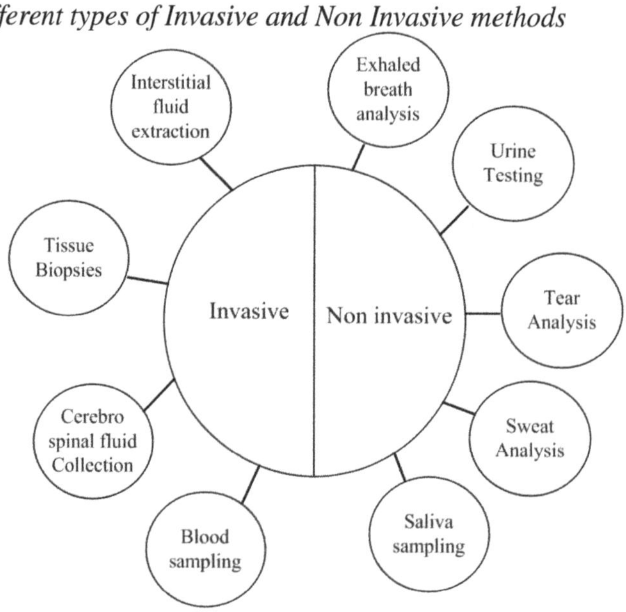

Table 2. SWOT Table analysis for Invasive and Non- Invasive technique

Strength		Weakness	
Invasive	**Non invasive**	**Invasive**	**Non invasive**
Enhanced Sensitivity and precision	Comfortability and compatibility with patient	Discomfortable to Patient due to anxiety and pain	Limited Biomarker Availability
Quick Diagnosis and less time consuming	Minimal complication and infection risk	Carries risks of infections	Environmental Factors can impact the accuracy
Provides Minute and Detailed Information	Involvement of simpler equipment.	Requires specialized equipments, and trained personnel, increasing the cost	May have lower Sensitivity and Accuracy as some biomarkers are less detectable in biofluids.
Direct Access to Biofluids.	Frequent and Continuous Monitoring	Sensors used are majorly single-use, so reusability is limited.	data interpretation can get influenced by various external factors
Opportunities		**Threat**	
Invasive	**Non invasive**	**Invasive**	**Non invasive**
Through Technological Advancements efficiency can be improved.	Can find Innovative solutions to improve sensitivity and specificity	Aversion of patient to diagnostic test may limit uptake of Biofluids.	Accuracy constraints as compared to Invasive Methods may limit the use
Can facilitate personalized treatment according to needs of patient.	Enhancement for advance monitoring solutions for health in real time	Rigid regulations for patient safety can limit the use invasive Biofluid sensing	Data of personal health metrics may raise concerns about data privacy and security,
Can achieve preventive Healthcare by reducing costs.	Preventive and Personalized Healthcare improving long-term patient outcomes.	Competition with rapidly advancing Non-Invasive Technologies may decrease demand. .	Competition in market from other technologies like advanced imaging methods can be a threat.
Can enhance diagnostic accuracy by Integrating with AI and Data Analytics	Integration with Digital Health Platforms for better tracking and personalized insights.	Risk of Misinterpretation	Regulatory approval and validation can be a challenge due to rigorous accuracy

Both of the techniques have distinct benefits, drawbacks and challenges in biofluid sensing. The preference to choose one over the other depends on the desired outcomes, accuracy and various other medical factors. Comparing both the techniques a SWOT analysis have been presented in Table 2.

NANOMATERIALS IN BIOFLUID SENSING

The incorporation of nanomaterials in biofluid sensing originated due to some unique properties possess by these nano sized materials that were successful to target the major drawbacks in biomarker detection in complex biofluids such as blood, urine, saliva, tear and sweat.

The early biosensors were based on enzymes (Arkhypova et al.,2023), these sensor systems used to encountered many constraints such as low sensitivity, low selectivity, limited lifespan and interference from complex biofluids. With the introduction of nanomaterials, came metal nanoparticles,, carbon nanotubes (CNT), graphene, nanorods, quantum dots and nanosheets which enhanced the interaction with biomolecules and bringing out the best result in diagnostics (Paramasivam et al., 2023). Nanomaterials have proven to be capable enough to hold a key position in various biomedical applications and hence in recent years they have gain much attention in scientific research and commercial purpose as well.

Emergence in Biofluid Sensing

Nanomaterials play a significant role in sensing technology because of their unique physical, chemical, electrical, thermal and optical properties. Their high surface to volume ratio, quantum effects, biocompatibility, optical and tunable properties make them suitable in detecting and analyzing chemical, biological, and electrical signals with excellent sensitivity and selectivity.

Scientists started exploring nanomaterials because of their capability of overcoming the challenges in traditional biofluid sensing, such as such as low sensitivity, low selectivity, low analyte concentration, interference from complex biofluid and the need for miniaturization. The main reasons for employing nanomaterials in biofluid sensing includes:

- Nanomaterials have a high surface to volume ratio yielding to their effective biomarker interaction enabling detection of minute concentration of substances, increasing sensitivity.
- The customization of nanomaterials allows selective binding for interactions with specific target biomarkers that enhances specificity in biofluids.
- Due to high reactivity and miniature size, nanomaterials are able to generate signals immediately and Metallic nanoparticles and quantum dots amplifies the generated electrochemical signals, improving detection efficiency.
- The nanoscale size of Nanomaterials facilitate the development of compact, portable sensors and wearable sensors that perfectly blends real-time monitoring systems with point-of-care settings.

Various nanomaterials such as Carbon-Based Nanomaterials, polymer nanomaterials, Metallic Nanoparticles, Quantum Dots and Metal Oxides have been incorporated in biofluid sensing. Carbon-Based Nanomaterials such as Graphene and Graphene Oxide are used to detect glucose, and proteins in biofluids (Das et al., 2023), (Zeng et al.,2024) due to high conductivity and biocompatibility. Researchers have also used Carbon Nanotubes (CNTs) in various forms like printable or combined with composites in electrochemical sensors in works (Tian et al., 2023), (Wali et al., 2024), (Ansari et al., 2024) and (Marchianò et al., 2024) for sweat and saliva analysis. Metallic Nanoparticles such as Gold Nanoparticles (AuNPs) are widely used in detection of glucose, antigens and cortisols in blood (Benedetti et al., 2024), (Kiio et al., 2023) and (Mani & Anirudhan, 2024). Also in detection of proteins like creatinine, uric acid and glutathione in urine, AuNPs have been used as reported in works (Chhillar et al., 2024), (Bayoumy et al., 2024) and (Qi et al., 2024). A paper based plasmonic nanosensor was designed in (Liu et al., 2025) for multiple metabolite detection, using a Fe^{2+} -catalyzed system (FeHOAuC) that prevents gold nanoparticle (AuNP) aggregation by oxidizing cysteine in the presence of H_2O_2. Pre-loaded oxidase enzymes convert each target analyte into H_2O_2, triggering AuNP color changes that are quantifiable via a smartphone camera using color algorithms. The sensor achieve a detection limit of ~5 μM for glucose, ~6 μM for cholesterol,~7 μM for uric acid,, ~10 μM for lactic acid within 40 minutes detection time. The recovery rates in serum ranged from 95.3% to 107.2%, indicating high accuracy and reliability.

Apart from Gold nanoparticles, Silver Nanoparticles have also been incorporated in sensing such as in surface-enhanced Raman spectroscopy (SERS), for detecting biofluid components (Al-Sammarraie et al., 2024) and for detecting antigens in human biofluids (Bahari et al., 2024). Some other nanomaterilas such as Quantum Dots (QDs) have also been explored in sensing of biomarkers in saliva and cerebrospinal fluid. In work by (Saedi et al., 2024) three carbon QD have been used in detection of A- synuclein in saliva. Cds QDs have also been used by researchers to detect Protein in saliva (Dong et al., 2022). Further metal oxide Nanostructures like ZnO are used for detection of glucose, lactate and pH in sweat (Hossain et al., 2024), (Shan & Zhang, 2024) and (Ghafouri & Manavizadeh, 2023), however detection of glucose in sweat is also done by incorporating other nanostructures such as TiO2 (Garcia Rey et al., 2023). Similarly there are numerous nanomaterials that are being employed as sensing element to target a specific biomarker in different biofluids. Nanomaterials have revolutionized biofluid sensing, offering unprecedented sensitivity, selectivity, and practicality. The nanomaterials used for biofluid sensing are listed in Table.3.

Table 3. Various Nanomaterials Employed in Biofluid Sensing

Sensing material	Biofluid	Target	Reference	Parameter metrics
AuNP	Breath	CH2SH (methanethiol)	(Bae et al., 2021)	Sensitivity ~ 4.99%
AuNP	urine	Uric acid	(Bayoumy et al., 2024)	LOD: 15.7 μM
AuNP	urine	Createnine	(Chhillar et al., 2024)	LOD: 0.02 μg/mL
AuNP	Breath	Glucose	(Jahangiri-Manesh et al., 2022)	LOD: 66 ppm
PtNP	Breath	H2S	(Yu et al., 2024)	Sensor response ~ 52% signal change.
TiO_2	Breath	NH3	(Brinza et al., 2023)	Concentration tested~100ppm
TiO_2	Sweat	glucose	(Garcia-Rey et al.,2023)	LOD: 7.7 μM
AgNP	CSF (cerebrospinal fluid)	CEA (Carcinoembryonic antigen) protein	(Bahari et al., 2024)	Limit of quantification: 1μg/mL
ZnO	Sweat	Glucose	(Hossain et al., 2024)	Sensitivity: 29.97μA per decade per cm^2
ZnO	Sweat	lactate	(Shan & Zhang,2024)	LOD: 2.3 μM
ZnO	Sweat	pH	(Ghafouri & Manavizadeh, 2023)	Detection range: pH 4-9
GOx	blood	glucose	(Das et al., 2023)	LOD: ~ 7.2mg/dL
GOx	Sweat	glucose	(Moulahoum et al.,2023)	LOD: 3-60 μM
GOx	Saliva	RNA	(Pitikultham et al.,2023)	LOD- miRNA-21: 3.85 fM

These Nanomaterial-Based Biofluid Sensors find application in various fields such as Healthcare, drug monitoring, Sports fitness and Point-of-Care Testing. However these nanomaterial have still not been utilized to their full potential, integrating with wearable devices, robotics and Internet of Things (IoT) for continuous monitoring is paving new ways for technical innovations and will act as a cornerstone for various emerging technologies, such as in case of robotic surgery, these nanomaterial will prove highly effective as nanomaterials can interact with tissues, cells, and individual molecules allowing ultra-precise targeting, making robotic surgeries more minimally invasive. Also,nanomaterials such as gold nanoparticles can act as contrast agents to enhance real-time imaging (MRI, CT, fluorescence). Coating robotic instruments with biocompatible nanomaterials such as graphene, carbon nanotubes improves durability reducing infection risk and extending lifespan of tools. Nanoscale actuators and haptic sensors improve robot sensitivity and movement control, mimicking the tactile feel of a surgeon's hand with greater accuracy (Abaszadeh et al., 2023), (Weerarathna et al., 2025).These factors made nanomaterials a transformative tool for next-generation minimally invasive surgical (MIS) techniques. Further, Developing multiplexed sensors using nanomaterials for simultaneous detection of multiple biomarkers integrating with AI to interpret sensor outputs in real-time can be a future prospect.

The major advantage of incorporating nanomaterials is its low cost. Its cost effectiveness makes it an attractive option to the widespread use in healthcare devices and systems. As nanoscale manufacturing processes are technologically advancing with more cost-effective techniques, such as nanostructured printing (Maafa, 2025) and automated fabrication (Sharmile et al., 2025), these are aiding in mass-scale nanosensor production at reduced costs increasing scalability.

The nanomaterial based device should have to be approved by medical regulatory bodies such as ICMR,CDSCO for ethical concern. As nanosensors interact directly with the human body so, the necessary tests and approvals must be performed to avoid any unknown risks and threats . Developing these regulatory frameworks and international standards in cooperation with stakeholders, health and government institutions can contribute to a general acceptance of this technology with a reduce patient's concern and thereby building nanomterial based intelligent robotic surgeries.

SENSORS IN WEARABLES

Biofluid sensing integrated with nanotechnology have extended to the field of wearables. These sensing mechanism in wearables analyzes bodily fluids such as sweat, saliva, tears and interstitial fluid (ISF) to monitor various biomarkers. These sensors are integrated into devices such as smartwatches, fitness trackers, smart glasses and wearables. Wearable devices utilizes these sensors to not only monitor health and fitness related data but also to track them. In recent years this field has gained momentum for non-invasive, continuous, and real-time health monitoring. Wearables provided with biofluid sensors are used in various applications like hydration monitoring, glucose tracking, stress tracking and electrolyte balance.

Sweat Sensors in Wearable

Sweat is one of the most commonly analyzed biofluid to detect and monitor biomarkers, sweat sensors analyses sweat and provides valuable health insights. Various sweat sensors like Electrochemical Sensors that Detect biomarkers like glucose, lactate, electrolyte. pH Sensors that indicate dehydration, Cortisol Sensor that Monitors stress levels have been employed in wearables. Abott freestyle libre is one of the finest example where sweat based monitoring is done for diabetes management (Yuan et al., 2023) Some of the other commercially used wearables are hexoskin smart skin, which is basically a shirt containing sensors to monitor sweat (Sakhare et al., 2023), Biolinq sweat sensor which is a disposable glucose monitoring patch (Mitsubayashi,2024,p.9) and Gatorade sweat patch (Patel et al., 2024) that measures electrolyte loss. Leveraging advancements in nanomaterials and biosensing, sweat sensors in wearables can revolutionize disease management. In a research work by (Garg et al., 2024) they have reported an imprinted wearable sensor for sweat biomarker analysis. Further in an another study (Ye et al., 2024) patterned gold Nanoparticle wearable sweat sensor have been suggested for hydration tracking. Wearable sweat sensors could also be used to monitor patients with heart failure providing an automated patient management (Brasier et al., 2024). An enzyme-free wearable sweat sensor was design by (Pei et al.,2025) using a copper-based MOF composite rather than enzyme-dependent catalysts. The sensor is designed for integration into flexible, skin-compatible patches, enabling continuous, real-time tracking of sweat lactate. As lactate is a key marker for muscle exertion and metabolic stress—this device could aid clinical monitoring of metabolic disorders. The sensor showed a linear Sensitivity of 118.55 mV per decade (logarithmic response) within the 1–10 mM lactate range The LOD is 1.09 μM which is exceptionally low, enabling early detection. Also the enzyme-free design enhances device durability and shelf-life. A non-invasive fingertip sweat biosensor for early kidney disease detection have been introduced in (Promphet et al., 2025), this introduces a cutting-edge, non-invasive wearable sensor that analyzes creatinine in fingertip sweat—allowing early detection of chronic kidney disease (CKD).The device is a sweat-based biosensor built on electrochemical principles. The wearable fingertip sensor quantifies creatinine levels in sweat, correlating strongly with blood serum creatinine. This sensor posses sensitivity of 0.133 $\mu A\ ng^{-1}\ mL^{-1}$ with LOD of 0.2 $ng\ mL^{-1}$ with a response time of 3 minutes. The sensor was able to retain $\geq$ 86% of initial sensor response after 4 months of storage. Clinical validation on real blood samples showed comparable results to the established Jaffe method

Saliva Sensors in Wearable for Next Generation Devices

Saliva, being the abundantly available biofluid, saliva sensors in wearables are the growing area of research offering a non invasive method to monitor health. Smart mouthguard (Matsumoto et al., 2023) is another tool that measure glucose fluctuations in body due to eating, sleeping etc. thereby helping in diabetes management. Wearable saliva analyzer detects glucose for personalized healthcare. Another research work where Stress biomarkers detection by saliva sensor is reported in (Pandit et al., 2024). Some other biosensing technologies in form of smart dentures and braces holds potential in providing personalized health management in future.

Interstitial Fluid (ISF) Sensing for Advanced Systems

ISF is the fluid surrounding cells and tissues, that can provide a rich source of biomarkers. ISF sensors in wearables are the cutting edge devices that are customized to monitor biomarkers in fluid that surrounds cells and tissues. ISF acts as a substitute for blood in wearable monitoring as concentrations of certain molecules may precede blood-level changes, making it ideal for early detection. The use of aptamer-based, enzymatic, or electrochemical nanosensors enables accurate ISF analysis in real time. Some of the microneedle systems are reviewed in (Xu et al., 2025) such as Balloon-anchored MN patch that Inflates to anchor MNs in wet internal tissues for drug delivery. Snake-inspired flexible MN that is designed to adapt to curved tissue surfaces like spinal cord or heart. MXene-integrated MNs that are Antibacterial and electroactive for wound monitoring. Aptamer-integrated MNs that detect inflammatory cytokines.In conclusion MN-based glucose sensors show limits of detection (LOD) around 40 μM, with sensitivities reaching 8 μA/mM and stable performance over 14 days, the aptameter based sensor deliver high specificity and reversible binding, offering real-time electrochemical detection in ISF.. These sensors are used for lactate monitoring, drug monitoring, hydration monitoring and hormone monitoring etc. Abbott frestyle libre is a widely used continuous glucose monitoring (CGM) device for measuring glucose level, worn on skin (Afeef et al., 2023), Eversense CGM (Almurashi et al., 2023) is also a long term implantable sensor that measures glucose in ISF. An ISF glucose sensor have been in builted in smartwatch PKvitality k'track (Mansuri et al., 2024). Various other ISF based wearable biosensors for healthcare have been investigated that can monitor electrolytes and metabolites (Wu et al., 2024)

Tear Sensing for Advance Medical Design

Tears are a valuable biofluid containing glucose, hormones, electrolytes, protein and other molecules that are helpful in providing body insights and for monitoring ocular health. Tear sensors in wearables is an emerging technology that analyses biomarkers in tears via non invasive way. Smart contact lens (Shetty et al., 2024) were nanosensors embedded contact lens use to measure glucose level. Another smart contact lenses Sensimed Triggerfish (Gaboriau et al., 2023) have been introduced to measure Intraocular Pressure (IOP) in glaucoma .A Wearable, biocompatible, ocular multisensor patch to monitor antibiotics in tears have been reported in (Yin et al., 2024). Metabolites are also detected as biomarkers in tear for sensing glucose and lactate. In a work (Ruan et al., 2017), authors have developed a novel contact lens with a hydro gel matrix attached for glucose sensing. Further, highly sensitive tear based smart eye wears are under research.

These biofluid based sensors blended with wearable, paved the way for advancement in various fields like disease diagnosis and monitoring, sports and fitness, mental Health, drug monitoring with overall health management.

ARTIFICIAL INTELLIGENCE IN SENSOR SYSTEM DESIGN

Intelligent sensor system have been designed with biofluid sensing that involves integrating cutting-edge approaches such as Machine Learning (ML) and Deep Learning (DL) with intelligent algorithms to analyze complex biofluid data for revolutionizing healthcare diagnostics and monitoring.

These intelligent systems incorporates advanced biosensors that are capable of detecting chemical, biological, and physical properties in biofluids such as- saliva, sweat, urine and blood with advanced computational models for precise data interpretation. The advanced integration with ML and DL based algorithms facilitates the system to process large amount of raw data from the sensor, extract patterns, and predict health conditions with optimum precision and reliability.

The raw data from the sensor is obtained in the form of electrical signals which are then processed and pre-processed to obtain the final outcome. The data collected through non invasive sensors can be evaluated using AI for development of next generations intelligent sensors. The Signal processing in an intelligent sensor system demands a sequence of steps shown in figure 4 in converting the raw data from the sensor to insightful information for analysis and precise decision-making. It assures data accuracy, data precision, reliability, and data usability for further computations.

The signal processing initiates with Signal Acquisition where the sensors detect any chemical, biological or physical stimuli such as bioanalytes and generates raw electrical signals in form of voltage, current, or resistance (Liu et al., 2022). For systems having multiple sensors, a multiplexer (MUX) is used to collect signals from various passages directing them to a single processor (Kumari et al., 2023). After the generation of signals, they are properly modified through the amplification of weak signals to match the input range of the ADC (Hu et al., 2024) filtration of signal from noise and unwanted frequencies using Low-pass filters, High-pass filters and Band-pass filters along with proper impedance matching to prevent any signal loss (Wu et al., 2023), (Setiadi et al., 2024). Once the required modifications are made, the signals are made digitized by passing through an ADC which gives output in discrete values representing the signal at timely intervals. From these digitized output for making analysis preprocessing is the vital step which is done by baseline Correction, Normalization or smoothing or data compression (Xu et al., 2024). The key features from the signal are then extracted which are relevant for analysis such as mean, variance or peak. Methods like Principal Component Analysis (PCA) or Recursive Feature Elimination (RFE) are used to select the most significant features. ML classification or regression models such as Support Vector Machines (SVM), Random Forests were trained to interpret biofluid signals and are validated using cross-validation techniques to ensure reliability. Now using deep learning (DL) or machine learning (ML) models signals are classified and patterns are detected such as Identifying health conditions based on biomarkers like glucose levels, electrolyte levels or pH levels and making predictive analysis from continous data (Rahman et al., 2023). Then the processed signal is used to generate actions by sending data to a cloud system for advanced analytics and providing information, alert or recommendations to end users through mobile apps or wearable interface for unusual readings. These systems also enables feedback mechanism to adjust the sensor parameters or signal processing algorithms to improvise performance over time.

Figure 4. Signal Processing in Intelligent Sensor Systems

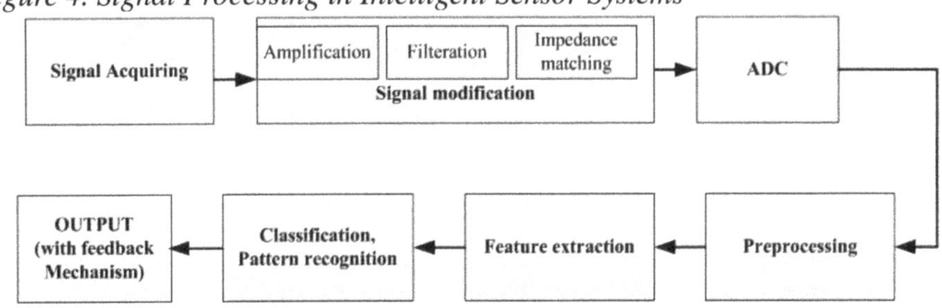

There are some advanced aspects of Signal Processing in Intelligent Sensor Systems specifically when integrating machine learning (ML) and deep learning (DL) such as Adaptive Filtering where Recursive Least Squares (RLS) or Least Mean Squares (LMS) algorithms can act as a tool for adjusting to changing noise patterns in real-time. In biofluid sensing, it helps to remove interference such as removing noise from electrical activity from the heart in sweat analysis (Prabakaran & Rufus, 2021). Machine Learning-Driven Preprocessing where algorithms like Isolation Forest identify and remove outliers in the raw sensor data prior to feature extraction (Vrazhnov et al., 2021) and Random Forest is helpful to reduce size by prioritizing most significant features retaining critical information. Further, techniques like Principal Component Analysis (PCA) helps in Signal Compression by compressing data for transmission without any information loss. Using Deep Learning models such as Convolution Neural Networks (CNNs), Recurrent Neural Networks (RNNs) (Mudireddy et al., 2024) temporal dependencies can be analyzed like trends in glucose levels over time. Lightweight ML models, such as TensorFlow Lite, are deployed on microcontrollers for Real-Time Processing.

By merging state-of-the-art biosensors with ML and DL algorithms, various intelligent sensor systems can be designed that further incorporates biofluid sensing to provide real-time, and personalized health monitoring solutions. Also, these cloud based sensing system brings powerful changes as offloading heavy tasks—like sensor data processing, environment mapping, or haptic signal interpretation—to cloud servers allows surgical robots to be lighter, faster, and more accurate. Further, the cloud integration decouples sensors, compute, and instruments. New sensing modalities (pressure strips, optical fibers, tactile e-skins) can be added seamlessly. As data is processed centrally, it enables robotic platforms can evolve without hardware overload(Rosa et al., 2022), (Gao et al.,2018).

ML models play significant role in classification and pattern recognition for enhance sensing result. In work (Patel et al., 2023) a graphene based H shaped biosensor is described for detection of urine molecules where ML based regression models are employed to predict the biosensor behavior with a very high sensitivity. The authors in (Ballard et al., 2020) have demonstrated DL assisted economical paper-based vertical flow assay for C-reactive protein detection where they have utilized ML-based model to measure an optimal configuration of immunoreactions spots to recognize the target biomolecule concentration. An intelligent paper-based colorimetric sensor have been prepared in (Tania et al., 2019) which is capable of performing a test automatically with 86% above precision rate. Here global thresholding, channel separation, and objection recognition have been used. Authors in (Kim et al., 2016) have proposed Smartphone based colorimetric detection of alcohol concentrations in saliva. ML algorithms LDA, SVM, and ANN are used for analyzing the color generated on a test strip with different alcohol concentrations, taken by Smartphone's Camera. In (Koh et al., 2016) a flexible microfluidic device is proposed to monitor sweat at exercise timing. It sticks with skin and was connected with a Smartphone to obtain and monitor the images for detection of glucose, lactate and chloride ion in sweat during exercise.

ML models can be utilized to assist in diagnosis, authors in (Jeon et al., 2017) proposed an ML model to predict the Unified Parkinson's Disease Rating Scale using a wearable sensing device where, a wrist-watch-type wearable gadget containing a gyroscope and accelerometer was used to gather the tremor signals of 85 Parkinson's disease patients. Using the informative features, a k-nearest-neighbor (kNN), support vector machine (SVM) and random forest (RF) model was utilized for computerized to determine disease severity in scores. More of some advancements in recent trends have been highlighted in work (Kadian et al., 2023).

With the merger of advanced signal processing with ML DL algorithms, intelligent sensor systems can further achieve extraordinary accuracy, and real-time analytics, making them indispensable in personalized healthcare solutions. However certain challenges are need to be overcome like data privacy, Limited training data for DL models and Real-time processing constraints in wearable devices (Krishnamoorthy & Sistla, 2023). Data privacy challenges should be addressed together by service providers, data handlers, and users through safe data sharing platform usage and rigid privacy policies. In case of DL models synthetic datasets can be use to expand the limited training data samples. Development of a safely assured patient friendly Intelligent sensor system can help patients and can transform the entire health management system. These systems finds applications in a diverse range of fields from chronic disease management to fitness tracking, revolutionizing how biofluid data is exploited for healthcare and diagnostics. However these system would rely extensively on the internet connection which can emerge as a critical issue for smooth and continuous operations of these systems in diverse geographical areas such as remote places with poor internet. It will also get compromised with the cost effectiveness as continuous need of internet services is a concern.

The intelligent system designing as requires AI for further enhancement, the associated ethical concerns are also a critical issue as inconvenience or absent regulation allows dual use and misuse of the tools. As AI system rely on large scale personal data which raises concern about privacy violation. Responsible AI should matter fo privacy, security and accountability of data. The stakeholders and government should come up together to form a definitive framework for building nanomaterial based Intelligent robotic system.

RECENT TECHNOLOGIES FOR NEXT GENERATION MEDICAL DEVICES AND ROBOTICS

IoT Integration Scope: Present and Future

In recent years with advancements in technological trends, nanomaterial aided sensors for biofluid sensing or nanobiosensors have been expanding to various domains. Now these nanobiosensors have been directed by researchers towards Internet of things (IOT) for biofluid analysis. The integration of IOT with nanobiosensors is an emerging field in disease diagnostics, healthcare and personalized medicine.

IOT plays a key role in enabling nanobiosensors to connect to digital scenario permitting remote data collection, processing and practical insights which in turn improves efficiency. The combination provides several benefits as remote monitoring and real time data analysis.

In a work (Mondal et al., 2024) authors have introduced a triboelectric nanosensor for real time urine analysis with precision of 95% where IOT can rapidly detect minute changes in concentration and character of urine components . An Aptameter based nanobiosensor is integrated in wearable sweat sensor connected to a Smartphone to track Oestradiol a female hormone, non invasively. This aims to provide sustainable solutions to female reproductive healthcare needs (Arduini, 2024). In another work (Kumar et al., 2023) the development of Smartphone based sensor for bull serum albumin (BSA) was studied. Authors in a work (Sun et al., 2024) have introduced feline biofluids IoT hub. They have used biofluids from pets and made connection to an IOT system via wifi network providing data visuals by mobile app. The goal is to monitor various illness by detecting analytes such as sodium, glucose in urine. In a work, (Hossain et al., 2023) authors have designed a non invasive sweat sensor to monitor potassium, calcium and pH levels in sweat with IOT connection. The role of iot in breath based nanosensor systems for disease diagnosis, as discussed in the paper (Taha et al., 2025), is crucial for transforming isolated sensing technologies into powerful, scalable healthcare tools as it allows continuous monitoring and wireless transmission of sensor data that can be uploaded in real time to cloud platforms or hospital servers for remote access. IoT networks enable scaling up breath diagnostics for public health by detecting early outbreaks like viral infections, monitoring air quality–health interactions and collecting epidemiological data across diverse populations.

There is a room for furthermore usage and exploration of IOT integration for biofluid sensing with faster connectivity and high speed communication of 5G faster data transmission and more impactful systems can be created.

Tiny ML Applications for Upgraded Medical System

Another significant emerging trend is the TinyML which is a sub discipline of AI dedicated to implementing machine learning models on ultra-low-power devices with limited computational resources. TinyML enables intelligent data processing directly on devices like sensors and to execute functions like as anomaly detection and speech recognition without relying on cloud data transmission. It is significant for battery-powered devices, including Wearable (Yammour & Lahcen, 2024) but posses tremendous potential in healthcare especially in biofluid sensors that analyzes biofluids like blood, sweat, urine, saliva, and interstitial fluids for diagnostic and monitoring purposes.

Employing TinyML models in biofluid sensing can provide subtle advantages like their Low Power Consumption, that makes them suitable for implantable biofluid sensors based on tiny batteries. Real-time Processing of data on device directly that boosts rapid decision-making and the Local data processing which will reduce risks associated with privacy of sensitive health data.

For next generation techniques like robotic surgeries require precise, real-time responses without delay and tinyML enables on-device processing of sensor data (from force sensors, accelerometers, vision systems), allowing the robot to react instantly without needing cloud or server communication.

In recent study (Filho et al., 2023) authors have reported on the use of TinyML in removing the background interference in complex solutions such as cerebrospinal fluid. Here, they have implemented TinyML in low-power, portable systems to make discrimination between uric and ascorbic acid. As a result the TinyML model obtained an accuracy of 98.1%. Further, in the work (Ali et al., 2023) have proposed a wearable fall detection system utilizing Tiny Convolution Neural Networks (TinyCNNs) on inertial sensors which successfully achieved a high accuracy and low latency in fall detection. This developed wearable system provides a practical solution for accurate fall detection in everyday scenarios. In (Gudiño-Ochoa et al., 2024) a portable, low power breath analysis system (an "electronic nose" or e nose) enhanced with TinyML is presented for non invasive detection of diabetes through breath acetone—a key biomarker of diabetes. Here 6 sensor array (MQ-series Metal Oxide Semiconductor) are attached inside a 3.5 L chamber. Tedlar bags used to collect 1 L exhaled breath samples. In order to reduce interference, a 24 V DC humidifier is used to lower the humidity. Processed on Arduino Nano 33 BLE Sense compatible with TensorFlow Lite for TinyML. Sensor data shown on an integrated LCD.Breath samples were calibrated, denoised, sampled, and preprocessed. Traditional ML: XGBoost and Deep learning: Dense Neural Network and 1D-CNN were optimized and converted to TensorFlow Lite for on-device inference. XGBoost achieved 95% classification accuracy and DNN/1D-CNN achieved 94.4% accuracy demonstrating a strong performance for real-time embedded breath-based diabetes detection.Some of the challenges need to be addressed here are small sample size (n=44) may limit generalization, sensor drift, variations in humidity, and hardware aging could impact accuracy.Breath sample standardization protocols need further refinement, future needs for larger datasets, robust calibration, and clinical validation

The studies suggested that TinyML can enhance the reliability, accuracy and real-time data processing abilities in future medical devices and can make a transformative impact in advancing healthcare monitoring via wearable sensors. Further, numerous AI based applications are expensive because it uses a lot of resources because it needs a lot of storage on the cloud to process and store the data whereas TinyML uses low-cost microcontroller devices to process data locally where the device itself can use AI locally to process the data with significant performance. Due to their low resource consumption microcontrollers are less expensive making it the highest cost effective technology (Njor et al.,2024).

Nanosensors and Robotic Surgery

Nanosensors, have the ability to accurately and timely identify molecular and cellular changes at the nano level, can very effectively help in the early diagnosis of diseases, especially in the early stages of diseases such as cancer. These sensors can provide more detailed information about the molecular and chemical structure of diseases, which causes more accuracy in diagnosing and differentiating diseases from similar conditions and hence elevating the quality of treatment. These nanosensors are applicable in various ways- invasively, non-invasively or minimal invasively.

The advantages of minimally invasive surgery have been extensively documented, including reduced complication rates, decreased length of hospital stay, diminished narcotic requirements, and expedited postoperative recovery. Robotic-assisted surgery, in particular, has gained widespread adoption in the 21st century as in figure 5, evolving from open surgery as shown in figure 6 offering enhanced range of motion, improved dexterity for intracorporeal suturing, ambidexterity, increased procedural safety, and reduced operator fatigue (South et al., 2025). Robotic surgery refers to a surgical technique that utilizes robotic systems as an aid to surgeons to perform complex procedures with increased precision, dexterity, and control. It is a minimal invasive surgery in which surgeons operate from a console equipped with robotic arms and instruments controlled by hand movements. with the advancement of technology, it has been upgraded to a smart surgery with incorporation of nanotechnology as nanosensors and nanobots

The incorporation of nanosensor in robotic surgery can boost up the performance of operations with an extraordinary degree of accuracy, allowing surgeons to access delicate areas of the brain or spine with a minimal disruption to surrounding tissues, like robotic surgery enhanced by nanosensors and nanorobots can target brain tumors with remarkable precision, reducing the need for traditional large incisions and minimizing post-operative recovery times (Society for Brain Mapping and Therapeutics, 2024). Also, nanosensors are able to track various parameters such as tissue temperature, chemical composition and pH that can help surgeon by providing a real time continuous information about the surgical environment (Ghorbian et al., 2025).Thus playing an important role by helping in minimizing surgical error and improving overall precision .Nanosensors can track even subtle changes in tissue or tumor characteristics, enabling surgeons to make more precise cuts and resections which is specifically important in minimally invasive procedures where small incisions are used, and the surgeon needs to be extremely precise. They can be also utilize into deliver drugs directly to the surgical site or to specific tissues, minimizing side effects and improving treatment outcomes as they can be designed to release drugs only when they encounter specific targets, such as tumor cells, ensuring that the medication is delivered only where it's required (Kong et al., 2023).

Nanosensors can be used to perform surgery at the cellular level, allowing for more precise tissue repair and regeneration

Robotic surgery is mostly used in Urology as shown in figure 7, however it is expanding to other domains as well .It is of different types- Da Vinci proceure, Cyberknife etc which are expanding very fast. The graph in fig v shows the number of surgical robots used from past few years (Dey, 2025). Studies comparing robotic surgery with open surgery for colorectal cancer treatment found that patients undergoing robotic-assisted surgery experienced significantly fewer complications of 14.1% as compared to open surgery with 21.2% complications and shorter hospital stays of 6.7 days as compared to 8.4 days. As there is a large room for advancement and widespread use of robotic surgeries, nanosensors can contribute a significant role in quality robotic surgery by providing real time surgical environment information, targeted drug delivery and tissue repair leading to next generation robotics

Figure 5. Bar diagram showing increasing rate of robotic surgery worldwide

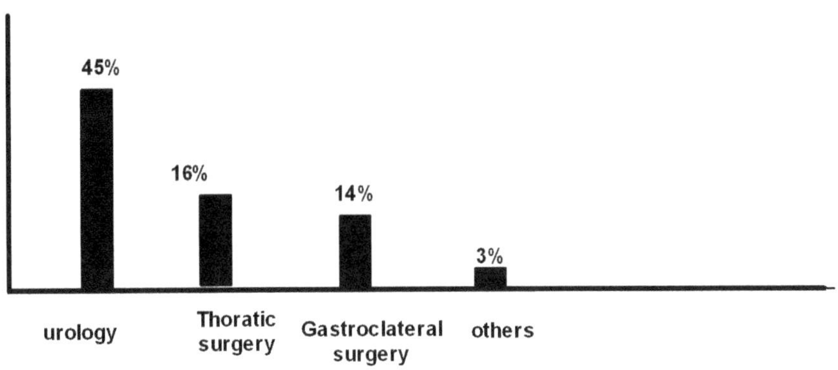

Figure 6. Generation and evolution of robotic surgery over years

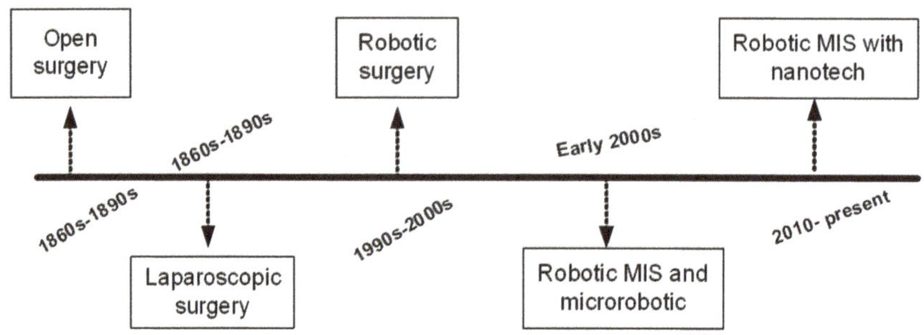

Figure 7. Different types of robotic surgeries emerging

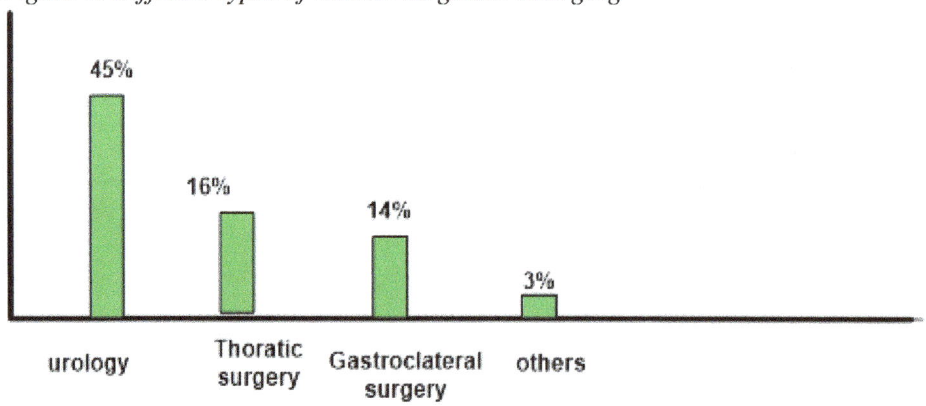

CHALLENGES AND OPPORTUNITIES

Nanobiosensors for biofluid sensing have made a notable growth in the past recent years. Furthermore, there is still tremendous potential unlocked which provides a huge space for research. With the ongoing research and development these will revolutionize the technological field to an unparallel zone. However their development and application possesses various challenges with dynamic opportunities such as:

Materials: Fabrication of stable, sensitive, and biocompatible nanomaterials will be a challenge as consistent performance of certain nanomaterials like metal nanoparticles, graphene or CNT is difficult. Also, the fabrication process is highly sophisticated and costly.

High Sensitivity: Obtaining high sensitivity in complex biofluids (saliva, urine or blood) is a challenge such as it contains various other interfering substances, also the selectivity for specific biomarkers is challenging because of the possible cross- sensitivity.

Validation Issues: Validation for biosensors in health monitoring to release in the market can be a challenge due to the rising ethical concerns about privacy and data security

Cost Effectiveness: The commercialization of the products is costly and time-demanding. Further, assuring affordability and accessibility of these devices for extensive use is a challenge.

Reuse: A lot of nanobiosensors are non reusable in nature and can be used for single time, where some of them have a very short duration use. So producing nanobiosensors with a long duration use with reusability is challenging.

Point-of-Care Diagnostics: Nanobiosensors can modernize the point-of-care testing with real-time, non-invasive, and portable diagnostics for diseases like diabetes, cancer or any other infectious diseases.

Advanced Personalized Treatment: With the ability to detect specific biomarkers in biofluids, nanobiosensors can revolutionize the personalized treatment upgrading therapeutic outcomes.

Early Detection: High sensitivity and specificity enables detection of diseases at an early stage, possibly improving conditions for treatment and survival chances ..

AI and IoT Integration: Combining nanobiosensors with AI can elevate data analysis, pattern recognition, and predictive modeling. Furthermore, fusion of nanobiosensors and IOT can generate real time and precise data that ensures to boost decision making and improve efficiency. So the AI and IOT integration with bionanosensors can unveil large opportunities for smarter and connected healthcare systems

Reduction of Cost Through Innovations: New innovations and development in manufacturing processes can however reduce the costs of nanobiosensors, making them cost effective and hence more accessible and affordable over time.

CONCLUSION

Nanomaterials has revolutionized the biosensing field, especially with the development of nanosensors for biofluids. These nanosensors for biofluids have become prominent in transforming healthcare by offering excellent sensitivity and specificity to detect or monitor biomarkers in real time.

The current trends emphasizes upon the integration of these nanosensors with advanced technologies such as machine learning (ML), Deep Learning (DL), TinyML, and the Internet of Things (IoT), that are redefining the capability horizons of these devices. The ML algorithm enhances the functionality of nanosensors by enabling real time analysis of complex datasets, making accurate pattern recognition and predictive diagnostics. For the large datasets formed by nanosensors, DL enables efficient analysis by utilizing complex Neural networks and thereby increasing accuracy in diagnostics and monitoring applications. In addition, integration with TinyML enables ML models on ultra low power devices, boosting the development for portable nanosensing systems for monitoring and wearable applications. Furthermore, IoT integration provides smooth data transmission along with remote monitoring, building a integrated healthcare system. The future scope of nanosensors in biofluids is huge. The combination of nanosensors with the cutting-edge technologies will address existing challenges, such as scalability, prolonged stability, biocompatibility and real-time decision-making. The potential to utilize nanosensors in wearable devices connecting to cloud-based platforms can transform personalized healthcare, and global health monitoring systems. Further, integration with robotics, will help in building next generation medical devices and systems by providing various advantages like high precision, minimal damage to body during surgeries etc. Also with the advance developments in nanomaterials, intelligent algorithms and IoT, self assisted nanosensors can be developed which will be able to function in limited resource environment. . These innovations are expected to redefine modern technologies by enabling more precise, accurate, affordable and predictive healthcare solutions to the society.

REFERENCES

Abaszadeh, F., Ashoub, M. H., Khajouie, G., & Amiri, M. (2023). Nanotechnology development in surgical applications: Recent trends and developments. *European Journal of Medical Research*, *28*(1). Advance online publication. DOI: 10.1186/s40001-023-01429-4 PMID: 38001554

Acharya, R., Patil, T. V., Dutta, S. D., Lee, J., Ganguly, K., Kim, H., Randhawa, A., & Lim, K. (2024). Single-Walled Carbon Nanotube-Based Optical Nano/Biosensors for biomedical applications: Role in bioimaging, disease diagnosis, and biomarkers detection. *Advanced Materials Technologies*, *9*(20). Advance online publication. DOI: 10.1002/admt.202400279

Afeef, S., Tolfrey, K., Zakrzewski-Fruer, J. K., & Barrett, L. A. (2023). Performance of the FreeStyle Libre Flash Glucose Monitoring System during an Oral Glucose Tolerance Test and Exercise in Healthy Adolescents. *Sensors (Basel)*, *23*(9), 4249. DOI: 10.3390/s23094249 PMID: 37177452

Al-Sammarraie, S. Z., Bratchenko, L. A., Tupikova, E. N., Skuratova, M. A., Wang, S., Lebedev, P. A., & Bratchenko, I. A. (2024). Human blood plasma SERS analysis using silver nanoparticles for cardiovascular diseases detection. *Journal of Biomedical Photonics & Engineering*, *10*(1), 010301. DOI: 10.18287/jbpe24.10.010301

Ali, Y. H., Chooralil, V. S., Balasubramanian, K., Manyam, R. R., Raju, S. K., Sadiq, A. T., & Farhan, A. K. (2023). Optimization system based on convolutional neural network and internet of medical things for early diagnosis of lung cancer. *Bioengineering (Basel, Switzerland)*, *10*(3), 320. DOI: 10.3390/bioengineering10030320 PMID: 36978711

Almurashi, A. M., Rodriguez, E., & Garg, S. K. (2023). Emerging Diabetes Technologies: Continuous Glucose Monitors/Artificial Pancreases. *Journal of the Indian Institute of Science*, *103*(1), 205–230. DOI: 10.1007/s41745-022-00348-3 PMID: 37362851

Altman, J., Jones, G., Ahmed, S., Sharma, S., & Sharma, A. (2023). Tear Film MicroRNAs as potential biomarkers: A review. *International Journal of Molecular Sciences*, *24*(4), 3694. DOI: 10.3390/ijms24043694 PMID: 36835108

Amal, H., Leja, M., Funka, K., Skapars, R., Sivins, A., Ancans, G., Liepniece-Karele, I., Kikuste, I., Lasina, I., & Haick, H. (2015). Detection of precancerous gastric lesions and gastric cancer through exhaled breath. *Gut*, *65*(3), 400–407. DOI: 10.1136/gutjnl-2014-308536 PMID: 25869737

Ansari, M. A., Mohd-Naim, N. F., & Ahmed, M. U. (2024). Electrochemical nanoaptasensor based on graphitic carbon Nitride/Zirconium Dioxide/Multiwalled carbon nanotubes for matrix metalloproteinase-9 in human serum and saliva. *ACS Applied Bio Materials*, *7*(3), 1579–1587. DOI: 10.1021/acsabm.3c01075 PMID: 38386014

Apoorva, S., Nguyen, N., & Sreejith, K. R. (2024). Recent developments and future perspectives of microfluidics and smart technologies in wearable devices. *Lab on a Chip*, *24*(7), 1833–1866. DOI: 10.1039/d4lc00089g PMID: 38476112

Arduini, F. (2024). Wireless real-time monitoring of oestradiol in sweat. *Nature Nanotechnology*, *19*(3), 271–272. DOI: 10.1038/s41565-024-01611-7 PMID: 38366226

Arkhypova, V., Soldatkin, O., Soldatkin, A., & Dzyadevych, S. (2023). Electrochemical biosensors based on enzyme inhibition effect. *Chemical Record (New York, N.Y.)*, *24*(2). Advance online publication. DOI: 10.1002/tcr.202300214 PMID: 37639188

Bae, G., Kim, M., Lee, A., Ji, S., Jang, M., Yim, S., Song, W., Lee, S. S., Yoon, D. H., & An, K. (2021). Nanometric lamination of zinc oxide nanofilms with gold nanoparticles for self-perceived periodontal disease sensors. *Composites. Part B, Engineering*, *230*, 109490. DOI: 10.1016/j.compositesb.2021.109490

Bahari, H., Hasanzadeh, M., Kohansal, F., Peirovi, B., & Shadjou, N. (2024a). Smartphone-assisted immunosensing of cancer biomarkers in human biofluids using poly (methyl methacrylate) decorated by triangular silver nanoparticles. *Journal of Photochemistry and Photobiology A Chemistry*, *457*, 115882. DOI: 10.1016/j.jphotochem.2024.115882

Bahari, H., Hasanzadeh, M., Kohansal, F., Peirovi, B., & Shadjou, N. (2024b). Smartphone-assisted immunosensing of cancer biomarkers in human biofluids using poly (methyl methacrylate) decorated by triangular silver nanoparticles. *Journal of Photochemistry and Photobiology A Chemistry*, *457*, 115882. DOI: 10.1016/j.jphotochem.2024.115882

Ballard, Z. S., Joung, H., Goncharov, A., Liang, J., Nugroho, K., Di Carlo, D., Garner, O. B., & Ozcan, A. (2020). Deep learning-enabled point-of-care sensing using multiplexed paper-based sensors. *NPJ Digital Medicine*, *3*(1). Advance online publication. DOI: 10.1038/s41746-020-0274-y PMID: 32411827

Bayoumy, R. E., El-Ragehy, N. A., Hassan, N. Y., & Mahmoud, A. M. (2024). Disposable Point-of-Care Electrochemical Sensor for Uric Acid Determination in Human Urine Utilizing a Pencil Graphite Electrode Modified with Polydopamine/Gold Nanoparticles. *Journal of the Electrochemical Society*, *171*(2), 027506. DOI: 10.1149/1945-7111/ad2281

Beatto, T. G., Gomes, W. E., Etchegaray, A., Gupta, R., & Mendes, R. K. (2023). Dopamine levels determined in synthetic urine using an electrochemical tyrosinase biosensor based on ZnO@Au core–shell. *RSC Advances, 13*(47), 33424–33429. DOI: 10.1039/d3ra06277e PMID: 38025875

Benedetti, T. M., Somerville, S. V., Wordsworth, J., Yamamoto, Y., Schuhmann, W., Tilley, R. D., & Gooding, J. J. (2024). An artificial enzyme: How nanoconfinement allows the selective electrochemical detection of glucose directly in whole blood. *Advanced Functional Materials, 34*(30). Advance online publication. DOI: 10.1002/adfm.202400322

Bi, Y., Sun, M., Wang, J., Zhu, Z., Bai, J., Emran, M. Y., Kotb, A., Bo, X., & Zhou, M. (2023). Universal fully integrated wearable sensor arrays for the multiple electrolyte and metabolite monitoring in raw sweat, saliva, or urine. *Analytical Chemistry, 95*(16), 6690–6699. DOI: 10.1021/acs.analchem.3c00361 PMID: 36961950

Bilsen, M. P., Treep, M. M., Aantjes, M. J., Van Andel, E., Stalenhoef, J. E., Van Nieuwkoop, C., Leyten, E. M., Delfos, N. M., Van Uhm, J. I., Sijbom, M., Akintola, A. A., Numans, M. E., Achterberg, W. P., Mooijaart, S. P., Van Der Beek, M. T., Cobbaert, C. M., Conroy, S. P., Visser, L. G., & Lambregts, M. M. (2023). Diagnostic accuracy of urine biomarkers for urinary tract infection in older women: A case-control study. *Clinical Microbiology and Infection, 30*(2), 216–222. DOI: 10.1016/j.cmi.2023.09.023 PMID: 37805035

Brasier, N., Frobert, O., De Ieso, F., Meyer, D., Kowatsch, T., & Ghaffari, R. (2024). The potential of wearable sweat sensors in heart failure management. *Nature Electronics, 7*(3), 182–184. DOI: 10.1038/s41928-024-01136-w

Brinza, M., Schröder, S., Ababii, N., Gronenberg, M., Strunskus, T., Pauporte, T., Adelung, R., Faupel, F., & Lupan, O. (2023). Two-in-One sensor based on PV4D4-Coated TIO2 films for food spoilage detection and as a breath marker for several diseases. *Biosensors (Basel), 13*(5), 538. DOI: 10.3390/bios13050538 PMID: 37232899

Cáceres, C., Heusser, B., Garnham, A., & Moczko, E. (2023). The major hypotheses of Alzheimer's disease: Related Nanotechnology-Based Approaches for its diagnosis and treatment. *Cells, 12*(23), 2669. DOI: 10.3390/cells12232669 PMID: 38067098

Chaudhary, V., Taha, B. A., Lucky, N., Rustagi, S., Khosla, A., Papakonstantinou, P., & Bhalla, N. (2024). Nose-on-Chip Nanobiosensors for early detection of lung cancer breath biomarkers. *ACS Sensors, 9*(9), 4469–4494. DOI: 10.1021/acssensors.4c01524 PMID: 39248694

Chhillar, M., Kukkar, D., Deep, A., Yadav, A. K., & Kim, K. (2023). Zn2+/GNPs nanocomposite for highly selective colorimetric detection of creatinine in urine samples of CKD patients. *Inorganic Chemistry Communications*, *158*, 111618. DOI: 10.1016/j.inoche.2023.111618

Chhillar, M., Kukkar, D., Yadav, A. K., & Kim, K. (2024). Nitrogen doped carbon dots and gold nanoparticles mediated FRET for the detection of creatinine in human urine samples. *Spectrochimica Acta Part a Molecular and Biomolecular Spectroscopy*, *321*, 124752. DOI: 10.1016/j.saa.2024.124752 PMID: 38945007

Cordas, C. M., Nunes, M. J., Valério, G. N., Samhan-Arias, A., Krippahl, L., Moura, J. J. G., Santos, G., Sousa, J. P., & Rouco, C. (2023). Sweat as a testing analytical fluid for emotions and stress biomarkers detection. In *Smart innovation, systems and technologies* (pp. 77–85). DOI: 10.1007/978-981-19-7689-6_7

Cruz, J. N., Da Silva Souza Filho, A. P., Oliveira, M. E. C., Pereira, D. S., & De Oliveira, M. S. (2021). Nanosensor for the detection of malaria parasite. In *Elsevier eBooks* (pp. 107–116). DOI: 10.1016/b978-0-12-821100-7.00024-8

Czarniak, N., Kamińska, J., Matowicka-Karna, J., & Koper-Lenkiewicz, O. (2023). Cerebrospinal Fluid–Basic Concepts Review. *Biomedicines*, *11*(5), 1461. DOI: 10.3390/biomedicines11051461 PMID: 37239132

Da Silva, S. M. S. D., Ferreira, C. L., Rizzato, J. M. B., Toledo, G. D. S., Furukawa, M., Rovai, E. S., Nogueira, M. S., & De Carvalho, L. F. D. C. E. S. (2024). Infrared spectroscopy for fast screening of diabetes and periodontitis. *Photodiagnosis and Photodynamic Therapy*, *46*, 104106. DOI: 10.1016/j.pdpdt.2024.104106 PMID: 38677501

Das, C., Das, S., Chugh, V., & Bhattacharjee, M. (2023). 3D Printed Design-Assisted Multilayered Graphene Oxide-Modified Polymer Glucose Sensor. *Advanced Engineering Materials*, *26*(1). Advance online publication. DOI: 10.1002/adem.202301067

De Jong, F. C., Iflé, I. G., Van Der Made, A. C., Kooper, D., De Jong, J. J., Franckena, M., Zuiverloon, T. C., Van Criekinge, W., Incrocci, L., Zwarthoff, E. C., & Boormans, J. L. (2024). A Genomic Urine Assay for Surveillance of Patients with Bladder Cancer Treated with Radiotherapy. *European Urology Open Science*, *62*, 131–139. DOI: 10.1016/j.euros.2024.02.009 PMID: 38496820

De Lima, L. T. F., Crawford, D. H., Broszczak, D. A., & Zhang, X., R, K. B., & Punyadeera, C. (2023). A salivary biomarker panel to detect liver cirrhosis. *iScience*, *26*(7), 107015. DOI: 10.1016/j.isci.2023.107015 PMID: 37360686

De Oliveira Filho, J. I., Faleiros, M. C., Ferreira, D. C., Mani, V., & Salama, K. N. (2023). Empowering Electrochemical Biosensors with AI: Overcoming Interference for Precise Dopamine Detection in Complex Samples. *Advanced Intelligent Systems, 5*(10). Advance online publication. DOI: 10.1002/aisy.202300227

Dey, M. (2025, January 28). *Surgical Robotics Statistics and Facts*. Electro IQ. https://electroiq.com/stats/surgical-robotics-statistics-and-facts/

Dong, T., Pires, N. M. M., Yang, Z., & Jiang, Z. (2022). Advances in electrochemical biosensors based on nanomaterials for protein biomarker detection in saliva. *Advancement of Science, 10*(6). Advance online publication. DOI: 10.1002/advs.202205429 PMID: 36585368

Ebersole, J. L., Hasturk, H., Huber, M., Gellibolian, R., Markaryan, A., Zhang, X. D., & Miller, C. S. (2024). Realizing the clinical utility of saliva for monitoring oral diseases. *Periodontology 2000, 95*(1), 203–219. DOI: 10.1111/prd.12581 PMID: 39010260

Emerging Nano-Theranostic Strategies against Non-Alcoholic Fatty Liver Disease: a review. (2023). *Iranian Journal Materials Science and Engineering* (Vols. 1–1, pp. 1–28). DOI: 10.22068/ijmse.2861

Gaboriau, T., Dubois, R., Foucque, B., Malet, F., & Schweitzer, C. (2023). 24-Hour monitoring of intraocular pressure fluctuations using a contact lens sensor: Diagnostic performance for glaucoma progression. *Investigative Ophthalmology & Visual Science, 64*(3), 3. DOI: 10.1167/iovs.64.3.3 PMID: 36862120

Ganesh, S., Dhinakaran, A. K., Premnath, P., Venkatakrishnan, K., & Tan, B. (2023). Label-Free Saliva Test for Rapid Detection of Coronavirus Using Nanosensor-Enabled SERS. *Bioengineering (Basel, Switzerland), 10*(3), 391. DOI: 10.3390/bioengineering10030391 PMID: 36978782

Gao, C., Liu, X., Peven, M., Unberath, M., & Reiter, A. (2018). Learning to See Forces: Surgical Force Prediction with RGB-Point Cloud Temporal Convolutional Networks. In *Lecture notes in computer science* (pp. 118–127). DOI: 10.1007/978-3-030-01201-4_14

Garcia-Rey, S., Gil-Hernandez, E., Gunatilake, U. B., Basabe-Desmonts, L., & Benito-Lopez, F. (2023). Development of an alginate/TiO2-based microfluidic biosystem for chrono-sampling and sensing of glucose in artificial sweat. *Sensors and Actuators. B, Chemical, 382*, 133514. DOI: 10.1016/j.snb.2023.133514

Garg, M., Guo, H., Maclam, E., Zhanov, E., Samudrala, S., Pavlov, A., Rahman, M. S., Namkoong, M., Moreno, J. P., & Tian, L. (2024). Molecularly Imprinted Wearable Sensor with Paper Microfluidics for Real-Time Sweat Biomarker Analysis. *ACS Applied Materials & Interfaces, 16*(35), 46113–46122. DOI: 10.1021/acsami.4c10033 PMID: 39178237

Ghafouri, T., & Manavizadeh, N. (2023). A 3D-printed millifluidic device for triboelectricity-driven pH sensing based on ZnO nanosheets with super-Nernstian response. *Analytica Chimica Acta, 1267*, 341342. DOI: 10.1016/j.aca.2023.341342 PMID: 37257971

Ghorbian, M., Ghobaei-Arani, M., Babaei, M. R., & Ghorbian, S. (2025). Nanotechnology and nanosensors in personalized healthcare: A comprehensive review. *Sensing and Bio-Sensing Research, 100740*. Advance online publication. DOI: 10.1016/j.sbsr.2025.100740

Ghosh, T. N., Rotake, D., Kumar, S., Kaur, I., & Singh, S. G. (2023). Tear-based MMP-9 detection: A rapid antigen test for ocular inflammatory disorders using vanadium disulfide nanowires assisted chemi-resistive biosensor. *Analytica Chimica Acta, 1263*, 341281. DOI: 10.1016/j.aca.2023.341281 PMID: 37225335

Guang, P., Huang, W., Guo, L., Yang, X., Huang, F., Yang, M., Wen, W., & Li, L. (2020). Blood-based FTIR-ATR spectroscopy coupled with extreme gradient boosting for the diagnosis of type 2 diabetes. *Medicine, 99*(15), e19657. DOI: 10.1097/md.0000000000019657 PMID: 32282717

Gudiño-Ochoa, A., García-Rodríguez, J. A., Ochoa-Ornelas, R., Cuevas-Chávez, J. I., & Sánchez-Arias, D. A. (2024). Noninvasive Diabetes Detection through Human Breath Using TinyML-Powered E-Nose. *Sensors (Basel), 24*(4), 1294. DOI: 10.3390/s24041294 PMID: 38400451

Hofman, P. (2024). Liquid and tissue biopsies for lung cancer: Algorithms and perspectives. *Cancers (Basel), 16*(19), 3340. DOI: 10.3390/cancers16193340 PMID: 39409960

Hooshiar, M. H., Moghaddam, M. A., Kiarashi, M., Al-Hijazi, A. Y., & Hussein, A. F., Aalrikabi, H., Salari, S., Esmaelian, S., Mesgari, H., & Yasamineh, S. (2024). Recent advances in nanomaterial-based biosensor for periodontitis detection. *Journal of Biological Engineering, 18*(1). Advance online publication. DOI: 10.1186/s13036-024-00423-6 PMID: 38637787

Hossain, G. M. M., Jalal, A. H., Pala, N., & Alam, F. (2024a). Advancements in Glucose Monitoring: A Thin Film ZnO-Nanoflakes Based Highly Sensitive Wearable Biosensor for Noninvasive Sweat-Based Point-of-Care Monitoring for Diabetes. *ECS Transactions, 113*(13), 35–42. DOI: 10.1149/11313.0035ecst

Hossain, N. I., Sharma, A., & Sonkusale, S. (2023a). A wearable and multiplexed electrochemical sensor suite for Real-Time sweat ionic content and pH monitoring with IoT integration. *IEEE Sensors Letters, 7*(9), 1–4. DOI: 10.1109/lsens.2023.3300827

Hu, B. (2023). Mass spectrometric analysis of exhaled breath: Recent advances and future perspectives. *Trends in Analytical Chemistry, 168*, 117320. DOI: 10.1016/j.trac.2023.117320

Hu, X., Mao, N., Yan, X., Huang, L., Liu, X., Yang, H., Sun, Q., Liu, X., & Jia, H. (2024). Non-invasive healthcare analytical platform based on organic electrochemical transistors. *Chemical Research in Chinese Universities*. Advance online publication. DOI: 10.1007/s40242-024-4176-4

Jahangiri-Manesh, A., Mousazadeh, M., & Nikkhah, M. (2022a). Fabrication of chemiresistive nanosensor using molecularly imprinted polymers for acetone detection in gaseous state. *Iranian Polymer Journal, 31*(7), 883–891. DOI: 10.1007/s13726-022-01044-w

Jahangiri-Manesh, A., Mousazadeh, M., & Nikkhah, M. (2022b). Fabrication of chemiresistive nanosensor using molecularly imprinted polymers for acetone detection in gaseous state. *Iranian Polymer Journal, 31*(7), 883–891. DOI: 10.1007/s13726-022-01044-w

Jeon, H., Lee, W., Park, H., Lee, H., Kim, S., Kim, H., Jeon, B., & Park, K. (2017). Correction: Automatic classification of tremor severity in Parkinson's disease using a wearable device. Sensors 2017, 17, 2067. *Sensors (Basel), 18*(1), 33. DOI: 10.3390/s18010033 PMID: 29295543

Jin, C., Yang, S., Zheng, J., Chai, F., & Tian, M. (2024). Paper-based triple-readout nanosensor for point-of-care detection of glucose in urine. *Biosensors & Bioelectronics, 269*, 116931. DOI: 10.1016/j.bios.2024.116931 PMID: 39549311

Jordaens, S., Zwaenepoel, K., Tjalma, W., Deben, C., Beyers, K., Vankerckhoven, V., Pauwels, P., & Vorsters, A. (2023a). Urine biomarkers in cancer detection: A systematic review of preanalytical parameters and applied methods. *International Journal of Cancer, 152*(10), 2186–2205. DOI: 10.1002/ijc.34434 PMID: 36647333

Kadian, S., Kumari, P., Shukla, S., & Narayan, R. (2023). Recent advancements in machine learning enabled portable and wearable biosensors. *Talanta Open*, *8*, 100267. DOI: 10.1016/j.talo.2023.100267

Kiio, L. K., Onyatta, J. O., Ndangili, P. M., Oloo, F., Santamaria, C., Montuenga, L. M., & Mbui, D. N. (2023). Ultrasensitive immunosensor for multiplex detection of cancer biomarkers carcinoembryonic antigen (CEA) and yamaguchi sarcoma viral oncogene homolog 1 (YES1) based on eco-friendly synthesized gold nanoparticles. *Talanta*, *266*, 124934. DOI: 10.1016/j.talanta.2023.124934 PMID: 37454512

Kim, H., Awofeso, O., Choi, S., Jung, Y., & Bae, E. (2016). Colorimetric analysis of saliva–alcohol test strips by smartphone-based instruments using machine-learning algorithms. *Applied Optics*, *56*(1), 84. DOI: 10.1364/ao.56.000084

Koh, A., Kang, D., Xue, Y., Lee, S., Pielak, R. M., Kim, J., Hwang, T., Min, S., Banks, A., Bastien, P., Manco, M. C., Wang, L., Ammann, K. R., Jang, K., Won, P., Han, S., Ghaffari, R., Paik, U., Slepian, M. J., & Rogers, J. A. (2016). A soft, wearable microfluidic device for the capture, storage, and colorimetric sensing of sweat. *Science Translational Medicine*, *8*(366). Advance online publication. DOI: 10.1126/scitranslmed.aaf2593 PMID: 27881826

Kong, X., Gao, P., Wang, J., Fang, Y., & Hwang, K. C. (2023). Advances of medical nanorobots for future cancer treatments. *Journal of Hematology & Oncology*, *16*(1). Advance online publication. DOI: 10.1186/s13045-023-01463-z PMID: 37452423

Krishnamoorthy, G., & Sistla, S. M. K. (2023). Exploring Machine Learning Intrusion Detection: Addressing security and Privacy Challenges in IoT - A Comprehensive review. *Journal of Knowledge Learning and Science Technology, 2*(2), 114–125. DOI: 10.60087/jklst.vol2.n2.p125

Kumar, D., Ram, R., & Sarkar, A. (2023). A smartphone enabled low-cost portable centrifuge integrated with a simple paper-based device for the estimation of plasma-albumin concentration. *Microchemical Journal, 197*, 109822. DOI: 10.1016/j.microc.2023.109822

Kumar, S., Singh, H., Feder-Kubis, J., & Nguyen, D. D. (2023). Recent advances in nanobiosensors for sustainable healthcare applications: A systematic literature review. *Environmental Research, 238*, 117177. DOI: 10.1016/j.envres.2023.117177 PMID: 37751831

Kumari, M., Kumar, D., Bhattacharyya, R., & Banerjee, D. (2024). Whether Dye-Based methods are ready for microalbuminuria detection: A review of research in the field. *Indian Journal of Clinical Biochemistry : IJCB*. Advance online publication. DOI: 10.1007/s12291-024-01213-z

Kumari, S., Islam, M., & Gupta, A. (2023). Paper-based multiplex biosensors for inexpensive healthcare diagnostics: A comprehensive review. *Biomedical Microdevices, 25*(2). Advance online publication. DOI: 10.1007/s10544-023-00656-0 PMID: 37133791

Kumari, S., Samara, M., Ramachandran, R. A., Gosh, S., George, H., Wang, R., Pesavento, R. P., & Mathew, M. T. (2023a). A review on Saliva-Based Health Diagnostics: Biomarker selection and future directions. *Deleted Journal, 2*(1), 121–138. DOI: 10.1007/s44174-023-00090-z PMID: 37363139

Lee, B., Lee, J., Lee, J., Hwang, Y., Bahn, H., Park, I., Jheon, S., & Lee, D. (2024). Breath analysis system with convolutional neural network (CNN) for early detection of lung cancer. *Sensors and Actuators. B, Chemical, 409*, 135578. DOI: 10.1016/j.snb.2024.135578

Liao, C., Chen, X., & Fu, Y. (2023). Salivary analysis: An emerging paradigm for non-invasive healthcare diagnosis and monitoring. *Deleted Journal, 1*(3). Advance online publication. DOI: 10.1002/inmd.20230009

Liu, T., Dong, Y., Chen, S., Zhou, J., Ma, Z., & Li, J. (2022). Battery-free, tuning circuit–inspired wireless sensor systems for detection of multiple biomarkers in bodily fluids. *Science Advances, 8*(27). Advance online publication. DOI: 10.1126/sciadv.abo7049 PMID: 35857473

Liu, Y., Wang, F., Hu, H., Zhang, Z., Yang, H., Yao, X., Liu, H., & Zheng, J. (2025). A paper-based label-free plasmonic nanosensor for portable pre-diagnosis of multiple metabolic diseases. *Biosensors & Bioelectronics, 275*, 117231. DOI: 10.1016/j.bios.2025.117231 PMID: 39946755

Lugonja, N., Marinković, V., Pucarević, M., Miletić, S., Stojić, N., Crnković, D., & Vrvić, M. (2024). Human Milk—The Biofluid That Nourishes Infants from the First Day of Life. *Foods, 13*(9), 1298. DOI: 10.3390/foods13091298 PMID: 38731669

Maafa, I. M. (2025). Potential of zinc oxide nanostructures in biosensor application. *Biosensors (Basel), 15*(1), 61. DOI: 10.3390/bios15010061 PMID: 39852112

Mani, A., & Anirudhan, T. (2024). Electrochemical sensing of cortisol by gold nanoparticle incorporated carboxylated graphene oxide based molecularly imprinted polymer. *Chemical Engineering Journal, 493*, 152654. DOI: 10.1016/j.cej.2024.152654

Mansuri, R., Hirpara, F., & Dudhat, K. (2024). Diabetes Mellitus: Prevalence, knowledge and future consideration for the development of technological innovation. DOI: 10.22034/abec.2024.713505

Marchianò, V., Tricase, A., Macchia, E., Bollella, P., & Torsi, L. (2024). Self-powered wearable biosensor based on stencil-printed carbon nanotube electrodes for ethanol detection in sweat. *Analytical and Bioanalytical Chemistry, 416*(24), 5303–5316. DOI: 10.1007/s00216-024-05467-7 PMID: 39134727

Matsumoto, H., Tomoto, K., Kawase, G., Iitani, K., Toma, K., Arakawa, T., Mitsubayashi, K., & Moriyama, K. (2023). Real-Time Continuous Monitoring of Oral Soft Tissue Pressure with a Wireless Mouthguard Device for Assessing Tongue Thrusting Habits. *Sensors (Basel), 23*(11), 5027. DOI: 10.3390/s23115027 PMID: 37299753

Memon, F. H., Inseok, K., Ahmed, F., Ali, W., Soomro, A. M., Memon, S. R., Memon, K. H., & Choi, K. H. (2023). A Comprehensive review of biosensor integration in microphysiological systems for online monitoring: Current challenges and future advancements. *ChemBioEng Reviews, 10*(5), 817–828. DOI: 10.1002/cben.202200066

Mitsubayashi, K. (2024). *Wearable biosensing in medicine and healthcare*. Springer Nature.

Mondal, I., Mansour, E., Zheng, Y., Gupta, R., & Haick, H. (2024). Self-Sustaining triboelectric nanosensors for Real-Time urine analysis in smart toilets. *Small, 20*(42). Advance online publication. DOI: 10.1002/smll.202403385 PMID: 39031720

Mottaghi, A., Nikkhah, M., & Masroor, M. J. (2023). Lable-Free LSPR-Based colorimetric detection of A-Synuclein, a biomarker of Parkinson's disease, in saliva. *IEEE Sensors Journal, 23*(6), 5713–5719. DOI: 10.1109/jsen.2023.3239887

Moulahoum, H., Ghorbanizamani, F., Beduk, T., Beduk, D., Ozufuklar, O., Celik, E. G., & Timur, S. (2023). Emerging trends in nanomaterial design for the development of point-of-care platforms and practical applications. *Journal of Pharmaceutical and Biomedical Analysis, 235*, 115623. DOI: 10.1016/j.jpba.2023.115623 PMID: 37542827

Mudireddy, D. R., Thakur, J., Vianney, N. J. M., Srivastava, S., Mathur, A., & Joseph, S. (2024). Prediction of blood glucose levels in diabetic and non-diabetic patients using Bi-RNN Transformers. *2021 IEEE International Conference on Electronics, Computing and Communication Technologies (CONECCT)*, 1–6. DOI: 10.1109/conecct62155.2024.10677194

Njor, E., Hasanpour, M. A., Madsen, J., & Fafoutis, X. (2024). A holistic review of the TinyML stack for predictive maintenance. *IEEE Access : Practical Innovations, Open Solutions, 1*. Advance online publication. DOI: 10.1109/access.2024.3512860

Paluszkiewicz, C., Pięta, E., Woźniak, M., Piergies, N., Koniewska, A., Ścierski, W., Misiołek, M., & Kwiatek, W. M. (2020). Saliva as a first-line diagnostic tool: A spectral challenge for identification of cancer biomarkers. *Journal of Molecular Liquids*, *307*, 112961. DOI: 10.1016/j.molliq.2020.112961

Pandit, P., Crewther, B., Cook, C., Punyadeera, C., & Pandey, A. K. (2024). Sensing methods for stress biomarker detection in human saliva: A new frontier for wearable electronics and biosensing. *Materials Advances*, *5*(13), 5339–5350. DOI: 10.1039/d3ma00937h

Paramasivam, G., Sanmugam, A., Palem, V. V., Sevanan, M., Sairam, A. B., Nachiappan, N., Youn, B., Lee, J. S., Nallal, M., & Park, K. H. (2023). Nanomaterials for detection of biomolecules and delivering therapeutic agents in theragnosis: A review. *International Journal of Biological Macromolecules*, *254*, 127904. DOI: 10.1016/j.ijbiomac.2023.127904 PMID: 37939770

Patel, S. K., Surve, J., Parmar, J., Armghan, A., Aliqab, K., Altahan, B. R., Ahmed, K., Bui, F. M., & Al-Zahrani, F. A. (2023). Graphene-based H-shaped biosensor with high sensitivity and optimization using ML-based algorithm. *Alexandria Engineering Journal*, *68*, 15–28. DOI: 10.1016/j.aej.2023.01.002

Patel, V., Bhatt, S., Daspoddar, A., Shirsekar, V., Kumari, R., Chandra, P., & Srivastava, R. (2024). Evolution of materials, geometries, and fabrication of sweat patches and their use in high-throughput point-of-care/onsite sensing. *Microchemical Journal*, *204*, 111165. DOI: 10.1016/j.microc.2024.111165

Pei, S., Ji, W., Yang, Y., Yang, S., Liu, T., Dai, J., Fu, C., Wu, J., Yin, Y., Wu, Q., Zheng, B., & Li, L. (2025). An enzyme-free wearable sweat sensor based on a Cu metal-organic frame composite material for monitoring lactate metabolism. *Sensors and Actuators. B, Chemical*, *137512*. Advance online publication. DOI: 10.1016/j.snb.2025.137512

Pitikultham, P., Putnin, T., Pimalai, D., Sathirapongsasuti, N., Kitiyakara, C., Jiang, Q., Ding, B., & Japrung, D. (2023). Ultrasensitive detection of MicroRNA in human saliva via rolling circle amplification using a DNA-Decorated graphene oxide sensor. *ACS Omega*, *8*(17), 15266–15275. DOI: 10.1021/acsomega.3c00411 PMID: 37151566

Polat, B., Rafeedi, T., Becerra, L., Chen, A. X., Chiang, K., Kaipu, V., Blau, R., Mercier, P. P., Cheng, C., & Lipomi, D. J. (2023). External measurement of swallowed volume during exercise enabled by stretchable derivatives of PEDOT:PSS, graphene, metallic nanoparticles, and machine learning. *Advanced Sensor Research*, *2*(4). Advance online publication. DOI: 10.1002/adsr.202200060

Prabakaran, A., & Rufus, E. (2021). Review on the wearable health-care monitoring system with robust motion artifacts reduction techniques. *Sensor Review*, *42*(1), 19–38. DOI: 10.1108/sr-05-2021-0150

Promphet, N., Akgönüllü, S., Moonla, C., Nandhakumar, P., Tanglertsampan, P., Laochai, T., Laichuthai, N., Wang, J., & Rodthongkum, N. (2025). Non-Invasive Fingertip Sweat biosensor for early kidney disease biomarker screening. *Sensors and Actuators. B, Chemical*, *441*, 137967. DOI: 10.1016/j.snb.2025.137967

Promphet, N., Thanawattano, C., Buekban, C., Laochai, T., Lormaneenopparat, P., Sukmas, W., Rattanawaleedirojn, P., Puthongkham, P., Potiyaraj, P., Leewattanakit, W., & Rodthongkum, N. (2024). Smartphone based wearable sweat glucose sensing device correlated with machine learning for real-time diabetes screening. *Analytica Chimica Acta*, *1312*, 342761. DOI: 10.1016/j.aca.2024.342761 PMID: 38834276

Qi, Y., Xu, M., Lu, H., Wang, X., Peng, Y., Wang, Z., Liang, F., Jiang, X., & Du, B. (2024). Hepatic biotransformation of renal clearable gold nanoparticles for noninvasive detection of liver glutathione level via urinalysis. *Angewandte Chemie International Edition*, *63*(36). Advance online publication. DOI: 10.1002/anie.202409477 PMID: 38877855

Ragavendran, L. T. P, A. P., & P, A. P. P. (2024). 1D Topological Photonic Crystal based Nanosensor for Tuberculosis Detection. *Nanotechnology*. Advance online publication. DOI: 10.1088/1361-6528/ad61ec

Rahman, S., Hasan, M., Sarkar, A. K., & Khan, F. (2023). Classification of Parkinson's Disease using Speech Signal with Machine Learning and Deep Learning Approaches. *European Journal of Electrical Engineering and Computer Science*, *7*(2), 20–27. DOI: 10.24018/ejece.2023.7.2.488

Rajan, A., Vishnu, J., & Shankar, B. (2024). Tear-Based Ocular Wearable biosensors for human health monitoring. *Biosensors (Basel)*, *14*(10), 483. DOI: 10.3390/bios14100483 PMID: 39451696

Rosa, M., Liu, R., Pitruzzello, G., & Tortora, G. (2022). A smart modular IoT sensing device for enhancing sensory feedbacks in surgical robotics. *Applied Sciences (Basel, Switzerland)*, *12*(16), 8083. DOI: 10.3390/app12168083

Rossi, F., Trakoolwilaiwan, T., Gigli, V., Tortolini, C., Lenzi, A., Isidori, A. M., Thanh, N. T. K., & Antiochia, R. (2024). Progress in Nanoparticle-based Electrochemical Biosensors for Hormone detection. *Nanoscale*, *16*(39), 18134–18164. DOI: 10.1039/d4nr02075h PMID: 39254475

Rossor, A. M., & Reilly, M. M. (2022). Blood biomarkers of peripheral neuropathy. *Acta Neurologica Scandinavica*, *146*(4), 325–331. DOI: 10.1111/ane.13650 PMID: 35611606

Ruan, J., Chen, C., Shen, J., Zhao, X., Qian, S., & Zhu, Z. (2017). A gelated colloidal crystal attached lens for noninvasive continuous monitoring of tear glucose. *Polymers*, *9*(4), 125. DOI: 10.3390/polym9040125 PMID: 30970805

Saedi, Z., Masroor, M. J., Jahangiri-Manesh, A., Rezaei, A., Siskova, K., & Nikkhah, M. (2024). A Label-Free sensor array based on carbon quantum dots for detection of A-Synuclein oligomers in saliva. *Analytical Chemistry*. Advance online publication. DOI: 10.1021/acs.analchem.4c00874 PMID: 39034918

Sakhare, N. S. A., Kale, N. a. A., More, N. D. G., Kumkar, N. P. A., Mirase, N. J. M., & Sahu, N. U. S. (2023a). Smart wearable safety jacket. *International Journal of Advanced Research in Science Communication and Technology*, 8–14. DOI: 10.48175/ijarsct-9311

Setiadi, R. N., Umar, L., & Arfianti, A. (2024). Low noise signal processing for electrochemical biosensor using narrow bandwidth filter. *Journal of Physics: Conference Series*, *2866*(1), 012032. DOI: 10.1088/1742-6596/2866/1/012032

Shan, L. L., & Zhang, Y. (2024). Preparation and application of ZnO-Ecoflex composite sensors for lactate detection during physical training. *Journal of Ovonic Research*, *20*(6), 763–778. DOI: 10.15251/jor.2024.206.763

Shanmugasundaram, A., & Lee, D. (2022). SnO2/rGO nanocomposite for the detection of biomarkers of lung cancer. *Micro and Nano Systems Letters*, *10*(1). Advance online publication. DOI: 10.1186/s40486-022-00154-7

Sharmile, N., Chowdhury, R. R., & Desai, S. (2025). A comprehensive review of quality control and reliability research in Micro–Nano technology. *Technologies*, *13*(3), 94. DOI: 10.3390/technologies13030094

Shetty, K. H., Desai, D. T., Patel, H. P., Shah, D. O., Willcox, M. D., & Maulvi, F. A. (2024). Contact lens as an emerging platform for non-invasive bio-sensing: A review. *Sensors and Actuators a Physical*, *376*, 115617. DOI: 10.1016/j.sna.2024.115617

Shreef, A., Shah, M., Habashy, A., & Mohamed, M. (2023). The Association of Microalbuminuria with Severity of Coronary Artery Disease Detected by Angiography in Type II Diabetes. *Zagazig University Medical Journal*. DOI: 10.21608/zumj.2023.224417.2830

Society for Brain Mapping and Therapeutics. (2024, December 18). *Role of nanotechnology in modern surgical techniques - Society for Brain Mapping and Therapeutics*. Society for Brain Mapping and Therapeutics - Breaking Boundries of Science, Technology, Medicine, Art & Healthcare Policy. https://www.worldbrainmapping.org/courses/lessons/role-of-nanotechnology-in-modern-surgical-techniques

South, C., Megafu, O., Moore, C., Williams, T., Hobson, L., Danner, O., & Johnson, S. (2025). Robotic surgery in Safety-Net Hospitals: Addressing health disparities and improving access to care. *The American Surgeon*. Advance online publication. DOI: 10.1177/00031348241312121 PMID: 39749432

Sreepada, A., Khasanov, R., Elkrewi, E. Z., De La Torre, C., Felcht, J., Abdulqader, A. A., Martel, R., Hoyos-Celis, N. A., Boettcher, M., Wessel, L. M., Schäfer, K., & Tapia-Laliena, M. Á. (2025). Urine miRNA signature as potential non-invasive diagnostic biomarker for Hirschsprung's disease. *Frontiers in Molecular Neuroscience, 17*. Advance online publication. DOI: 10.3389/fnmol.2024.1504424 PMID: 39872605

Suarez-Ortegón, M. F., Del Pilar Zea-León, M., Astudillo-Gironza, A. M., Garzón, S., Portela, G. F., & Villarreal-Nieto, O. D. (2024). Sweat rate, sweat sodium losses, and body composition in professional male soccer players in Southwest Colombia. *Medicina*, *60*(1), 113. DOI: 10.3390/medicina60010113 PMID: 38256373

Sun, S., Reagan, K., Seker, E., & Vega, K. (2024). GLUCAT: a feline Biofluids IoT hub for electrochemical glucose biosensing. *TEI '24: Proceedings of the Eighteenth International Conference on Tangible, Embedded, and Embodied Interaction*, 70. DOI: 10.1145/3623509.3635250

Taha, B. A., Addie, A. J., Haider, A. J., & Arsad, N. (2025). Nanosensors Based on Breathomics for Human Disease Diagnosis: A New Frontier in Personalized Healthcare. *BioNanoScience*, *15*(2). Advance online publication. DOI: 10.1007/s12668-025-01876-9

Tania, M. H., Lwin, K. T., Shabut, A. M., Najlah, M., Chin, J., & Hossain, M. (2019). Intelligent image-based colourimetric tests using machine learning framework for lateral flow assays. *Expert Systems with Applications*, *139*, 112843. DOI: 10.1016/j.eswa.2019.112843

Tasnim, T., Sugireng, S., Imran, I., & Akib, N. I. (2024). Analysis of differences in early detection of chronic kidney disease with urine creatinine, proteins and individual health status based on behavioural, stress and genetic factors in Kendari City, Indonesia. *Public Health of Indonesia*, *10*(2), 203–213. DOI: 10.36685/phi.v10i2.801

Tian, L., Jiang, M., Su, M., Cao, X., Jiang, Q., Liu, Q., & Yu, C. (2022). Sweat cortisol determination utilizing MXene and multi-walled carbon nanotube nanocomposite functionalized immunosensor. *Microchemical Journal, 185*, 108172. DOI: 10.1016/j.microc.2022.108172

Van De Sande, N., Ramakers, I. H. G. B., Visser, P. J., Verhey, F. R. J., Verbraak, F. D., Bouwman, F. H., Berendschot, T. T. J. M., Nuijts, R. M. M. A., Webers, C. B., & Gijs, M. (2023). Tear biomarkers for Alzheimer's disease screening and diagnosis (the TearAD study): Design and rationale of an observational longitudinal multicenter study. *BMC Neurology, 23*(1). Advance online publication. DOI: 10.1186/s12883-023-03335-y PMID: 37543602

Vrazhnov, D. A., Ovchinnikova, D. A., Kabanova, T. V., Paulish, A. G., Kistenev, Y. V., Nikolaev, N. A., & Cherkasova, O. P. (2024). Terahertz Time-Domain spectroscopy of blood serum for differentiation of glioblastoma and traumatic brain injury. *Applied Sciences (Basel, Switzerland), 14*(7), 2872. DOI: 10.3390/app14072872

Wali, R., Moulaee, K., Qasymeh, M., Maalej, R., & Neri, G. (2024). Atomic layer deposition of NiO-Coated CNT nanocomposites: Tailoring electrochemical properties for salivary lactate detection. *Journal of Electroanalytical Chemistry (Lausanne, Switzerland), 971*, 118594. DOI: 10.1016/j.jelechem.2024.118594

Wang, T., Huang, X., Huang, H., Luo, P., & Qing, L. (2022). Nanomaterial-based optical- and electrochemical-biosensors for urine glucose detection: A comprehensive review. *Advanced Sensor and Energy Materials, 1*(3), 100016. DOI: 10.1016/j.asems.2022.100016

Wasilewski, T., Kamysz, W., & Gębicki, J. (2024). AI-Assisted detection of biomarkers by sensors and biosensors for early diagnosis and monitoring. *Biosensors (Basel), 14*(7), 356. DOI: 10.3390/bios14070356 PMID: 39056632

Weerarathna, I. N., Kumar, P., Dzoagbe, H. Y., & Kiwanuka, L. (2025). Advancements in Micro/Nanorobots in Medicine: Design, actuation, and Transformative Application. *ACS Omega, 10*(6), 5214–5250. DOI: 10.1021/acsomega.4c09806 PMID: 39989765

Wiewiora, M., Jopek, J., Świętochowska, E., Sławomir, G., Piecuch, J., Gąska, M., & Piecuch, J. (2023). Blood-based protein biomarkers and red blood cell aggregation in pancreatic cancer. *Clinical Hemorheology and Microcirculation, 85*(4), 371–383. DOI: 10.3233/ch-231814 PMID: 37718785

Wu, W., Yang, J., Zhou, Y., Zheng, Q., Chen, Q., Bai, Z., & Niu, J. (2023). Chemometrics-based signal processing methods for biosensors in health and environment: A review. *Electroanalysis*, *36*(7). Advance online publication. DOI: 10.1002/elan.202300207

Wu, Z., Qiao, Z., Chen, S., Fan, S., Liu, Y., Qi, J., & Lim, C. T. (2024). Interstitial fluid-based wearable biosensors for minimally invasive healthcare and biomedical applications. *Communications Materials*, *5*(1). Advance online publication. DOI: 10.1038/s43246-024-00468-6

Xu, C., Wu, F., Duan, Z., Rajbanshi, B., Qi, Y., Qin, J., Dai, L., Liu, C., Jin, T., Zhang, B., & Zhang, X. (2025). Microneedle-aided nanotherapeutics delivery and nanosensor intervention in advanced tissue regeneration. *Journal of Nanobiotechnology*, *23*(1). Advance online publication. DOI: 10.1186/s12951-025-03383-1 PMID: 40319333

Xu, R., Zi, Y., Dai, L., Yu, H., & Zhu, M. (2024). Advancing Medical Diagnostics with Deep Learning and Data Preprocessing. *International Journal of Innovative Research in Computer Science & Technology*, *12*(3), 143–147. DOI: 10.55524/ijircst.2024.12.3.24

Yadav, N., Narang, J., Chhillar, A. K., Rana, J. S., Siddique, M. U. M., Kenawy, E., Alkahtani, S., Ahsan, M. N., Nayak, A. K., & Hasnain, M. S. (2023). Diagnostic methods employing kidney biomarkers clinching biosensors as promising tools. *Sensors International*, *5*, 100253. DOI: 10.1016/j.sintl.2023.100253

Yammouri, G., & Lahcen, A. A. (2024). AI-Reinforced wearable sensors and intelligent Point-of-Care tests. *Journal of Personalized Medicine*, *14*(11), 1088. DOI: 10.3390/jpm14111088 PMID: 39590580

Yang, Y., Sheng, C., Dong, F., & Liu, S. (2024). An integrated wearable differential microneedle array for continuous glucose monitoring in interstitial fluids. *Biosensors & Bioelectronics*, *256*, 116280. DOI: 10.1016/j.bios.2024.116280 PMID: 38603840

Ye, H., Chen, X., Huang, X., Li, C., Yin, X., Zhao, W., & Wang, T. (2024). Patterned gold nanoparticle superlattice film for wearable sweat sensors. *Nano Letters*, *24*(35), 11082–11089. DOI: 10.1021/acs.nanolett.4c03254 PMID: 39171663

Yin, S., Chen, X., Li, R., Sun, L., Yao, C., & Li, Z. (2024). Wearable, biocompatible, and Dual-Emission ocular multisensor patch for continuous profiling of fluoroquinolone antibiotics in tears. *ACS Nano*, *18*(28), 18522–18533. DOI: 10.1021/acsnano.4c04153 PMID: 38963059

Yu, W., Mou, S., Zhang, X., Sun, J., Xue, Y., Xiong, H., Hsia, K. J., Wan, H., & Wang, P. (2024). Application of sensing devices in the detection of oral, pulmonary, and gastrointestinal diseases. *Chemosensors (Basel, Switzerland)*, *12*(4), 57. DOI: 10.3390/chemosensors12040057

Yuan, X., Ouaskioud, O., Yin, X., Li, C., Ma, P., Yang, Y., Yang, P., Xie, L., & Ren, L. (2023). Epidermal wearable biosensors for the continuous monitoring of biomarkers of chronic disease in interstitial fluid. *Micromachines*, *14*(7), 1452. DOI: 10.3390/mi14071452 PMID: 37512763

Zeng, Z., Li, W., Zhang, J., Hu, Z., Wu, J., Ye, G., & Luo, Y. (2024). Highly sensitive and specific graphene oxide-based FRET aptasensor for quantitative detection of human soluble growth stimulating gene protein 2. *Talanta*, *271*, 125629. DOI: 10.1016/j.talanta.2024.125629 PMID: 38245955

Zhang, M., Wang, Y., You, B., Qi, Z., Wang, Y., & Zhang, Z. (2024). Nickel oxide decorated popcorn derived biochar as a non-invasive electrochemical sensor for sensitive detection of glucose in saliva. *Journal of Alloys and Compounds*, *1010*, 177427. DOI: 10.1016/j.jallcom.2024.177427

Zhang, Y., Bi, K., Zhou, L., Wang, J., Huang, L., Sun, Y., Peng, G., & Wu, W. (2024). Advances in blood biomarkers for Alzheimer's Disease: Ultra-Sensitive Detection Technologies and Impact on clinical diagnosis. *Degenerative Neurological and Neuromuscular Disease*, *14*, 85–102. DOI: 10.2147/dnnd.s471174 PMID: 39100640

Zhang, Y., Yan, P., Tang, H., & Zhang, J. (2023). Rapid detection of tear lactoferrin for diagnosis of dry eyes by using fluorescence polarization-based aptasensor. *Scientific Reports*, *13*(1). Advance online publication. DOI: 10.1038/s41598-023-42484-5 PMID: 37704755

Zhang, Z., Li, Z., Wei, K., Cao, Z., Zhu, Z., & Chen, R. (2024). Sweat as a source of non-invasive biomarkers for clinical diagnosis: An overview. *Talanta*, *273*, 125865. DOI: 10.1016/j.talanta.2024.125865 PMID: 38452593

Zhao, H., Zhao, H., Wang, J., Ren, J., Yao, J., Li, Y., & Zhang, R. (2023). Bovine OMASUM-Inspired Interfacial Carbon-Based nanocomposite for saliva metabolic screening of gastric cancer. *Analytical Chemistry*, *95*(30), 11296–11305. DOI: 10.1021/acs.analchem.3c01358 PMID: 37458487

Chapter 8
Medical Robots Applications in Surgery

Jyoti R. Munavalli
https://orcid.org/0000-0002-0811-1499
BNM Institute of Technology, Bangalore, India

Rajeshwari B. S.
Institute of Health Management Research, Bangalore, India

Sunil Kumar C. N.
Narayana Health, India

Pradeep Narayan
Narayana Health, India

ABSTRACT

Medical robots are sophisticated machines designed to assist healthcare professionals in performing complex medical procedures with precision, accuracy, and minimal invasiveness. Medical robots utilize cutting-edge technologies such as artificial intelligence, machine learning, and sensor systems to enhance surgical outcomes, reduce recuperation periods, and ultimately enhance patient care and happiness. Medical robots are adept at handling even the most delicate jobs. Thus, the use of medical robots in a variety of surgical specialties has grown, including cardiology, urology, neurology, and orthopedics. The real-time data and visualization capabilities of medical robots help surgeons to make more educated decisions, lower the risk of complications, and ultimately improve patient outcomes. This chapter explains different kinds of medical robots, their parts, surgical uses, advantages,

DOI: 10.4018/979-8-3373-1514-0.ch008

challenges, and upcoming developments in surgical medical robots. Lastly, the authors present a case study of Narayana Health in Bangalore, India, where every day robotic procedures are carried out.

1. INTRODUCTION TO MEDICAL ROBOTS

Robots are intelligent machines that blend physical capabilities with mental processing, empowering them to undertake tasks autonomously or under human direction. Robots are used in applications such as security, agriculture, disaster management, manufacturing, military, food preparations, healthcare, and entertainment (Gyles, 2019; O. Mohan Banur, Feb 2024; Sindhwani, 2024; Singh, 2024). The robots when used in medical field are referred as medical robots. Medical robots leverage robotic technology to optimize healthcare delivery, supporting medical professionals and elevating patient outcomes (Leung & Vyas, 2014; Rivero-Moreno et al., 2023). Unlike traditional medical instruments, these systems combine fine-tuned mechanical components with smart sensing and control, allowing them to carry out delicate and complex procedures with remarkable precision. Robotics has diverse applications, including diagnostic robotics, surgical robotics, rehabilitation and assistive robotics, hospital automation and service robots, as well as remote and preventive care. AI powered diagnostics reduce clinician burnout and improve precision and reduce wait times. Examples are Babylon Health's AI Chatbot, Da Vinci robotic surgeries. Elderly care and assistive robots aide the aging population and declining healthcare workforce. Examples are Paro, Cyberdyne HAL and Japan METI. A major breakthrough came with the ROBODOC system, which was among the first used in orthopaedic surgeries. This was followed by the widely known da Vinci Surgical System, which opened new possibilities in minimally invasive surgery. This chapter focusses on surgical robots/robotic surgery.

The global demand for robotic surgeries have increased in recent years. By 2030, this market is projected to exceed $25 billion. This demand is driven by increase in adoption of minimally invasive procedures, aging populations, and surgical precision requirements (Fortune Business Insights, 2024). In the United States alone, in 2023, more than 1.8 million robotic-assisted surgeries were performed.

North America continues to dominate the global medical robotics market due to its early adoption of advanced technologies, structured reimbursement frameworks, and the availability of highly skilled surgical professionals. In contrast, Europe and the Asia-Pacific region are emerging as high-growth markets, fuelled by increasing investments in healthcare robotics. Countries such as India, China, and Japan are making significant progress in this domain. According to Fortune Business Insights

(2023), India has experienced a nearly 400% rise in robotic surgeries over the past five years, with more than 100 robotic platforms deployed across leading hospitals.

This growth underscores the critical role of medical robots in transforming healthcare delivery worldwide. As global demand for these procedures continues to rise, there is a pressing need to investigate the capabilities and challenges of these evolving technologies. Despite this momentum, significant gaps remain in the areas of system design, contextual adaptability, affordability, and large-scale deployment, particularly in developing regions (Mehta et al., 2022).

While the potential of medical robotics is widely acknowledged, a structured exploration is essential to evaluate its real-world applications, implications, and future trajectories.

Study objectives:

- To trace the historical evolution of medical robots and analyze their current and emerging roles within the frameworks of Industry 4.0 and Healthcare 5.0.
- To classify medical robots based on their functions and components, and evaluate how these classifications impact their levels of autonomy and operational performance.
- To examine the applications of medical robots across rehabilitative, diagnostic, remote care settings and particularly surgical applications, highlighting real-world use cases.
- To assess the advantages and clinical outcomes of medical robotic systems for patients, healthcare professionals, and overall health system efficiency.
- To identify key limitations and adoption barriers associated with medical robots.
- To explore the potential of emerging technologies, such as artificial intelligence, cloud computing, and nanotechnology, in enhancing the functionality of future medical robotic systems.

By addressing these questions, this chapter aims to offer a holistic understanding of next-generation medical robotics—from foundational technologies and classification to impact analysis, case-based insights, and strategic foresight.

The idea of automata dates back to ancient Greece and China. The rise of mechanical engineering and industrial automation in 18th century resulted in the formation of machine control logic. In the 20th century, the evolution of robotics began, combining mechanical ingenuity, electrical innovation, and computational intelligence. Table 1 shows the evolution of modern robots from 1960 to till date.

Table 1. Timeline of Innovation

Year	Robot Evolutions	Innovation
1985	Robotics 1.0	The PUMA 560 robot assists in a delicate neurosurgical biopsy—one of the first uses of robotics in surgery
1992	Robotics 2.0	ROBODOC becomes the first robot to assist in orthopaedic hip replacement procedures.
2000	Robotics 3.0	The **da Vinci Surgical System** receives FDA approval, changing the landscape of minimally invasive surgery.
2020	Robotics 4.0	Robots are increasingly used in rehabilitation, telemedicine, and even hospital logistics, such as medicine delivery and disinfection.

The period from 1960 to 1980 was the early stage of robotics that involved controllers, motors. From 1990 to 2000, it was a transforming stage and called as Robotics 2.0 that included sensors, 2D/3D machines. Big Bang Stage is from 2010 to 2020 which is Robotics 3.0 involved ROS, ROS2, NLP for natural interaction between human and robot, connectivity, high processing and AI were major part of this evolution. From 2020 onwards is termed as prosperous stage termed as Robotics 4.0 that uses Brain-on-cloud, Artificial Intelligence of Things, 5G communications, hybrid intelligence and perception (Gao, Wanyama, Singh, Gadhrri, & Schmidt, 2020).

Medical robots are the convergence of Industry 4.0 technologies (Sulaiman et al., 2021) (Ahsan & Siddique, 2022; Castro & Faria Araújo, 2020), Robotics and Healthcare 5.0 (Basulo-Ribeiro & Teixeira, 2024). Fig.1 shows how Industry 4.0 empowers Robotics and in turn robotics enables the Healthcare 5.0 transformations. Industry 4.0 refers to the fourth industrial revolution that focuses on connected technologies thereby providing digital infrastructure. Robotics provide multi arm robots capable of performing tasks like telepresence, mobility and assistance. Healthcare 5.0 is human-centric and personalized. It focusses on accessibility, sustainability and inclusivity. The synergy between these three domains shows a paradigm shift towards intelligent, integrated and patient centric healthcare. This convergence is vast and transformative.

Figure 1. Convergence of Industry 4.0, Robotics and Healthcare 5.0

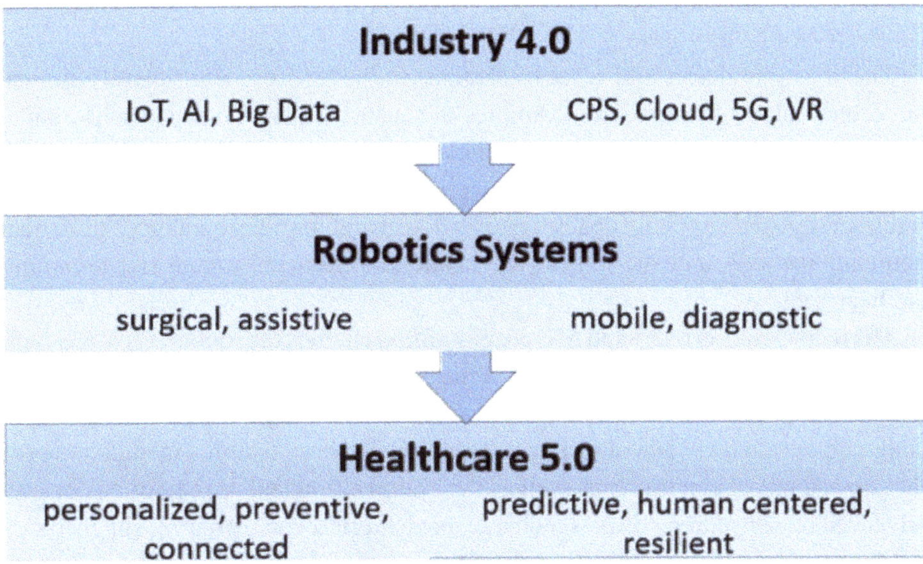

2. CHARACTERISTICS OF MEDICAL ROBOTS

Medical robots make use of robotic innovations along with medical expertise to boost patient care and streamline medical processes. Robots have different characteristics as shown in Fig. 2. The physical characteristics include the physical body/structure, the size - micro or large, weight that depends on materials and what types of materials to be used – metal, plastic or composites that do not cause infection and are sterile. These characteristics enable medical robots to interact effectively with patients and hospital environments. Their appearance is sleek with compact designs so that their navigation in constrained spaces become easier. They are flexible with their movements as advanced materials are used in building medical robots. Titanium and aluminium have light weight properties and provide strength and durability. High resolution cameras, sensors and displays are used to capture critical information that are useful during surgeries.

The key features of functional characteristics are precision, autonomy, speed and power. Precision allows the medical robots to perform delicate procedures with high accuracy and minimum errors. The functional features include the capacity to function autonomously, where advanced navigation is required to move efficiently and safely in complex environments. These robots are designed to be adaptable, reprogrammed and reconfigured so that they can be used for applications like surgery, rehabilitation and health education. The robots have advanced control systems and use electric or battery power.

The ability to detect and react to changes in the environment, identify things, and detect touch and sound are examples of sensory traits. Advanced sensors like ultrasound sensors, cameras, tactile sensors, pressure sensors, vibration sensors and electromagnetic sensors assist robots in visualizing, tracking and monitoring. Force sensors and haptic feedback systems detect and mimic the nuances of human tactile interaction/ Acoustic sensors detect and interpret vital sounds like breathing and heartbeat.

The incorporation of AI and ML programming enables the robots to learn, adapt, and make effective decisions, is what is meant by the cognitive features. Complex information is processed to take informed decisions. Large datasets are analysed using computer vision and algorithms. Additional energy features include the production and use of electricity as well as the optimization and upkeep of power use. Advanced power sources such as rechargeable batteries, energy harvesting methods and super-capacitors are utilized to minimize energy consumption. Medical robots can be wirelessly charged, flexible and portable.

Interaction, adaptation, and cooperation with people are all part of the behavioural features. Medical robots exhibit social behaviour by engaging with patients and healthcare professionals. For this, facial recognition, natural language processing and emotional intelligence are used. Ultimately, the performance attributes include safety, dependability, efficiency, and precision. Additionally, the robots have to be affordable, scalable, adaptable, and simple to maintain (Albustanji, Elmanaseer, & Alkhatib, 2023; Bai et al., 2023; Flatebø, Tran, Wang, & Bongo, 2024; Richert, Shehadeh, Müller, Schröder, & Jeschke, 2016; Warnecke & Schiele, 1985).

Figure 2. Characteristics of Medical Robots

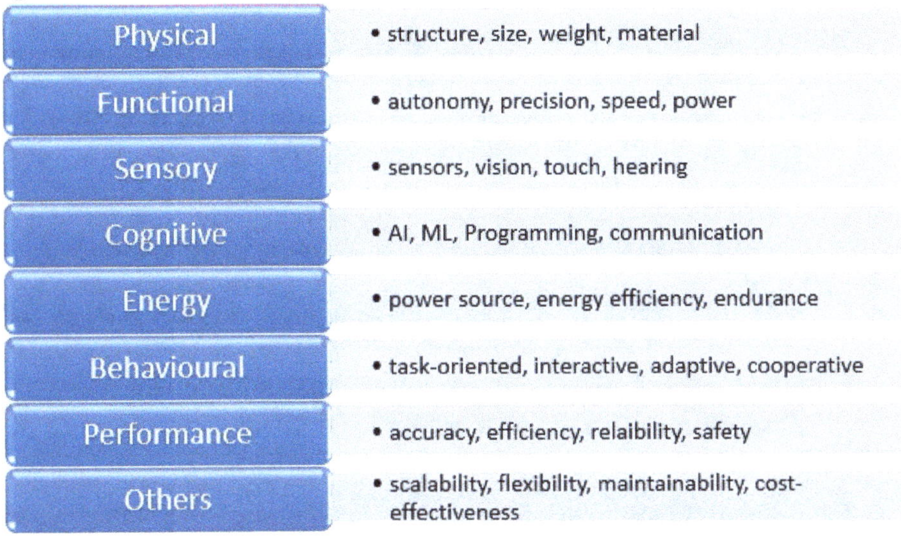

3. Classification of Medical Robots

Generally, robots are classified based on their functionality, applications, design, specialization and emerging categories. The different types of robots are Industrial robots, Service robots, Autonomous Robots, humanoid robots, social robots and flying robots (Fig. 3) (Javaid et al., 2025). All these robots find their applications in medical field as follows:

1. **Industrial robots**: These are programmable mechanical arms that perform repetitive tasks. These are used as surgical robots for their precise movements, high accuracy, speed, endurance and automation. The industrial robots are used in robotic surgery, medical device manufacturing, hospital logistics, lab automation, rehab robotics and pharma robotics. The surgical robots require sterile environments and accurate navigation (Rivero-Moreno et al., 2023; Urrea & Kern, 2025; Zenati & Mahvash, 2012). Few industrial robots used in medical robotics are KUKA, ABB, Universal Robots, Fanuc, Staubli and Yaskawa. These robots make use of AI, ML and sensor integration thereby reducing assembly times around 30% and improving the quality by 15%. These also minimize the errors and energy usage.

Figure 3. Classification based on Applications

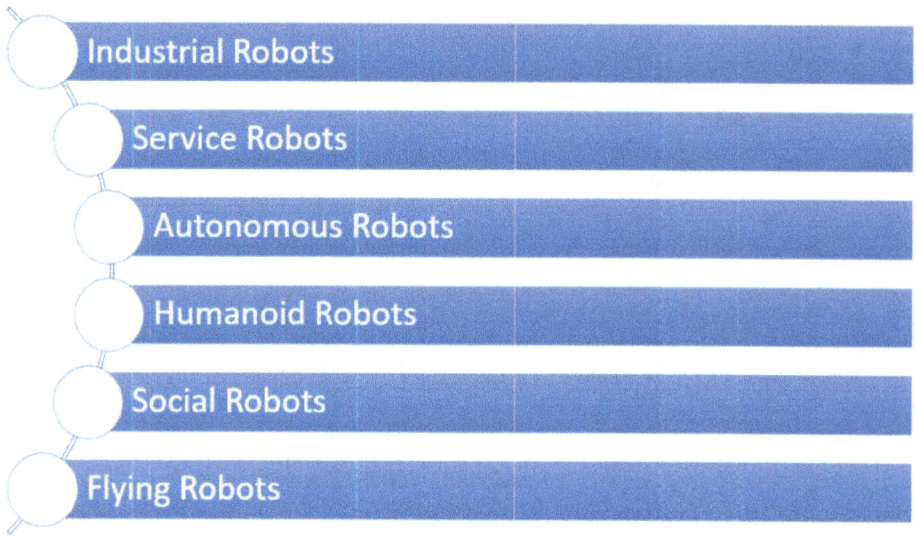

2. **Service robots**: The service robots are machines designed to assist people by performing useful tasks, often in environments like homes, hospitals, hotels, or offices. Unlike industrial robots, which are typically confined to manufacturing settings, service robots interact more directly with humans in everyday situations. These robots are used as hospital service robots for assistance with tasks and interactions with humans. These focus on healthcare tasks and patient transportation and other logistics (Zhang, Liu, Qiao, & Fan, 2023). The service robots can perform various tasks like delivering food, equipment and medications, cleaning floors, rehabilitation exercises etc. These robots are equipped with various kinds of sensors and cameras. The collected data is processed using AI algorithms that help in navigating through a defined area, recognizing faces and understanding audio commands. Robots like *TUG* and *Robear* have been implemented to reduce physical strain on healthcare workers.
3. **Autonomous robots**: These robots in medical field are designed to operate with minimal human intervention, basically depend on Artificial Intelligence, Computer Vision and sensor technology. Most prominent applications of autonomous robots is in surgical assistance. Most of them are tele-operated robots which perform independent operations and navigations. These robots are specifically for remote communication through video conferencing. The robots perform tasks based on pre-programmed rules or real-time imaging These robots also

assist in patient monitoring through vital measurements, mobility support and reminder systems for patients (Kubota, Ogawa, Yoshikawa, & Ishiguro, 2022).

4. **Humanoid robots**: These robots look like humans in physical structure and interaction. These robots find their applications as rehabilitation robots. These robots perform human-like interactions with patients. These are used for elderly care, physio-therapies, and recoveries after surgery and so on. These are also employed as receptionists in hospital environments by greeting patients, check-in processes. Robots such as *PEPPER* and *NAO* are programmed to engage patients in conversation, lead them through physical therapy exercises, or offer cognitive stimulation through games and memory tasks.
5. **Social robots**: These robots are the assistive robots that aide in providing human interactions and assist on daily activities of patients. These are impactful in mental health, autism therapy support and paediatric care (Flatebø et al., 2024; Richert et al., 2016). Robots like *MEDi* and *NAO* can engage young patients through storytelling, games, or guided breathing exercises, creating a more relaxed and positive clinical experience. Robots such as *PARO*, a therapeutic seal robot, have been deployed in eldercare facilities and psychiatric wards to provide comfort and reduce feelings of loneliness or anxiety.
6. **Flying robots**: Often called as drones are unmanned vehicles. Drones are used in emergency medical delivery, to transport medical supplies and blood samples. In poor infrastructure regions, these drones reduce delivery times. Drones equipped with automated external defibrillators (AEDs) have been tested to reach victims faster than ambulances. In pilot programs across Europe and North America, AED drones have been shown to arrive several minutes ahead of traditional emergency services.

All these types of medical robots prioritize precision, sterility, and patient safety with all the guidelines provided by regulatory associations. Few examples of medical robots are Da Vinci Surgical System (Intuitive Surgical) (Fig. 4), Robear (RIKEN), REEM (Pal Robotics), Pepper (SoftBank Robotics), Mako (Stryker), Medtronic's Mazor X, Brain-Computer Interface (BCI) robots (Leung & Vyas, 2014; Rivero-Moreno et al., 2023).

Figure 4. Photograph of Da Vinci Surgical System

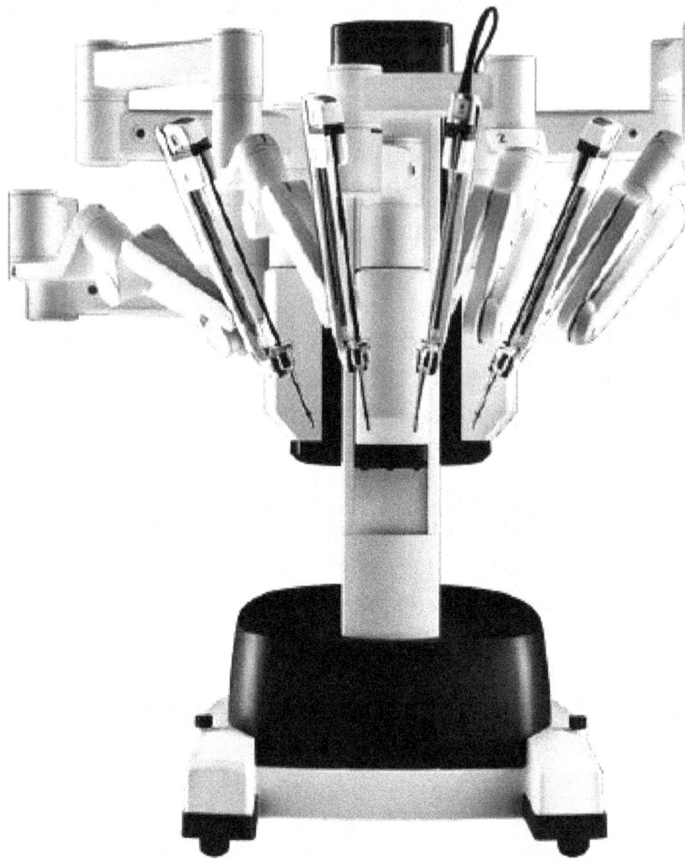

Another way of classification of medical robots is based on model of operations which mainly highlights the human intervention, safety, and decision-making control (Fig. 5).(Kubota et al., 2022; Seppänen, Vepsäläinen, Ojala, & Tammi, 2022; Trivino, Mengual, & van der Heide, 2009)

Figure 5. Classification based on mode of operations

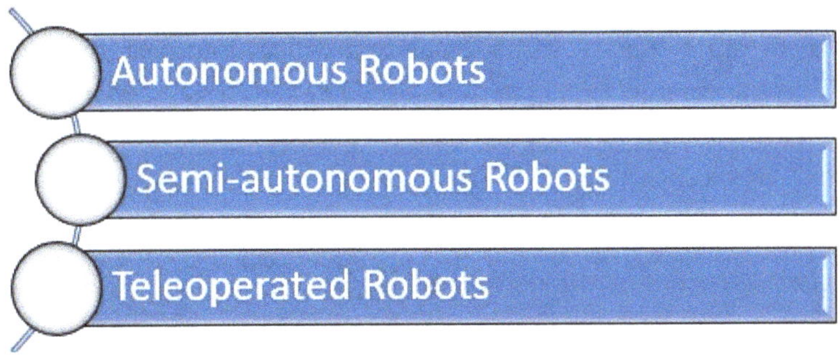

1. Autonomous robots

These robots operate independently with any intervention of humans. These robots are programmed in such a way using AI and ML algorithms that these are capable of taking decisions depending on the sensor data. These robots are highly adaptive to their changing environment. Autonomous medical robots can handle very efficiently. These types of robots have high efficiency and reduced labor costs but developmental cost will be high.

2. Semi-Autonomous robots

These robots are monitored by human though these have all autonomous capabilities. Critical decisions are taken by human whereas the tasks are performed by robots. The design mainly focuses on efficiency and safety. These types of medical robots are used for surgery in hospitals. These have balanced autonomy and human control so it has improved human safety. There is possibility of communication errors.

3. Teleoperated robots

These robots are controlled remotely by humans via communication systems. The sensors and camera act as input based on which doctors take decisions and communicate back to the robots to perform the tasks.

4. MEDICAL ROBOT COMPONENTS & TECHNOLOGIES

The medical robot consists of hardware and software to perform the tasks intelligently. It is a special robotic system that is designed to assist doctors in medical tasks like diagnostics, surgery, patient care and logistics. The core components of medical robot are as shown in the Fig. 6.

Figure 6. Components of Medical Robots

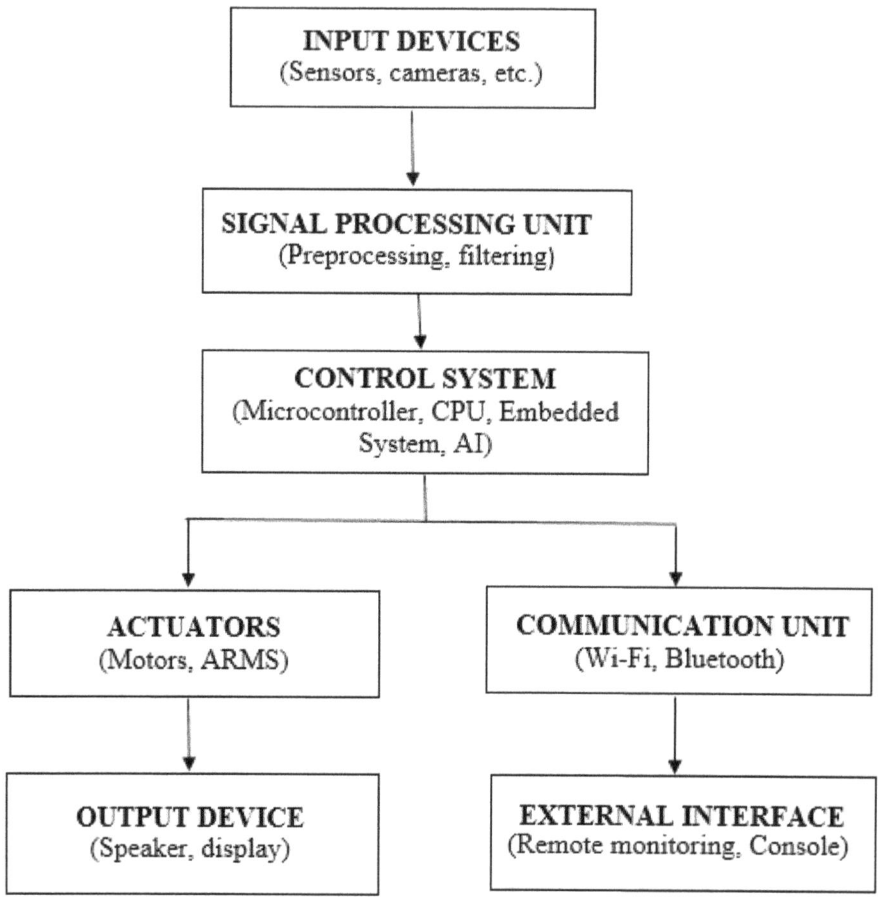

The input devices collect real time data like patient vitals, positions and images through sensors like camera, optical sensors, force, pressure and vibration sensors and microphones are used for visualization and proximity detection. The Signal processing unit prepares and processes the data such as pre-processing techniques, filtering for noise removal, that help robot to take control decisions. The control system consists of microcontroller, embedded systems, CPU and AI models that makes decisions based on the processed data. The control unit acts as a brain of the robot and processes all the information. Actuators are the physical components that actually performs the actions like arm movement, leg movement etc. The mechanical components are the arms, end effectors, actuators and frames and chassis used in all the movements for the robot.

The communication unit sends and receives data from/to external systems. The navigation system consists of GPS, localization, and mapping for the robot to navigate correctly without collision. Output devices displays the information using speakers or display units/screens. They also provide feedbacks. External interface is the user interaction that is performed through Human Machine interface unit. The robot also has real-time operating system, AI components for data analytics and decision making, and communication and networking protocols. Medical specific components like medical imaging, patient monitoring, sterilization systems (UV, radiation, chemical), disinfection systems, surgical instruments and pharmacological systems are also included (Adiuku, Avdelidis, Tang, & Plastropoulos, 2024; Gul, Rahiman, & Nazli Alhady, 2019; Kapoor, Deguet, & Kazanzides, 2006).

The key technologies used in medical robots are Artificial Intelligence (AI), Robot Operating Systems (ROS), Internet of Things (IoT), Sensor Fusion and Human-Machine Interface (HMI). (Fig. 7).

Figure 7. Key technologies used in Medical Robots

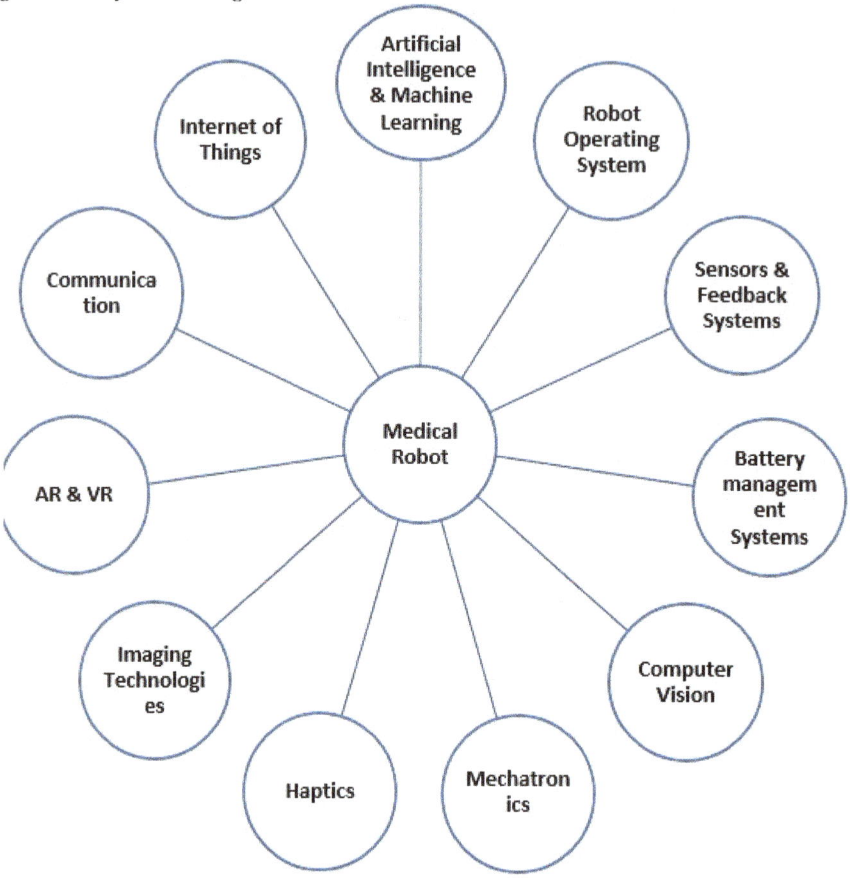

AI & ML has transformed medical robots in a big way. These are used in decision-making, image analysis, diagnosis support and surgical planning. These help to improve precision and enhance tool positioning and tremor reduction. They provide better accuracy and faster recovery. ML models detect anomalies through scans. ML models also monitor the patient's vitals and alert doctors thereby reducing mortality. AI analyses patient history and provide personalised medicines and schedules. Commonly used techniques in medical robotics are Convolutional Neural Networks, RNN, Reinforcement Learning, supervised learning and unsupervised learning. Motion smoothing, supervised learning and image guided tool tracking are used in Da Vinci Surgical System. Moxi Robot uses reinforcement learning and behaviour cloning for hospital logistics, particularly workflow automation.

Robot Operating System is a flexible framework for writing robot software to provide communication between components, simulation and visualization tools. The

ROS provides modular development, real-time data exchange, AI & ML integration (TensorFlow,PyTorch, OpenCV), multiple sensor combination and obstacle detection and path planning. ROS tools used are RViz, Gazebo, ros_control, Movelt! And TF.

Sensors provide continuous data in real-time and feedback systems adjust actions accordingly. Temperature sensors, proximity sensors, force sensors, infrared sensors, ECG and EMG sensors, pressure sensors, cameras, ultrasonic sensors and inertial measurement unit are used in medical robots. Feedback systems use sensor data and adjust arm position, grip pressure, detect obstruction and so on. All these sensors are integrated with ROS.

Battery management is a critical aspect in medical robots as these robots must be reliable, available and safe. Battery Management System (BMS) should monitor voltage, current and temperature, protect from overheating, send battery health through CAN or UART to microcontroller and estimate battery runtime using AI and ML algorithms.

Computer vision helps the robots to see and understand the environment around it. With this, robots can interpret visual data and make decisions. It uses AI, deep learning and image processing techniques. Different types of cameras are used such as RGB cameras, depth cameras, infrared cameras, endoscopic and stereo vision cameras. DICOM and NIFTI images are used.

Mechatronics is a combination of mechanical and electronics. Mechanical systems like joints, arms, gears and structures are used for robotic arms and exoskeleton frames that hep robots to move precisely. Da Vinci uses mechanical arms, servo motors, camera vision and haptic feedback where surgeons control the micro-scale precision.

Haptics deals with the sense or touch. This helps doctors to feel the force during operation. Haptic interfaces are joysticks, gloves and styluses.

Imaging techniques use the modalities like endoscopy, ultrasound, x-ray, CT Scan, PET, 3D surface scanning, Optical Coherence Tomography and MRI. Imaging techniques provide visual guidance, intraoperative navigation and postoperative analysis. Medical robots use tools like 3D slicer, OpenCV, MITK, ROS+rviz for implementing the imaging techniques. Recent innovations in this domain are fused imaging where CT, MRI and ultrasound are integrated for real-time surgery and use of augmented reality.

AR & VR are the technologies that make training more immersive and interactive. AR implementation uses cameras, tracking systems and haptic feedback. It also uses tools such as HoloLens, Oculus Rift, Quest, Unity, Vuforia, ARKit,ARCore and Leap Motion. Real world examples are Medivis SurgicalAR which uses AR guided robotic neurosurgery and MindMaze where VR rehab robots for stroke patients.

Communication technologies facilitates exchange of data between robots and doctors/humans, sensors and controllers and robots to other robots. For internal communication, that is inside the robots, technologies used are UART, RS-485,

CAN Bus, I2C and SPI. For external communication, we use the technologies like Wi-Fi, Bluetooth, 5G, Zigbee, Ethernet, MQTT and HL7. These technologies must also provide security so the sensitive data should be encrypted, authenticated and reliable. Da Vinci uses CAN for ARM control and Ethernet for camera feeding, and hospital network for remote access.

Internet of Things (IoT) is integration of sensors, actuators, cloud systems and communication systems so that medical robots can interact with each other to send/ receive data or commands. IoT aides in scalable solutions where multiple robots can be managed remotely.

5. SURGICAL APPLICATIONS OF MEDICAL ROBOTS

Robotic technology has transformed the field of surgery, enabling healthcare professionals to perform procedures with greater precision, accuracy, and minimal invasiveness. The integration of robotic systems in surgical procedures has led to remarkable advancements in healthcare, marked by rapid growth. Robotic-assisted surgery overcomes human limitations, enhancing precision and optimizing patient outcomes (Biswas, Sikander, & Kulkarni, 2023; Bora et al., 2020; Lengyel, Chinnadurai, Corr, Lumsden, & Bavare, 2024; Zenati & Mahvash, 2012). India's journey with robotic surgery began in 2006 with the introduction of the da Vinci S system at the All-India Institute of Medical Sciences (AIIMS), New Delhi. Since then, the country has witnessed significant expansion: 66 specialized robotic surgery centres, over 500 trained robotic surgeons and more than 12,800 successful procedures performed as of July 2019.

The surgeries performed by robots should be distinguished from the traditional surgery and the laparoscopic surgery. Traditionally, surgeries are performed by opening the human body, doing the procedure, and suturing the body. Laparoscopic surgery is performed by smaller incisions and inserting scopes to visualize the internal organs. Surgery is performed by manually articulating instruments inserted through these small incisions of a centimetre in dimension. In robotic surgery the articulation of these instruments is by the robots which are controlled by the surgeon. These instruments are inserted with the incision of about eight millimetres. The surgeon articulates the instruments through a console that provides three-dimensional images. Depending on the complication of the case and the reach of surgical area, one can choose laparoscopic or robotic surgery.

The medical robots are commonly used in the following surgeries.

- **Orthopaedic Surgery**: This is a minimally invasive surgical procedure where robots assist surgeons in total knee arthroplasty, partial knee arthroplasty, soft tissue surgery, joint replacement, joint resurfacing and fracture surgery thus by improving accuracy and reducing recovery time (Fan et al., 2025; Hu, Longo, Pittman, & Nazarian, 2025; Ram, Jeyaraman, Jeyaraman, Yadav, & Venkatasalam, 2023; Vanderstappen, van Ochten, & Verborgt, 2025; Wu, Zheng, & Zhang, 2024). The robotics systems used in orthopaedic surgery are Mako, Navio and Robodoc.

- **Neurosurgery**: This type of surgery utilizes robots to assist surgeons to enable precise dissection, resection, and implant placement in delicate brain and spinal procedures. Surgeries like Stereo-Electroencephalography, brain tumour resection, deep brain stimulation and cerebrovascular surgeries. The robotics systems used in neurosurgery are Medtronic's Rosa -Spine & Brain, Renishaw's neuromata, Brainlab's Cirq and Zeiss's OPMI Pentero. These robots use AI along with haptic for tactile feedback (Doulgeris et al., 2015; Jha & Chaurasia, 2024; Liu, Liu, Jin, & Wu, 2024).
- **Urologic Surgery**: The urinary tract includes the kidneys, bladder, and associated connective tissues and muscles. The male reproductive system encompasses the prostate gland, penis, testicles, and associated connective structures. Conditions that cause problems of these systems include, but are not limited to, enlarged prostate, benign tumours, and cancer and may require medical attention. Doctors perform many urologic procedures using minimally invasive laparoscopic or robotic-assisted surgery, possibly with da Vinci technology. The robotic-assisted prostatectomy, nephrectomy, and bladder surgery improve accuracy and reduce complications (Cuevas, Alvarado, González, Peña, & Castro, 2025; Koukourikis & Rha, 2021; Pokhrel et al., 2025).
- **Cardiothoracic Surgery**: Robotic-assisted surgery is a leading-edge procedure. It is minimally invasive which means that large surgical incisions are not required and the precision of the technology can be an ideal option for delicate and complex surgeries around the heart and in the chest. Robots enhance precision in coronary artery bypass grafting, mitral valve repair, and other complex procedures. Cardiothoracic surgeons also perform mediastina tumour resections, oesophageal resection and repair and diaphragmatic procedures. Wet lab simulation accelerates the learning process for robotic cardiac surgery (Harky & Hussain, 2019; Mori & Geirsson, 2024; Stuart, Meguid, & Rove, 2025; Zenati & Mahvash, 2012).
- **Ophthalmic Surgery**: In the field of ophthalmology, robotics is increasingly being used in surgical procedures and interventions. Robotic assistance provides significant advancements in distance sensing, improved visualization, tremor cancellation, and movement control. The development is still in its early phases because robotic technology has only lately been incorporated

into ophthalmology. In the field of ophthalmology, robotic technologies like the da Vinci Surgical System are being used to help surgeons perform intricate eye surgeries. Robotic-assisted eye surgery improves precision in cataract removal, retinal detachment repair, and glaucoma treatment (Gerber, Pettenkofer, & Hubschman, 2020; Madadi et al., 2024; Pandey & Sharma, 2019).

- **Reconstructive Surgery**: A state-of-the-art specialty that frequently sets the standard for surgical technical innovation is plastic and reconstructive surgery. Furthermore, it collaborates with many other surgical specialties, so practitioners are likely to come across advancements in robotic surgery in these other specialties. Plastic surgeons must thus embrace this new surgical platform, research its potential uses, and learn from those who have already incorporated robotics into their surgical toolbox. Robots assist with reconstruction, tissue transfer, and microsurgery (Dobbs, Cundy, Samarendra, Khan, & Whitaker, 2017; Nehme, Neville, & Bahsoun, 2017; Rojas Burbano et al., 2025; Seth, Lim, Chang, Rozen, & Ng, 2025).
- **Paediatric Surgery**: Compared to adult robotic surgery, paediatric robotic surgery is still in its infancy. Due to their smaller abdomens than adults, children present a challenge for paediatric robotic surgery. Because there is limited space for robotic arms, the cramped workspaces present a problem for robotic surgery. The typical adult instruments are used in paediatrics; no specialized robots or robotic instruments are available. The same tools and robot will be used by the robotic surgeon for both children and the elderly. Indeed, paediatric robotic surgery has advanced significantly over the last 20 years. Despite having success rates comparable to those of standard laparoscopy, a significant number of surgical procedures were carried out on children with the aid of robots. It's a new field, so there are still a lot of challenges (Ballouhey et al., 2025; Boscarelli et al., 2023; Esposito et al., 2025; Mei & Tang, 2023; Sutyak & Tsao, 2024).

6. IMPACT OF ROBOTIC SURGERIES

Robots offer many benefits in the field of Medicine ranging from simple drug delivery to advanced minimally invasive surgery in the compact areas of human body with vital organs. The benefits of robotic surgery can be distinguished as clinical and nonclinical benefits.

6.1. Clinical Outcomes

Clinical benefits can be further distinguished into benefits for the doctor delivering care and that for the patients. Enhanced precision, minimally invasive procedure, enhanced visualization and access, standardization, reduced surgeon fatigue, ergonomic strain and reduced risks of infections and complications are the benefits to using medical robots in surgeries. Reduced trauma and shorter recovery are the benefits the patients.

Benefits for the Surgeons

- **Improved Precision**: Enhanced dexterity and accuracy by the robots are the advantages that the robots provide for the surgeon operating the patients. The robots have extended arm length and can perform intricate movement. These movement can be for accessing remote areas in the closed cavities in the body from the back the organs leading to improved access for the surgery, thus giving better success and surgical outcomes (Rojas Burbano et al., 2025; Wah, 2025).
- **Enhanced Visualization**: The visualization of the surgical areas is enhanced using robots. This is possible using a High-definition two or even three-dimensional imaging. This enhanced visualization will aid in better analysis and characterisation of the surgical site during complex procedures. This will lead to lesser complications during surgery thereby enhancing surgical skills of the surgeon(Rahman, Bristi, Yesmin, & Islam, 2025).

Benefits for the Patients

- **Reduced Trauma**: Robotic surgery involves minimal incisions to access the body cavities which leads to less tissue damage including blood loss. As less raw tissue is exposed there are lesser infections and thus minimization of the pain experienced by the patients. As a result of minimal incision, the cosmetic outcome of robotic surgery is enormous for the patient's point of view.
- **Shorter Recovery**: The robotic surgery needs minimal incision, leading to lesser exposure, reduced tissue damage and disruption leading to minimal scarring, as a result the patients experience less pain. Less pain means the patients can mobilize sooner leading to quicker recovery. This also translates to less time spent in hospitals and earlier return to normal activities.

6.2. Non-Clinical Outcomes

The medical robots offer certain advantages to the organization in terms of improved productivity and revenue due to medical value travel.

- **Improved productivity:** The increased ability to perform better surgeries and minimal complications by the surgeons transforms into better productivity. A surgeon can treat more patients bringing revenue to the organization. This also translates into earlier breakeven of the investment by the organization, furthering the investments and technological advancement to the next phases.
- **Medical Value Travel**: Earlier known as Medical Tourism is providing medical and surgical care to patients of foreign origin who visit Indian hospitals as cost of care is less in India. Robotic surgery provides an opportunity for organisations to increase their revenue by catering to a larger patient population from around the world. This high-end care boosts the revenue to the hospital by attracting patients seeking quality care from overseas. This also builds on the organization's reputation in foreign soil as the centre for advanced care. Thus, robotic surgery not only enhances revenue but provides the opportunity to enhance organizations credibility leading to further growth.

7. CHALLENGES AND LIMITATIONS

Though robotic surgeries provide enormous benefits, these are accompanied by certain challenges that comes as a result of the being the high-end technology. The challenges include technical limitations, regulatory framework for use of such technologies, need for additional training and education, cost of surgery and affordability by the patients, acceptance by the patients, and availability of this surgery in various locations.

Technical Limitations: The robotic surgeries can be used in abdominal cavities needing extensive manoeuvring with obtuse digitization, but they cannot be used in biological area with limited spaces like cranium. Other challenges are the cost of maintaining the equipment. The equipment being a of high-end, needs equipment specific environment to be maintained for optimum functionality. They also need to be maintained as per the company specifications, which adds up to the cost of maintaining such equipment by the organization. Challenges include limited space in wearable devices, the need for medical-grade batteries, adaptation to sterile environments, and the risk of overengineering.

Regulatory Framework: The equipment should meet all the specifications of the nation and also international regulatory bodies to ensure Safety and Efficacy of care standards. This calls for consistent efforts in negotiating complex compliance standards that are paramount for maintaining patient safety. Thus dedicated resources would have to be developed and maintained by the organization.

Training and Education: The robotic surgery calls for the steep learning curve in surgeon's training to use and excel in performing surgeries to precision. Surgeons require extensive training in vitro and in vivo using simulation exercises so that they can excel in the procedures. This ongoing education to keep up with the technological advancements calls for additional time and resources adding to the overall costs.

Patient Acceptance: The details of the robotic surgery can be overwhelming to the patients. Gaining the trust of the patients is essential for increased patient acceptance. This apprehension on part of the patients would lead to them gravitating towards conventional methods or even laparoscopic surgery. Comfort and trust in robotic surgery should be enhanced with effective communication about the benefits and safety associated with robotic surgery. Thus, their concerns can be mitigated to increase the acceptance of robotic surgery.

Cost of surgery and affordability: The cost of equipment, infrastructure needed, the surgeon training costs all leads to high cost of performing surgery on the patients. These costs can limit the access and deter patients from robotic surgery. These disparities will have to be considered in patient care. Collaboration with insurance companies and other cost sharing or cost cutting mechanisms like subsidies will have to be considered to ensure affordability to advanced surgical technology.

Availability of services: The nature of robotic surgery ensures that not all the organizations are able to provide robotic surgical services. This means that these robotic surgeries are concentrated in tier-I or tier-II cities leading to inequitable access to advanced robotic surgical technology for the needy patients. This means one has to travel to distinct locations to access advanced surgery, enhancing the overall cost of care.

There are hospitals that have embraced this robotics technology to leverage its benefits to patients, doctors and hospital operations. In this chapter, we bring to you the case study of Narayana Health that has actively adopted digital transformations and advanced technologies to enhance patient care.

8. INTERNATIONAL CASE STUDY ON ROBOTIC SURGERY FROM NARAYANA HEALTH (INDIA)

India's leading healthcare provider, the Narayana Health (NH), has embraced a technology first model to provide high quality healthcare that is affordable and accessible to both rural and urban population. The hospital is in Bangalore, Karnataka.

8.1. Operational Highlights of NH:

- Modern infrastructure: The Bangalore campus, which covers 30 acres, has 3,000 beds, round-the-clock emergency services, and state-of-the-art diagnostic and treatment technologies.
- Multispecialty care: NH provides thorough care in a number of specialties, such as orthopaedics, neurology, nephrology, cardiology, and oncology.
- Reasonably priced: The goal of NH is to ensure that everyone has access to healthcare. Through creative financing methods, effective operations, and economies of scale, it does this.
- Skilled medical staff: NH's team consists of highly qualified physicians, nurses, and other support personnel, guaranteeing top-notch patient care.
- Research and education: NH performs clinical studies, works with foreign institutions, and offers medical professionals training programs.

Quote from Dr. Devi Shetty (Founder):
"Technology is the only way to scale healthcare delivery while maintaining quality."

The Narayana Health, Bangalore is a shining example of innovative healthcare delivery, making high-quality medical care accessible and affordable for millions of people. Its commitment to excellence, research, and social responsibility has transformed the healthcare landscape in India. It has embraced technology and implemented AI & bigdata, telemedicine platform, hospital automation and robotic surgery, predictive analytics for cardiac care, cloud enabled diagnostics, RFID tracking of resources, eHealth services and autonomous delivery robots. This centre recently became the fastest in the country and the second fastest in the world to successfully perform 100 robotic-assisted cardiac surgeries, by completing it in 147 days.

Urology, Gynaecology, Cardiothoracic Surgery, General Surgery, Head and Neck Surgery, and Colorectal Surgery are among the common surgical specialties where robotic surgery offers a practical benefit. The da Vinci Surgical System, produced by Intuitive Surgical Inc., is the most widely used robotic system in the world. The Hugo RAS System from Medtronic and the Versius Surgical Robotic System from CMR Surgical (UK) are the other robotic systems on the market. The SSi Mantra robotic system from SS Innovations is another robotic system that is becoming more and more well-liked both domestically and internationally. Its goal is to offer a sophisticated, reasonably priced surgical robotic system.

8.2. Traditional Surgery Vs Robotic Surgery

While traditional surgery relies on the surgeon's direct manual control of instruments, robotic surgery employs a computerized system where the surgeon manipulates controls to guide robotic arms equipped with surgical tools. This system provides enhanced precision, 3D visualization, and the ability to perform complex manoeuvres in tight spaces.

The surgeon remains close to the patient while doing the operation, seated at a control station. Beside the patient on the bed is an auxiliary surgeon. The operating surgeon monitors the surgical area via a video camera and manipulates multiple robotic arms from a console, simulating the surgeon's hand movements. Unprecedented surgical precision is made possible by the three computers at the console, which digitize the information and track those motions 1,000 times per second (Fig. 8 and 9).

Figure 8. Actual Photographs from the hospital

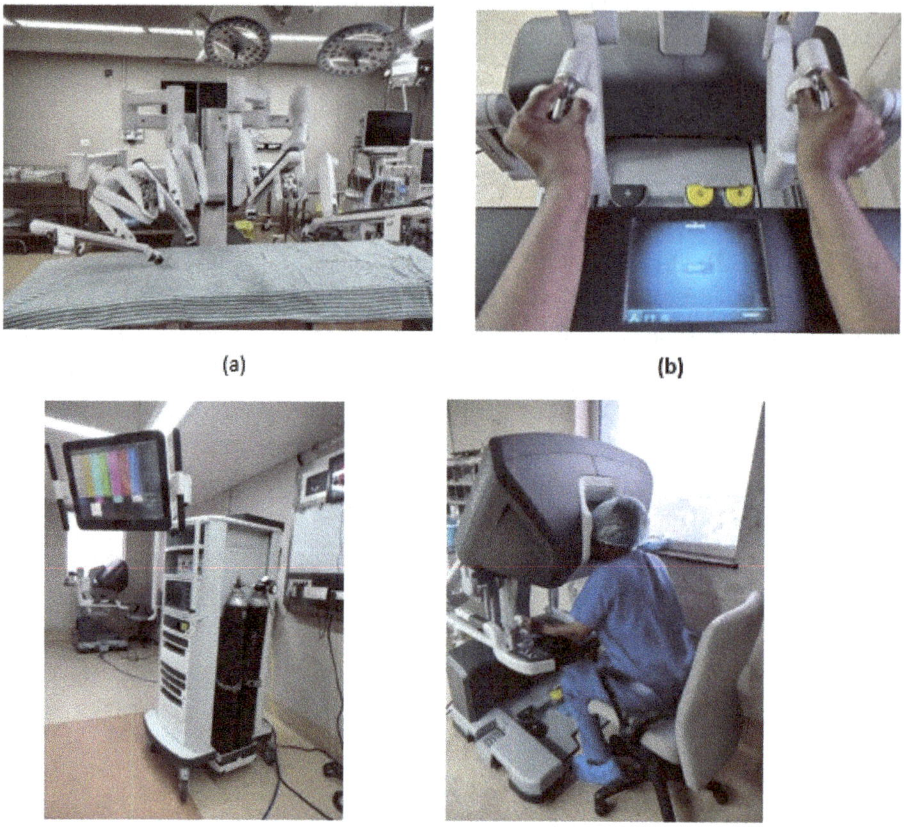

(a) (b) (c) (d)

Figure 9. Actual Photographs during surgery

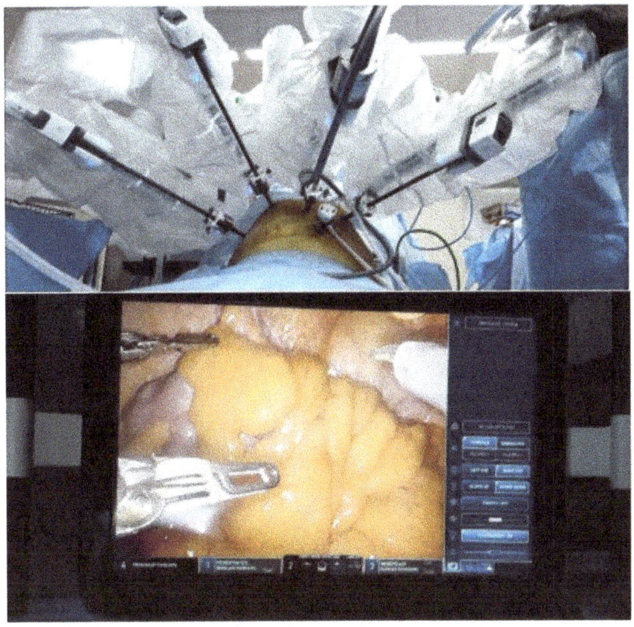

- **Procedure Time**

Procedure time in robotic surgery versus traditional surgery can vary. Generally, robotic surgeries may take longer due to setup time and the learning curve for surgeons. However, as surgeons gain experience, the time difference often becomes negligible, and in some cases, robotic surgeries can be faster, especially for complex procedures.

- **Healing time**

Healing time for robotic surgery is typically shorter compared to traditional surgery. The minimally invasive nature of robotic procedures usually results in smaller incisions, less tissue trauma, and reduced blood loss. This often leads to faster recovery, shorter hospital stays, and quicker return to normal activities for patients.

- **Surgery statistics**

There is a substantial difference in the daily surgical volume between robotic and non-robotic procedures. In contrast to non-robotic situations, where the daily totals are greater at 4-6 big cases or 6-8 small cases, there are typically 2 major cases or 3-4 minor cases per day.

These disparities are caused by a number of variables. Even while early learning curve surgery frequently takes far longer than conventional surgery, there is also lost time between cases as the robot must be undocked before being setup and docked for the subsequent case. Additionally, the figures differ according on the surgical specialty. In general, conventional surgery allows for higher daily case loads, but as surgical teams gain experience with robotic systems, the productivity gap narrows dramatically. Fig. 10(a) shows the statistics of the total surgery performed and number of robotic surgery performed in one of the departments during 2024 from January to December. When compared the robotics surgeries account to less than 5% of the total surgeries performed (Fig. 10(b)).

Figure 10. (a) Comparison of number of robotics vs traditional surgeries in 2024 (b) percentage of robotics surgeries in 2024

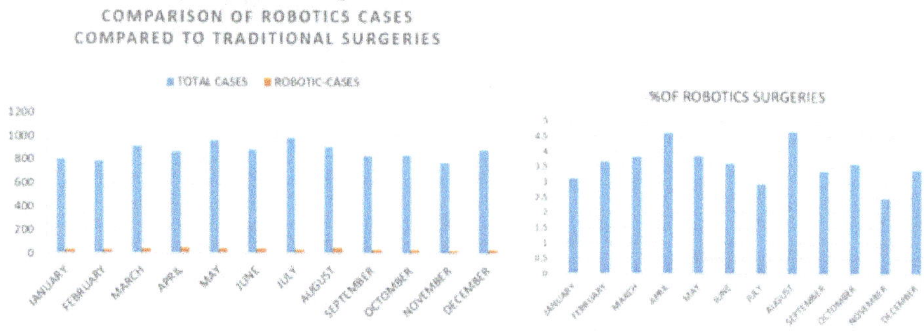

- **Reasons for Patients opting for robotic surgery**

It is not possible to give an accurate number of patients opting for robotic surgery. Some of the available data suggests

- India performs more than 60,000 robotic-assisted surgeries annually. [https://www.medicalbuyer.co.in/over-60000-robotic-assisted-surgeries-performed-in-india-annually/#:~:text=Over%2060%2C000%20robotic%2Dassisted%20surgeries%20performed%20in%20India%20annually,-Headlines%20of%20The]
- In 2022, India performed 12,000 robotic surgeries, which is 0.15% of all surgeries. [https://www.venkateshwarhospitals.com/blog/robotic-surgery-a-medical-revolution-or-just-a-trend/]

Patients choose robotic surgery for a number of reasons. Most important being a minimally invasive technique. Robotic systems allow for smaller incisions that lead to less pain and faster recovery and shorter hospital stays.

- **Reasons for patients not opting for robotic surgery**

It is not possible to provide exact number of patients do not opt for robotic surgery. However, the uptake is less than 1%. The likely reasons include cost, availability of expertise and lack of awareness. Robotic surgeries are more expensive than traditional methods. Not all hospitals or surgical centres have robotic systems and patients prefer surgeons with extensive experience in traditional techniques over those newer to robotic systems. Many patients may not be fully informed about robotic surgery as an option. There is also limited long-term data confirming its superiority over traditional surgery.

- **Opinion of surgeons regarding robotic surgery v/s traditional one**

When surgeons were interviewed for the feedback on the robotic surgery, they shared few opinions. Surgeons' opinions on robotic surgery are mixed. Many appreciate the enhanced precision and visualization it offers, particularly for complex procedures. However, challenges include the steep learning curve, significant time investment for training, and the high cost of equipment. Some surgeons also note the lack of tactile feedback as a drawback. Availability of training can be limited, especially in smaller hospitals or rural areas.

- **The opportunity cost for the company to have robotic surgery**

The opportunity cost for a company to implement robotic surgery is substantial. It involves significant upfront investment in equipment, ongoing maintenance costs, and extensive staff training. There's also the potential loss of revenue during the transition period as surgeons and staff learn the new system. However, this may be offset by potential increases in surgical volume, improved patient outcomes, and enhanced reputation as a cutting-edge facility.

- **Advantages and disadvantages of surgical robots**

While the robot provides superior visualization, provides better ergonomics, enhanced dexterity in tight spaces and reduces physical strain for the surgeon there is a high initial capital investment that results in high per-procedure costs.

Robotic surgical systems eliminate natural hand tremors leading to improved accuracy. The articulating instruments provide greater freedom than the human wrist and thus the robot can manoeuvre in tight spaces with precision. Combined with the stable positioning of robotic arms that can maintain the same position indefinitely without fatigue, this technology enables surgeons to perform delicate procedures with superior precision.

9. FUTURE DIRECTIONS OF SURGICAL ROBOTS

The Robotics in surgery is revolutionizing the treatments and outcomes of the patients to a great extent. This can be further improvised through the incorporation of emerging trends.

- AI integration with enhanced Automation-The surgical precision and the decision-making capabilities can be enhanced by integration of robotics surgical systems with Artificial Intelligence (AI). The AI would analyse the vast datasets from various systems on the disease condition and the surgical techniques leading to cumulative knowledge and better approaches to surgery, thus better patient outcomes (Yang et al., 2017).
- Miniaturization leading to portability of the surgical systems-With the advancement of technology, the large surgical setups is expected to reduce in the bulk become more portable thus making it a minimally invasive surgeries with possibilities of remote operations. This could leverage the availability of experts on site of the surgery.
- Haptic feedback to surgeons
    - o The future breakthrough in robotic surgery could be incorporation of haptic feedback to surgeons to enhance the tactile sensation during the surgical procedures aimed at better dexterity and precision (Marbán, Casals, Fernández, & Amat, 2014).
- Remote Surgery
    - o With the advancement of the technology the robot surgical procedures can follow the path of tele-medicine leading to remote surgery, thereby leveraging the availability of trained specialist at multiple locations (Choi, Oskouian, & Tubbs, 2018).
- Concurrent use of robotic surgery with other technologies
    - o Integration of multiple technologies for performing robotic surgery could also be explored in the future. These technologies could be augmented reality, virtual reality which can be used for training the sur-

geons for steep learning curve. This can also be achieved by immersive simulation and real-time data monitoring for remote location.

- o Use of bioluminescent glucose uptake probe for real-time, non-invasive longitudinal imaging can be used to locate cancers in the body by fluorescent tagging. This can be used along with robotic surgery to deliver precision procedures for better patient outcomes. Robotic surgery in collaboration with Neuro-navigation using infrared and electromagnetic radiations can be explored to enhance the precision (Maric et al., 2019; Orringer, Golby, & Jolesz, 2012; Williams, McVeigh, Handa, & Lee, 2020).

10. CONCLUSION

The integration of robotics into modern healthcare marks a significant advancement in medical science and technology. From surgical procedures and rehabilitation support to hospital logistics and remote consultations, robotic systems are playing a growing role in reshaping clinical workflows and improving patient outcomes.

Throughout this chapter, we have examined how medical robots are categorized based on function and autonomy, and how their components—both hardware and software—contribute to their capabilities. The minimally invasive surgery applications demonstrate the versatility and value these technologies bring to patient care.

At the same time, there are several limitations and challenges like high implementation costs, lack of uniform standards, limited access in under-resourced areas, and the need for specialized training continue to pose challenges to broader adoption. Nevertheless, examples like Narayana Health showcase how innovative healthcare models can successfully integrate robotic technologies while maintaining affordability and scalability.

Looking to the future, continued developments in robotics such as miniaturized systems, enhanced autonomy, and improved connectivity are likely to push the boundaries of what is possible in patient care. As these tools become more refined and accessible, they have the potential to contribute significantly to more personalized, efficient, and equitable healthcare delivery.

In conclusion, medical robotics is steadily becoming an essential part of the healthcare ecosystem, offering new possibilities to improve quality, access, and safety in medical services worldwide.

REFERENCES

Adiuku, N., Avdelidis, N. P., Tang, G., & Plastropoulos, A. (2024). Advancements in Learning-Based Navigation Systems for Robotic Applications in MRO Hangar [Review]. *Sensors (Basel), 24*(5), 1377. https://www.mdpi.com/1424-8220/24/5/1377 PMID: 38474913

Ahsan, M. M., & Siddique, Z. (2022). Industry 4.0 in Healthcare: A systematic review. *International Journal of Information Management Data Insights, 2*(1), 100079. DOI: 10.1016/j.jjimei.2022.100079

Albustanji, R. N., Elmanaseer, S., & Alkhatib, A. A. A. (2023). Robotics: Five Senses plus One—An Overview. *Robotics (Basel, Switzerland), 12*(3), 68. https://www.mdpi.com/2218-6581/12/3/68

Bai, N., Xue, Y., Chen, S., Shi, L., Shi, J., Zhang, Y., & Guo, C. F. (2023). A robotic sensory system with high spatiotemporal resolution for texture recognition. *Nature Communications, 14*(1), 7121. DOI: 10.1038/s41467-023-42722-4 PMID: 37963866

Ballouhey, Q., Esposito, C., Taghavi, K., Lardy, H., Berte, N., Abbo, O., & Blanc, T. (2025). Robot-assisted Surgery in Pediatric Patients: Results of a French Multicenter Study on 1401 Patients. *Journal of Pediatric Surgery, 60*(8), 162397. DOI: 10.1016/j.jpedsurg.2025.162397 PMID: 40472888

Basulo-Ribeiro, J., & Teixeira, L. (2024). The Future of Healthcare with Industry 5.0: Preliminary Interview-Based Qualitative Analysis. *Future Internet, 16*(3), 68. https://www.mdpi.com/1999-5903/16/3/68

Biswas, P., Sikander, S., & Kulkarni, P. (2023). Recent advances in robot-assisted surgical systems. *Biomedical Engineering Advances, 6*, 100109. DOI: 10.1016/j.bea.2023.100109

Bora, G. S., Narain, T. A., Sharma, A. P., Mavuduru, R. S., Devana, S. K., Singh, S. K., & Mandal, A. K. (2020). Robot-assisted surgery in India: A SWOT analysis. *Indian Journal of Urology : IJU : Journal of the Urological Society of India, 36*(1). https://journals.lww.com/indianjurol/fulltext/2020/36010/robot_assisted_surgery_in_india__a_swot_analysis.1.aspx PMID: 31983817

Boscarelli, A., Giglione, E., Caputo, M. R., Guida, E., Iaquinto, M., Scarpa, M. G., & Schleef, J. (2023). Robotic-assisted surgery in pediatrics: What is evidence-based?-a literature review. *Translational Pediatrics, 12*(2), 271–279. DOI: 10.21037/tp-22-338 PMID: 36891357

Castro, E. M. J., & Faria Araújo, N. M. (2020). Impact of the Fourth Industrial Revolution on the Health Sector: A Qualitative Study. *Healthcare Informatics Research, 26*(4), 328–334. DOI: 10.4258/hir.2020.26.4.328 PMID: 33190467

Choi, P. J., Oskouian, R. J., & Tubbs, R. S. (2018). Telesurgery: Past, Present, and Future. *Cureus, 10*(5), e2716. DOI: 10.7759/cureus.2716 PMID: 30079282

Cuevas, C. A. G., Alvarado, G. A. D., González, C. J., Peña, C. F. P., & Castro, L. E. C. (2025). Scientific evolution of robotic surgery in urogenital diseases: Bibliometric analysis. *Journal of Robotic Surgery, 19*(1), 219. DOI: 10.1007/s11701-025-02359-5 PMID: 40377820

Dobbs, T. D., Cundy, O., Samarendra, H., Khan, K., & Whitaker, I. S. (2017). A Systematic Review of the Role of Robotics in Plastic and Reconstructive Surgery-From Inception to the Future. *Frontiers in Surgery, 4*, 66. DOI: 10.3389/fsurg.2017.00066 PMID: 29188219

Doulgeris, J. J., Gonzalez-Blohm, S. A., Filis, A. K., Shea, T. M., Aghayev, K., & Vrionis, F. D. (2015). Robotics in Neurosurgery: Evolution, Current Challenges, and Compromises. *Cancer Control : Journal of the Moffitt Cancer Center, 22*(3), 352–359. DOI: 10.1177/107327481502200314 PMID: 26351892

Esposito, C., Masieri, L., Di Mento, C., Cerulo, M., Del Conte, F., Coppola, V., & Escolino, M. (2025). Seven years of pediatric robotic-assisted surgery: Insights from 105 procedures. *Journal of Robotic Surgery, 19*(1), 157. DOI: 10.1007/s11701-025-02257-w PMID: 40232570

Fan, X., Wang, Y., Zhang, S., Xing, Y., Li, J., Ma, X., & Ma, J. (2025). Orthopedic surgical robotic systems in knee arthroplasty: A comprehensive review. *Frontiers in Bioengineering and Biotechnology, 13*, 1523631. DOI: 10.3389/fbioe.2025.1523631 PMID: 40051834

Flatebø, S., Tran, V. N., Wang, C. E. A., & Bongo, L. A. (2024). Social robots in research on social and cognitive development in infants and toddlers: A scoping review. *PLoS One, 19*(5), e0303704. DOI: 10.1371/journal.pone.0303704 PMID: 38748722

Gao, Z., Wanyama, T., Singh, I., Gadhrri, A., & Schmidt, R. (2020). From Industry 4.0 to Robotics 4.0 - A Conceptual Framework for Collaborative and Intelligent Robotic Systems. *Procedia Manufacturing, 46*, 591–599. DOI: 10.1016/j.promfg.2020.03.085

Gerber, M. J., Pettenkofer, M., & Hubschman, J.-P. (2020). Advanced robotic surgical systems in ophthalmology. *Eye, 34*(9), 1554–1562. DOI: 10.1038/s41433-020-0837-9 PMID: 32152518

Gul, F., Rahiman, W., & Nazli Alhady, S. S. (2019). A comprehensive study for robot navigation techniques. *Cogent Engineering, 6*(1), 1632046. DOI: 10.1080/23311916.2019.1632046

Gyles, C. (2019). Robots in medicine. *The Canadian Veterinary Journal = La Revue Vétérinaire Canadienne, 60*(8), 819–820. PMID: 31391598

Harky, A., & Hussain, S. M. A. (2019). Robotic Cardiac Surgery: The Future Gold Standard or An Unnecessary Extravagance? *Braz J Cardiovasc Surg, 34*(4), xii-xiii. DOI: 10.21470/1678-9741-2019-0194

Hu, R., Longo, U. G., Pittman, J., & Nazarian, A. (2025). Robotic Innovations in Orthopedics: A Growing Landscape, Challenges, and Implications for Care. *Osteology, 5*(2), 13. https://www.mdpi.com/2673-4036/5/2/13

Javaid, M., Haleem, A., Pratap Singh, R., Rab, S., Suman, R., & Kumar, L. (2025). Utilization of Robotics for Healthcare: A Scoping Review. *Journal of Industrial Integration and Management, 10*(01), 43–65. DOI: 10.1142/s2424862222500154

Jha, P., & Chaurasia, B. (2024). The art of neurosurgery: Precision beyond machines. *Annals of Medicine and Surgery (London), 86*(8), 4325–4326. DOI: 10.1097/ms9.0000000000002280 PMID: 39118761

Kapoor, A., Deguet, A., & Kazanzides, P. (2006). Software components and frameworks for medical robot control. *Proceedings 2006 IEEE International Conference on Robotics and Automation, 2006. ICRA 2006.*

Koukourikis, P., & Rha, K. H. (2021). Robotic surgical systems in urology: What is currently available? *Investigative and Clinical Urology, 62*(1), 14–22. DOI: 10.4111/icu.20200387 PMID: 33381927

Kubota, T., Ogawa, K., Yoshikawa, Y., & Ishiguro, H. (2022). Alignment of the attitude of teleoperators with that of a semi-autonomous android. *Scientific Reports, 12*(1), 10473. DOI: 10.1038/s41598-022-13829-3 PMID: 35760935

Lengyel, B. C., Chinnadurai, P., Corr, S. J., Lumsden, A. B., & Bavare, C. S. (2024). Robot-assisted vascular surgery: Literature review, clinical applications, and future perspectives. *Journal of Robotic Surgery, 18*(1), 328. DOI: 10.1007/s11701-024-02087-2 PMID: 39174843

Leung, T., & Vyas, D. (2014). Robotic Surgery: Applications. *American Journal of Robotic Surgery*, *1*(1), 1–64. PMID: 26501128

Liu, X., Liu, F., Jin, L., & Wu, J. (2024). Evolution of Neurosurgical Robots: Historical Progress and Future Direction. *World Neurosurgery*, *191*, 49–57. DOI: 10.1016/j.wneu.2024.08.008 PMID: 39116942

Madadi, Y., Delsoz, M., Khouri, A. S., Boland, M., Grzybowski, A., & Yousefi, S. (2024). Applications of artificial intelligence-enabled robots and chatbots in ophthalmology: Recent advances and future trends. *Current Opinion in Ophthalmology*, *35*(3), 238–243. DOI: 10.1097/icu.0000000000001035 PMID: 38277274

Marbán, A., Casals, A., Fernández, J., & Amat, J. (2014). Haptic Feedback in Surgical Robotics: Still a Challenge. In Armada, M. A., Sanfeliu, A., & Ferre, M. (Eds.), *ROBOT2013: First Iberian Robotics Conference: Advances in Robotics,* Vol. 1 (pp. 245-253). Cham: Springer International Publishing.

Maric, T., Mikhaylov, G., Khodakivskyi, P., Bazhin, A., Sinisi, R., Bonhoure, N., & Goun, E. (2019). Bioluminescent-based imaging and quantification of glucose uptake in vivo. *Nature Methods*, *16*(6), 526–532. DOI: 10.1038/s41592-019-0421-z PMID: 31086341

Mehta, A., Cheng Ng, J., Andrew Awuah, W., Huang, H., Kalmanovich, J., Agrawal, A., & Isik, A. (2022). Embracing robotic surgery in low- and middle-income countries: Potential benefits, challenges, and scope in the future. *Annals of Medicine and Surgery (London)*, *84*, 104803. DOI: 10.1016/j.amsu.2022.104803 PMID: 36582867

Mei, H., & Tang, S. (2023). Robotic-assisted surgery in the pediatric surgeons' world: Current situation and future prospectives. *Frontiers in Pediatrics*, *11*, 1120831. DOI: 10.3389/fped.2023.1120831 PMID: 36865692

Mohan, O., Banur, B. K. P., & Pawar, S. (2024, February). Integration of robotics and automation in supply chain: A comprehensive review. *Robotic Systems and Applications*, *4*(1), 1–19. DOI: 10.21595/rsa.2023.23349

Mori, M., & Geirsson, A. (2024). The way forward in research on robotic cardiac surgery: The need for transatlantic robotic cardiac surgery registry. *Annals of Cardiothoracic Surgery*, *13*(4), 376–378. https://www.annalscts.com/article/view/17105 PMID: 39157188

Nehme, J., Neville, J. J., & Bahsoun, A. N. (2017). The use of robotics in plastic and reconstructive surgery: A systematic review. *JPRAS Open*, *13*, 1–10. DOI: 10.1016/j.jpra.2017.03.005

Orringer, D. A., Golby, A., & Jolesz, F. (2012). Neuronavigation in the surgical management of brain tumors: Current and future trends. *Expert Review of Medical Devices*, *9*(5), 491–500. DOI: 10.1586/erd.12.42 PMID: 23116076

Pandey, S. K., & Sharma, V. (2019). Robotics and ophthalmology: Are we there yet? *Indian Journal of Ophthalmology*, *67*(7), 988–994. DOI: 10.4103/ijo.IJO_1131_18 PMID: 31238393

Pokhrel, G., Wang, Z., Cui, J., Jin, B., Zheng, H., Tao, J., & Zhang, X. (2025). Initial experience with the novel modular robotic system Carina in urology: A prospective study on safety feasibility and surgical settings. *Scientific Reports*, *15*(1), 12686. DOI: 10.1038/s41598-025-97411-7 PMID: 40221629

Rahman, M. A., Bristi, S. A., Yesmin, T., & Islam, M. T. (2025). *Application of robotics in modern surgery and critical operations: Current status, challenges, and future directions*. ITPS. DOI: 10.36922/itps.4664

Ram, P. R., Jeyaraman, M., Jeyaraman, N., Yadav, S., & Venkatasalam, R. (2023). Revolutionizing Orthopedic Healthcare: The Role of Robotics. *Cureus*, *15*(9), e44820. DOI: 10.7759/cureus.44820 PMID: 37809251

Richert, A., Shehadeh, M. A., Müller, S. L., Schröder, S., & Jeschke, S. (2016). Socializing with robots: Human-robot interactions within a virtual environment. Paper presented at the 2016 IEEE Workshop on Advanced Robotics and its Social Impacts (ARSO).

Rivero-Moreno, Y., Echevarria, S., Vidal-Valderrama, C., Pianetti, L., Cordova-Guilarte, J., Navarro-Gonzalez, J., & Acero-Alvarracín, K. (2023). Robotic Surgery: A Comprehensive Review of the Literature and Current Trends. *Cureus*, *15*(7), e42370. DOI: 10.7759/cureus.42370 PMID: 37621804

Rojas Burbano, J. C., Ruiz, N. I., Rojas Burbano, G. A., Guacho Inca, J. S., Arragan Lezama, C. A., & González, M. S. (2025). Robot-Assisted Surgery: Current Applications and Future Trends in General Surgery. *Cureus*, *17*(4), e82318. DOI: 10.7759/cureus.82318 PMID: 40376327

Seppänen, A., Vepsäläinen, J., Ojala, R., & Tammi, K. (2022). Comparison of Semi-autonomous Mobile Robot Control Strategies in Presence of Large Delay Fluctuation. *Journal of Intelligent & Robotic Systems*, *106*(1), 28. DOI: 10.1007/s10846-022-01711-3

Seth, I., Lim, K., Chang, E., Rozen, W. M., & Ng, S. K.-H. (2025). Evaluating the Clinical Utility of Robotic Systems in Plastic and Reconstructive Surgery: A Systematic Review. *Sensors (Basel)*, *25*(10), 3238. https://www.mdpi.com/1424-8220/25/10/3238 PMID: 40432030

Sindhwani, N., Anand, R., George, A., & Pandey, D. (Eds.). (2024). *Robotics and Automation in Industry 4.0: Smart Industries and Intelligent Technologies* (1st ed.). CRC Press.

Singh, P. (2024). Role Of Automation And Robotics In Transforming The Food Industry. *Revista Electrónica de Veterinaria*, *25*(1), 1119–1125. DOI: 10.69980/redvet.v25i1.809

Stuart, C. M., Meguid, R. A., & Rove, J. Y. (2025). Noteworthy in Cardiothoracic Surgery 2024. *Seminars in Cardiothoracic and Vascular Anesthesia*, *29*(2), 126–133. DOI: 10.1177/10892532251332455 PMID: 40198923

Sulaiman, N. b., binti Mahmud, N. P. N., Nazir, U., binti Abdul Latib, S. K. K., Muhammad Hafidz, H. F. b., & Abid, S. K. (2021). The Role of Autonomous Robots in Fourth Industrial Revolution (4IR) as an Approach of Sustainable Development Goals (SDG9): Industry, Innovation and Infrastructure in Handling the Effect of COVID-19 Outbreak. *IOP Conference Series. Earth and Environmental Science*, *775*(1), 012017. DOI: 10.1088/1755-1315/775/1/012017

Sutyak, K. M., & Tsao, K. (2024). Pedi-Bots: Innovations and progress in robotic pediatric general surgery. *Journal of Pediatric Surgery Open*, *7*, 100156. DOI: 10.1016/j.yjpso.2024.100156

Trivino, G., Mengual, L., & van der Heide, A. (2009). Towards an architecture for semiautonomous robot telecontrol systems. *Information Sciences*, *179*(23), 3973–3984. DOI: 10.1016/j.ins.2009.08.007

Urrea, C., & Kern, J. (2025). Recent Advances and Challenges in Industrial Robotics: A Systematic Review of Technological Trends and Emerging Applications. *Processes (Basel, Switzerland)*, *13*(3), 832. https://www.mdpi.com/2227-9717/13/3/832

Vanderstappen, M., van Ochten, J. H. M., & Verborgt, O. (2025). Robotics in arthroplasty: How good are they? *JSES International*, *9*(3), 968–973. DOI: 10.1016/j.jseint.2024.09.005 PMID: 40486812

Wah, J. N. K. (2025). Revolutionizing surgery: AI and robotics for precision, risk reduction, and innovation. *Journal of Robotic Surgery*, *19*(1), 47. DOI: 10.1007/s11701-024-02205-0 PMID: 39776281

Warnecke, H. J., & Schiele, G. (1985). Performance Characteristics and Performance Testing of Industrial Robots — State of the Art. Academic Press.

Williams, M. A., McVeigh, J., Handa, A. I., & Lee, R. (2020). Augmented reality in surgical training: A systematic review. *Postgraduate Medical Journal*, *96*(1139), 537–542. DOI: 10.1136/postgradmedj-2020-137600 PMID: 32229513

Wu, Z., Zheng, Y., & Zhang, X. (2024). Safety and efficacy of orthopedic robots in total hip arthroplasty: A network meta-analysis and systematic review. *Journal of Orthopaedic Surgery and Research*, *19*(1), 846. DOI: 10.1186/s13018-024-05279-6 PMID: 39696343

Yang, G. Z., Cambias, J., Cleary, K., Daimler, E., Drake, J., Dupont, P. E., & Taylor, R. H. (2017). Medical robotics-Regulatory, ethical, and legal considerations for increasing levels of autonomy. *Science Robotics*, *2*(4). Advance online publication. DOI: 10.1126/scirobotics.aam8638 PMID: 33157870

Zenati, M. A., & Mahvash, M. (2012). 4 - Robotic systems for cardiovascular interventions. In Gomes, P. (Ed.), *Medical Robotics* (pp. 78–89). Woodhead Publishing.

Zhang, Y., Liu, X., Qiao, X., & Fan, Y. (2023). Characteristics and Emerging Trends in Research on Rehabilitation Robots from 2001 to 2020: Bibliometric Study. *Journal of Medical Internet Research*, *25*, e42901. DOI: 10.2196/42901 PMID: 37256670

Chapter 9
Robotic Medication and Water Delivery:
A Solution for Independent Living in Seniors

Mohammad Salah Uddin
https://orcid.org/0000-0002-4180-2355
East West University, Bangladesh

Anisur Rahman
https://orcid.org/0009-0006-0359-1207
East West University, Bangladesh

ABSTRACT

Lack of medication and dehydration are major health problems among older people living alone. Often, these problems result in unnecessary hospital visits. Sometimes these problems worsen chronic diseases and reduce the quality of life. As the elderly population grows rapidly, innovative solutions to support their independent living have become important. This chapter presents a robotic system designed to deliver medication (medicines) and water to older people in a home environment. The system integrates robotic systems, various sensing technologies, and the internet of things (IoT). It consists of a wheeled robot that delivers pills and water directly to users, a robot unit that stores, organizes, and prepares medications, and a user-friendly smartphone app for remote monitoring and management. The robotic system ensures accurate and timely delivery of medication and water using a navigation system, infrared sensors, and vision-based person detection algorithms. The robot is connected to an IoT-cloud, which provides personalized schedules, timely reminders to users.

DOI: 10.4018/979-8-3373-1514-0.ch009

1. INTRODUCTION

As the global population continues to grow, the number of older adults living alone is increasing rapidly. According to the World Health Organization (WHO), the population aged 60 years and above is expected to reach 2.1 billion by 2050 (WHO, 2021). A significant portion of this population (older) lives independently, without regular contact with caregivers or regular clinical supervision.

In the Asia-Pacific region, this trend is particularly striking:

- In Japan, more than 28% of the population is already over 65. This is the highest proportion worldwide, with more than 6 million elderly people living alone (UNIVERSAL, 2022).
- In South Korea, the proportion of elderly people living alone reached 19.6% in 2022 and is expected to increase to 23% by 2035 (Statistics Korea, 2023).
- In China, the number of "empty-nest elderly" (elderly people living without children or close relatives) has exceeded 118 million (Zhao, 2023).
- The European Union is in a similar situation. In EU, almost a third of people aged 65 and above live alone, with Sweden, Denmark and the Netherlands having the highest rates of elderly people living alone (Eurostat, 2020).

Independence can be empowering, but it also poses serious health risks. Two of the most overlooked but important issues are medication mismanagement and inadequate hydration. These issues may seem minor on the surface, but their impact can be life-threatening. Older adults may miss essential medications or forget to drink enough water due to cognitive impairment, memory loss, and reduced physical mobility. The following subsections present the impact of medication mismanagement and dehydration risks on older adults worldwide and discuss several statistics.

1.1 Medication Mismanagement

Most elderly people take multiple medications daily—for chronic conditions like high blood pressure, diabetes, arthritis, and heart disease. Managing these medications is complex: different dosages, varying times, and specific instructions (with food, without food, etc.). Without proper support, mistakes are common. Some statistics are listed below:

- Nearly 90% of adults over age 65 take at least one prescription drug. Around 36% take five or more daily (Cohen & Mykyta, 2024).
- Studies show that at least 1 in 4 older adults have reported forgetting to take medications or taking them incorrectly (Albee & Hunter, 2022).

- According to Unnissa et al. (2024), medication errors account for approximately 700,000 emergency department visits and 100,000 hospitalizations each year in the U.S. alone.

And some common problems (due to medication mismanagement) are also listed here:

- Missed doses due to forgetfulness or confusion.
- Double dose when they forget they've already taken it.
- Mix-ups between medications that look or sound similar.
- Expired medications that are still being taken.
- Lack of understanding of what each drug does or why it's prescribed.

These errors can result in grave consequences—falls from low blood pressure, heart complications, dangerous drug interactions, or worsening of the very conditions they're trying to treat. For seniors living alone, these mistakes often go unnoticed until a health crisis occurs.

1.2 Risk of Dehydration

Many elderly people simply don't drink enough water. This isn't just about forgetting; it's also about decreased thirst sensation, limited mobility, and fear of incontinence. Some may avoid drinking fluids to reduce trips to the bathroom, especially at night or when help is not nearby.

- Research shows that over 30% of older adults, particularly those in care homes or living alone, experience chronic low-intake dehydration (Alsanie et al., 2024).
- Dehydration is a leading cause of hospitalization for people over age 65, particularly during warmer months (Dhar et al., 2023).
- Mild dehydration can increase the risk of falls by more than 50%, according to clinical studies (WellMed Medical Management, 2023).

The consequences of drinking less water are given below,

- Confusion and dizziness, often mistaken for dementia or stroke.
- Urinary tract infections, which can escalate quickly.
- Constipation, impacting appetite and digestion.
- Kidney problems, including considerable risk of kidney stones or failure.
- Falls, due to dizziness or lightheadedness from dehydration.

Like medication issues, dehydration is often under-diagnosed in elderly individuals, especially those living alone—because symptoms are subtle until they become dangerous. Without someone checking in daily, there's no backup system. If a senior forgets a medication or hasn't had a glass of water all day, no one may notice until they become visibly ill or are rushed to the hospital. Even when home health aides or family visit occasionally, problems can slip through the cracks. A full medicine cabinet doesn't guarantee that pills are being taken correctly. An empty water bottle doesn't mean it was recently filled. However, some existing digital tools, such as alarm-based pillboxes and mobile app-based reminders for pill reminders and other devices for hydration reminders, are not suitable for older adults due to limited accessibility and customization. Given the limitations of traditional eldercare and devices, smart solutions are not just helpful, they are essential. Robotics and IoT (Internet of Things) technology now offer practical ways to support the elderly at home in a reliable and effective way.

Focusing on these two critical issues facing older adults, this chapter explores how next-generation assistive medical robots can enhance safety, reduce caregiver burden, and improve the quality of life of older populations worldwide. This chapter presents a robotic system specifically designed for that purpose. It consists of three main components: a mobile robot that delivers medication and water, a stationary unit that stores and prepares the correct dose of medicine, and a smartphone app that connects and monitors everything. The mobile robot moves around the home on its own, bringing water and medication directly to the user (older adults). The stationary robot manages safe storage and ensures that each dose is measured correctly. Using sensor fusion based indoor localization, the system navigates safely through the home. Lidar sensors help avoid obstacles, and a user identification algorithm ensures that the right person gets the right medication at the right time. The entire setup works within a home system, providing personalized reminders, scheduling, and emergency alerts. With built-in sensors and IoT integration, caregivers or family members can monitor medication intake and hydration levels in real-time, even from a distance. Additional safety features like fall detection and obstacle avoidance make the system more reliable and safer for everyday use.

The rest of the chapter is divided into several sections. Section 2 provides a comprehensive review of the related literature. After the review, Section 3 explains the design methodology of the proposed system. This section covers multiple aspects such as the functional requirements of the robot and the simulation environment used. It also describes the design specifications of the robot in detail. Various control methods and algorithms are also discussed. This section covers how robots are integrated with IoT systems and mobile applications. It explains the step-by-step mobile app development process as well. After the design methodology section, Section 4 presents the results of the tests and evaluation. The testing section includes multiple scenarios testing, robot performance tests, and stress tests under different conditions. The evaluation subsection presents a user survey using a Likert-scale chart to evaluate usability and satisfaction. The comparison section compares the performance of the robot with traditional methods. In addition, the potential applications of this robot in different areas of the medical field are also included. The conclusion section ends the chapter.

2. LITERATURE REVIEW

The global increase in the elderly population has shown the need for supportive technologies. Older adults, especially those living alone, often struggle with medication adherence, hydration, mobility, and safety. Researchers have explored robotic and smart home technologies to address these challenges. This review focuses on existing robotic elderly care solutions, particularly for medication and hydration support. It also identifies current limitations motivating the development of integrated home-care robots. Many studies emphasize the importance of assistive technology in helping elderly people maintain independence. Nearly 22% of the global population is projected to be over 60 by 2050 (WHO, 2024). Most seniors prefer to age at home rather than in care facilities. However, traditional home care is often insufficient due to high costs, caregiver shortages, or geographic access barriers (Wikipedia contributors, n.d.). Smart home and IoT solutions offer scalable alternatives. Recent advances in ambient sensors and wearable devices have enhanced fall detection, vital monitoring, and activity tracking in older adults. However, most systems still lack interactivity for delivering hydration or medications (Guarducci et al., 2025). Moreover, medication non-adherence remains a critical issue, with up to 50% of older adults failing to take prescriptions as directed (Hart et al., 2025). Common reasons include forgetfulness, complicated medication schedules, cognitive decline, and physical limitations. Several automated pill dispensers exist, including MedMinder, Philips Medication Dispenser, and TabSafe. However, these devices are usually stationary and require user action, such as pressing buttons or retrieving pills. This can be challenging for individuals with mobility or memory problems. Recent research by Kostavelis, Ioannis, et al. (2022) explored robotic arms to deliver medication. But these solutions are typically fixed and too expensive for average homes. Dehydration is another serious, yet often overlooked, issue. Chronic dehydration may affect over 30% of older adults due to age-related changes in thirst perception, reduced mobility, and behavioral factors like fear of incontinence (Jang et al., 2024). Smart water bottles, like HidrateSpark and Ulla, exist but typically require manual interaction. They do not guarantee water reaches the user. Smart reminders alone are insufficient without direct delivery. Few studies have explored proactive automated hydration systems for home use. Domestic service robots have shown promise in supporting elderly users with various tasks. Robots like Toyota's Human Support Robot (HSR) and Willow Garage's PR2 can fetch objects, open doors, and interact with people. However, their excessive cost, complexity, and large size make them impractical for common home settings. More compact robots, such as Germany's Care-O-bot and France's Buddy, provide reminders and navigation assistance. Yet, most lack integrated medication or hydration functions. Additionally, IoT-enabled robots can potentially combine mobility, automation, and remote monitoring. Bathirappan et al. (2022) proposed a robotic system for monitoring and treating patients in hospitals. It also delivers pills to the patients automatically based on schedule. However, such integrated setups are rare for home use. Currently, home solutions are fragmented: one device handles reminders, another dispenses medication, and a separate one tracks health.

Several gaps emerge from the existing literature, which are listed below:

- Medication systems often rely on user-initiated interaction, problematic for seniors with mobility or cognitive issues.
- Hydration monitoring typically depends on self-reporting or passive sensors.
- Current robotic solutions are either overly complex or unsuitable for the home environment.
- Few integrated solutions exist combining medication, hydration, mobility, and remote caregiver communication.

These gaps highlight the need for a low-cost, reliable, integrated robotic solution. Such a system would autonomously deliver medication and water, verify user interaction, and provide real-time caregiver updates, especially beneficial for elderly individuals living alone.

3. DESIGN METHODOLOGY

Elderly individuals who live alone face daily challenges. Simple health tasks can become difficult. These include taking medication on time and drinking enough water. With reduced mobility and memory issues, managing routines becomes harder. The absence of caregivers adds to the struggle. To address this, a service robot is introduced in this study. It assists with two key tasks—timely medication reminders and water delivery. The robot functions autonomously. It is built to navigate a structured home environment safely. It follows a set schedule and adapts to obstacles. The robot detects objects in its path. It avoids collisions. It physically carries pills and water to ensure proper delivery. These features help meet the daily needs of elderly individuals. Key challenges are modeled in simulation. These include moving through rooms, rccognizing spaces, managing items, and engaging with users. The system is evaluated in a realistic home setup. The goal is to prove that such a robot can support aging in place. This solution offers more than reminders. It provides active, physical assistance. With thoughtful design, it supports independence and improves daily quality of life for older adults.

3.1 System Functional Requirements

The robot must satisfy the following key functional requirements to support its intended assistive role in elderly care:

- **Autonomous Navigation and Localization**: The robot should move independently between rooms while identifying its own position within the home layout.
- **Time-Based Task Scheduling**: Daily care routines, such as medication reminders and hydration prompts, must be executed at specific simulated times.
- **Environmental Awareness**: The robot must detect and respond to static and dynamic obstacles, as well as closed doors that obstruct its path.
- **Reminder-Based Interaction**: The robot must alert the user at scheduled times with clear prompts for taking medication or drinking water.
- **Integrated Pill Box**: A compact pill carrying unit should be mounted on the robot's body, allowing the system to bring pills directly to the user.
- **Integrated Water Dispenser**: The robot must carry a water container onboard and simulate a dispensing action upon interaction.

Figure 1. A simplified home layout in webots simulation

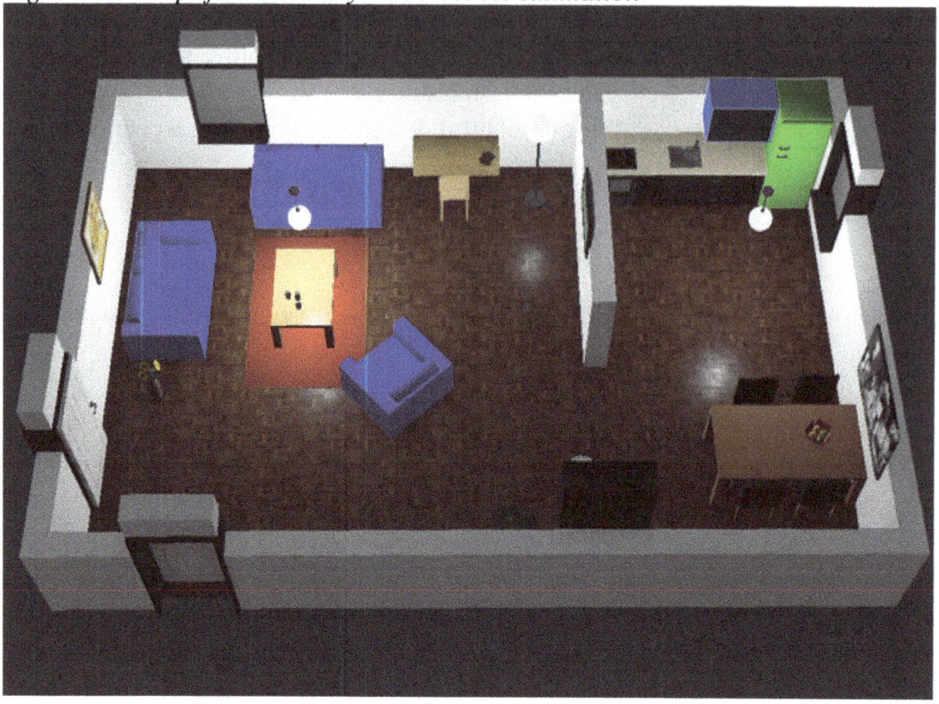

3.2 Simulation Environment Setup

To develop and evaluate the robot, a virtual home environment was created using the Webots simulation platform (Michel, 2025 and Farley et al., 2022). The simulation environment was designed to reflect the layout of a simplified home presented in Figure 01. On the left, there is a cozy living room. It has three blue sofas surrounded by a red carpet. A small wooden coffee table is located. There is a floor lamp next to one of the sofas. A flowerpot is placed in the corner. A picture hangs on the wall near the entrance. In the middle section, there is a small workspace. It has a desk and a chair. A tall lamp is placed next to the desk. A television is mounted on the wall above the desk. A compact kitchen is shown in the upper right corner. It has a stove, a sink, and a countertop. There are green and blue kitchen cabinets above the counter. At the end, a refrigerator is placed. In the lower right corner is the dining area. There is a rectangular wooden table placed there. There are four black chairs around it. A bowl of fruit is placed in the middle. A large photo frame hangs on the wall. The apartment has two doors. One is the main entrance on the lower left. The second door is on the upper left wall. The floor has a wood pattern. This setup enables controlled evaluation of navigation, task execution, and user interaction scenarios.

3.3 Specification of the Robot

The robot used in the simulation has a four-wheeled, rectangular design. The robot has a thick red body (body pose) measuring 0.2 m (width) × 0.2 m (depth) × 0.3 m (height). On top of this main body, a flat yellow platform (top base) measuring 0.2 × 0.2 × 0.01 m serves as the mounting area for sensors and objects. The robot is shown in Figure 02.

Figure 2. Conceptual model of a robot for a simulated environment. The robot consists of a four-wheeled vehicle with a water container, pill storage, camera, and several sensors

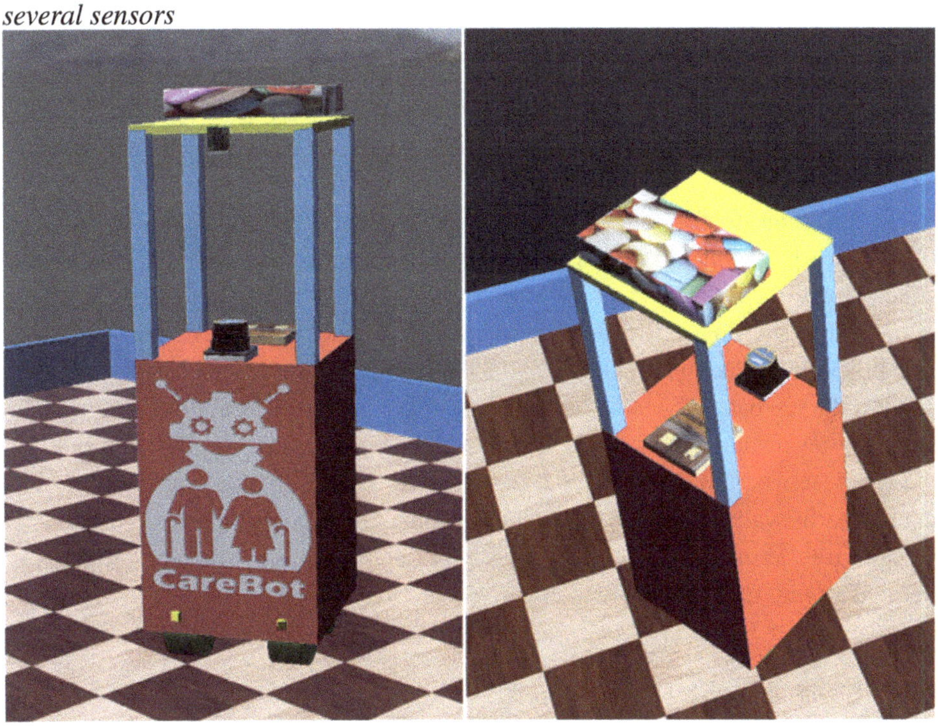

3.4 Sensors and Components of the robot

1. Camera
   - Size: Default Webots camera size (small box shaped).

- Position: Mounted at the front-center of the top panel, facing forward.
- Purpose: Captures visual data for object detection and path tracking.

2. LiDAR Sensor
    - Size: Approx. 0.04 meters (diameter), 0.03 meters (height) (cylinder).
    - Position: Placed in the center of the top panel.
    - Purpose: Scans surroundings to build a 2D/3D map for obstacle avoidance and SLAM.
3. Water Pot
    - Size: 0.05 meters (diameter) × 0.06 meters (height).
    - Position: Placed on the back-left of the top panel (translation -0.06 -0.06 0.55).
    - Purpose: Represents delivery or caregiving functionality (e.g., carrying water).
4. Pill Box
    - Size: 0.05 meters (width) × 0.03 meters (depth) × 0.02 meters (height) (a small rectangular box).
    - Position: Back-right of the top panel (translation 0.06 -0.06 0.55).
    - Purpose: Simulates the robot's ability to carry medicine or small objects.

The robot has four independently controlled wheels. Each wheel is a cylinder of 0.04 meters in height and radius, placed at each corner of the base. The wheels are attached with HingeJoints and powered by RotationalMotors (wheel1 to wheel4), allowing full mobility—forward, backward, and in-place rotation. Four blue vertical side pillars, each measuring 0.02 × 0.02 × 0.24 meters, are placed at the corners to support the top panel. These pillars give the robot a solid and balanced frame. Two small yellow distance sensors (ds_left and ds_right) are placed on the front sides of the robot (translation 0.1 ±0.06 0.02). They are slightly rotated outward and help detect nearby walls or objects to avoid collisions. The robot is placed slightly above ground (translation z ≈ 0.04 m) and has a total mass of 3 kg. The bounding box is defined around the main body to ensure correct physical interactions.

Table 1. The simulated robot specification

Component	Specification
Body	Box shape, size: 0.2 m (W) × 0.2 m (D) × 0.3 m (H), color: red
Top Platform	Box shape, size: 0.2 m × 0.2 m × 0.01 m, color: yellow
Wheels (4 pcs)	Cylinder shape, radius: 0.04 m, height: 0.04 m, color: green
Pillars (4 pcs)	Box shape, size: 0.02 m × 0.02 m × 0.24 m, color: blue
Camera	Mounted at front-center on top, default Webots camera, facing forward

continued on following page

Table 1. Continued

Component	Specification
LiDAR	Cylinder shape, radius: 0.04 m, height: 0.03 m, center-top placement
Water Pot	Rectangle shape, radius: 0.025 m, height: 0.06 m, position: back-left of top
Pill Box	Box shape, size: 0.05 m × 0.03 m × 0.02 m, position: top
Distance Sensors	2 units (left & right front), box size: 0.01 m × 0.01 m × 0.01 m, yellow
Motors	4 RotationalMotors (wheel1 to wheel4), independently drive each wheel
Bounding Box	Covers main body; used for collision and physics
Mass	3 kg
Position	Placed ~0.04 m above ground (Z-axis), centered on X and Y
Purpose	Indoor navigation, delivery of water and pills, sensing environment

This simulation configuration allows comprehensive testing of all required functionalities, particularly the integration of physical pill/water carrying capabilities with autonomous task execution.

3.5 Control Methods and Algorithmic Modules

3.5.1 Navigation and Path Planning Algorithm

The robot operates in a predefined indoor environment and requires safe, intelligent movement from one place to another. A path planning method is implemented using a grid-based A* (star) path finding algorithm. Obstacles are detected using range sensors such as LiDAR or distance sensors. The steps are given below:

1. Define key waypoints for each room or target zone.
2. Check for obstacle-free paths between waypoints using sensor data.
3. If blocked, select alternate waypoint or wait.
4. Control robot's wheel motors to move toward the next waypoint.
5. Continuously re-evaluate the path if dynamic obstacles are encountered.

3.5.2 Time-Based Task Scheduling

To complete tasks like medication and hydration reminders on schedule, a time-based scheduler is implemented. The robot uses the simulation clock to trigger these tasks. The steps are,

1. Maintain a task queue sorted by simulation timestamps.
2. At each simulation step, check the current time against the next scheduled task.

3. If a task is due, interrupt current operation if allowed and execute the reminder.
4. Log the reminder as completed and schedule the next instance if periodic.

3.5.3 Reminder and Interaction Logic

The interaction logic is managed through a finite state machine (FSM) to guide the robot through the reminders, and the delivery steps are as follows,

```
   4.1 IDLE: Waiting for a task.
   4.2 NAVIGATE_TO_USER: Moving toward the user location.
   4.3 REMINDER_ACTIVE: Delivering the reminder (beep/audio
prompt).
   4.4 WAIT_FOR_ACK: Pause for user acknowledgment.
   4.5 RETURN_TO_IDLE: Resetting for next task.
```

This structure ensures predictable and easily debug able task flow.

3.5.4 Human Localization

In the simulation, human presence is estimated using fixed or random target locations within the home. In a real deployment, this would be replaced by computer vision or beacon tracking. The methodological steps are:

1. Load or generate person position based on scenario.
2. Move to that position using navigation logic.
3. Confirm arrival using distance to target threshold.

3.5.5 Interaction Procedure

The robot's body has a pill box and a water container. During work, the robot makes audio beeps. The steps are,

1. On task trigger, highlight the object (e.g., open pill drawer).
2. Play reminder message as audio beep sound.
3. Wait for simulated user response or continue after delay.

3.5. 6 Obstacle Avoidance

To avoid collisions during navigation, the robot uses a reactive algorithm based on sensor thresholds. The methods are,

1. Continuously monitor the left, right, and front sensors.
2. If an obstacle is detected in front, stop and move slightly in the opposite direction.
3. Move away from the nearest obstacle.

This method ensures real-time responsiveness in confined spaces.

3.6 Mobile App Integration with IoT

The mobile app was developed as a supporting tool to monitor and manage the robot's pill and water supply. The control system is not included. Instead, it enables users – such as caregivers and family members – to access important data and schedule service appointments via an IoT-based architecture. The details framework is given in Figure 03.

Figure 3. The details diagram of the IoT based connectivity with robot

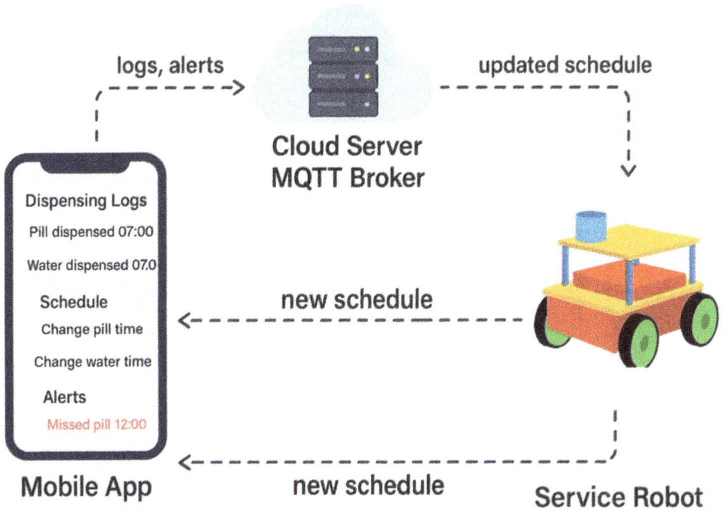

3.6.1 System Architecture

The system consists of three main components:

1. **Service Robot**: Operates autonomously in a simulated environment. It performs tasks such as pill and water delivery based on its internal schedule.

2. **Cloud Server (or Local MQTT Broker)**: Facilitates secure data exchange between the robot and the mobile application using the MQTT protocol.
3. **Mobile App**: Provides a user-friendly interface to view logs, update dispensing schedules, and receive alerts.

3.6.2 Communication Protocol

- MQTT protocol was used due to its lightweight and real-time capabilities.
- The robot publishes logs to specific MQTT topics, including timestamps of pill or water delivery, sensor feedback, and alert messages.
- The mobile app subscribes to these topics to stay updated.
- Users can update pill or water dispensing schedules by publishing new settings to robot-listening topics.

Figure 4. The several screenshots of mobile application

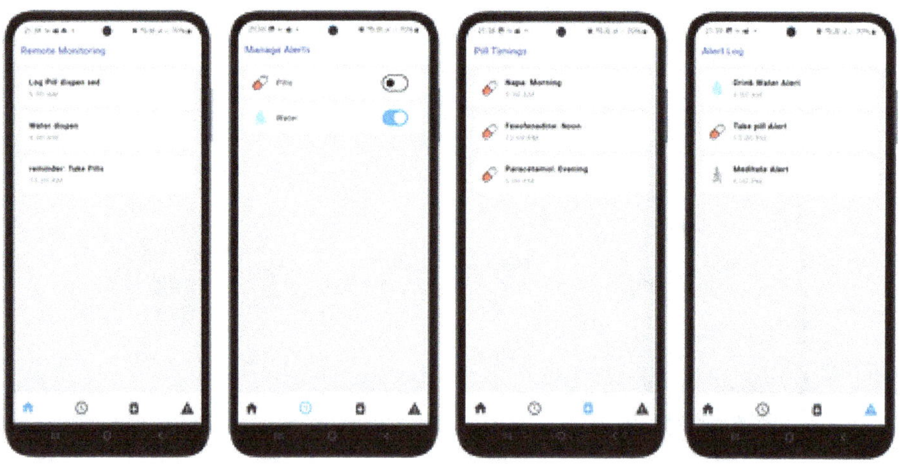

3.6.3 App Features and Interface

The app is designed for Android users. The image of Figure 04 below shows several screenshots of the mobile apps. Its primary features include:

- **Dispensing Log Viewer**: Displays timestamps of pill and water dispensing events.
- **Schedule Editor**: Allows users to change the times for pill and water delivery.

- **Alert Log**: Shows missed doses or delays.
- **Notifications**: Sends alerts when a scheduled task is executed or missed.
- **Security**: Ensures only authorized users can access or update schedules.

4. TESTING AND EVALUATION

To verify the functionality and performance of the elderly care service robot, a series of tests were conducted within the Webots simulation environment. The evaluation process was conducted entirely in this virtual (simulation) setting. This section presents the testing methods used, which include specific test cases and simulated scenarios. Additionally, user evaluations were included to assess both the technical capabilities of the robot and its effectiveness in user interaction. Details of the test pipeline are presented in the appendix section.

4.1 Functional Testing

Functional testing checks whether the robot is performing its tasks correctly. Each feature was evaluated one by one. The robot was asked to move forward, backward, and turn. It was evaluated to avoid obstacles. The camera was evaluated for object detection. The LiDAR was assessed for scanning the area. The robot carried a water container and pill box. These objects were tested to check whether they were stable. The distance sensor was tested for edge detection. The following test cases were included for functional testing:

- **Navigation test:** The robot moved from kitchen to living room. It avoided walls, potted plants and furniture.
- **Reminder test**: The robot gave reminders at the correct simulated times.
- **Object delivery test**: The robot reached the user. It initiated the interaction of the pill and water.
- **Obstacle avoidance test:** The robot changed its path when it suddenly encountered an obstacle.
- **Data Sync with cloud:** All the logs are uploaded to IoT-cloud and reflected in caregiver or family members mobile apps.

Figure 5. The functional testing results of the robot across five key features

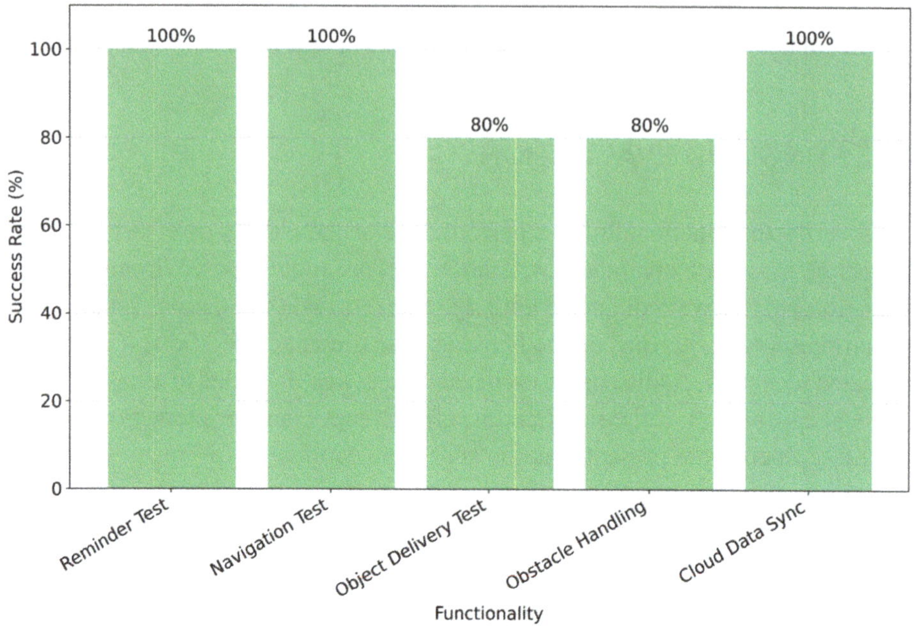

Functional testing ensures that the robot delivers pills and water correctly. It (the robot) automatically detects and navigates to the user. It triggers reminders at scheduled times. It logs events and triggers alerts for missing tasks. During navigation robots must deal with obstacles as well. The benefits of functional testing are:

- It validates all feature works as designed.
- Catches logical or sequence errors.
- Confirms integration between modules (navigation, scheduling, alert, interface).

Each test confirmed that the robot performed its task as expected. The bar chart in Figure 05 summarizes the results of the robot's functional testing across several key features. According to the charts, reminder trigger, navigation test and cloud data sync all achieved 100% success rates. Object delivery test and obstacle handling showed slightly lower success rates (80%).

4.2 Scenario Testing

Scenario testing examines how the robot behaves in real-life daily routines. It focuses on multi-step tasks. These tasks are based on how the robot will be used in a real home. Example scenarios include:

- The robot finds the user in the room. It delivers medication and water.
- The robot moves to the living room. It gives a reminder to drink water.
- The robot performs many tasks one after another. It follows the right order and avoids obstacles.

Figure 6. Screenshots of several test cases in simulated environment

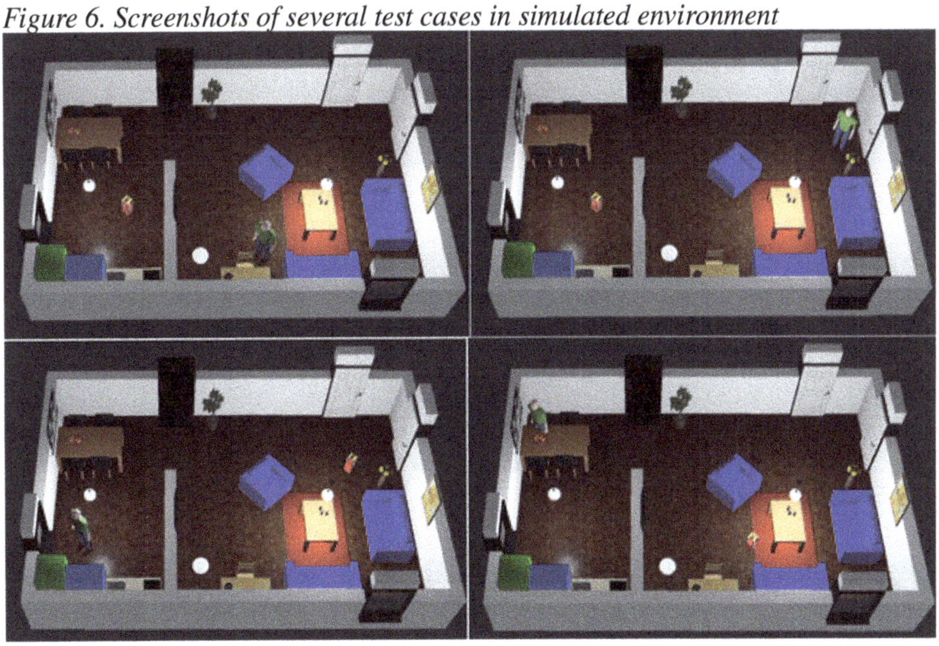

These tests help ensure that the robot can manage daily care activities. Screenshots of several test cases are provided in Figure 06. In the first scene, the person is sitting at the living room table reading or writing something and the robot is in the kitchen. The robot's goal is to find the person and give him water, because the water intake schedule has been activated. During the experimental test, the robot will complete the test smoothly. In the second scene, both the robot and the person have changed their positions. At this time, the robot will give the person a pill because the pill intake time has started. Here the robot performs the task beautifully. In the remaining scenes, the robot has completed its task correctly. The amount of time the robot took for each task or scenario was measured and then plotted. In Figure 07, each bar represents a task sequence like water delivery, pill delivery, or combined routines. This chart clarifies the efficiency and reliability of the robot.

Figure 7. Scenario testing chart: time taken per scenario

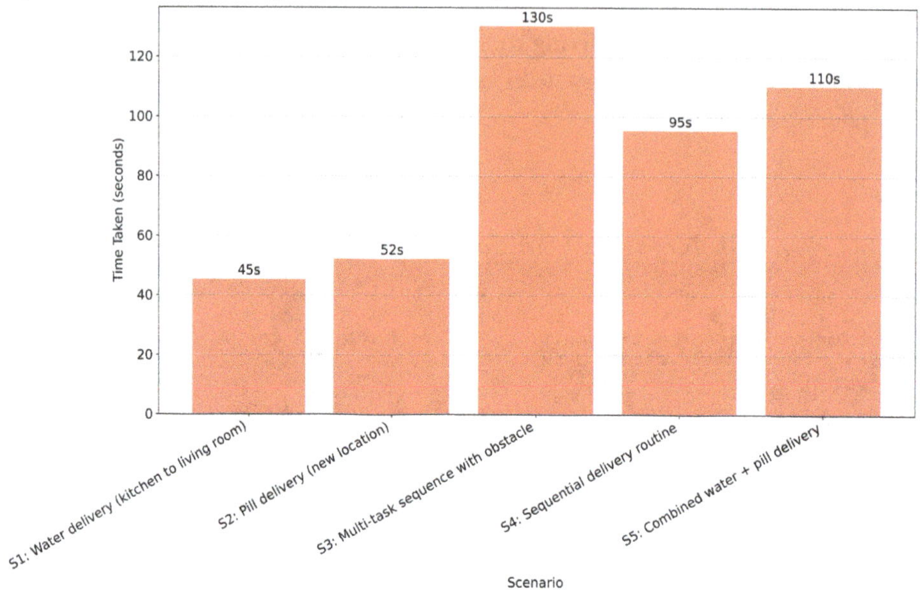

4.3 Stress Testing

To test the robot's reliability and robustness over time, stress testing was performed by accelerating the simulation clock and running the robot for extended periods of time. This allowed for multiple reminder and navigational tasks to be simulated over several minutes. The robot was monitored for task accuracy, collision frequency, and timing accuracy.

Figure 8. Stress testing results

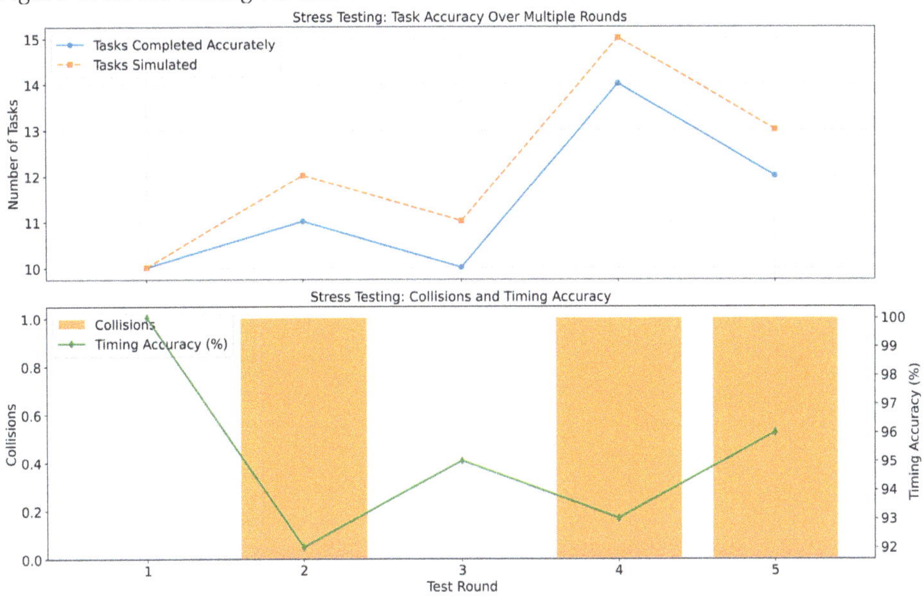

Two charts that visualize the stress testing performance of the robot in Figure 08. The task accuracy chart (in top) shows how many tasks were simulated vs. how many were completed accurately across multiple test rounds. Collisions and timing accuracy (in button) displays the number of collisions (bars) and timing precision (line) per test round. Stress tests highlight both the safety and schedule reliability of the robot.

4.4 User Evaluation

To assess the usability and acceptability of the robot from the perspective of potential users, video demonstrations of the simulated robot were shown to selected individuals, including:

1. Elderly users
2. Family caregivers
3. Healthcare professionals

Participants completed a Likert-scale survey assessing crucial factors such as ease of use, perceived helpfulness, trust in reminders, and level of comfort with the robot's interaction. Qualitative feedback was also collected to refine the design and functionality. We tested how users felt about the robot. A total of 30 participants took part. They included elderly users, family caregivers and healthcare workers. Each watched a video of the robot. Then they filled out a survey. The survey used a scale of 1 to 5. It focused on four key areas.

1. Ease of Use
2. Helpfulness
3. Trust in Reminders
4. Comfort with Interaction

Users gave high scores in all areas. "Helpfulness" scored the highest with 4.60. This means people found the robot useful. "Ease of Use" and "Comfort" both scored 4.53. Most users felt the robot was easy and friendly. "Trust in Reminders" scored 4.47. This shows users mostly trusted the alerts/ notifications. The questions and scores are listed in Table 02.

Table 2. Survey questions and average scores

Category	Question	Average Score (out of 5)
Ease of Use	The robot's functions were easy to understand.	4.53
Ease of Use	I could use the robot with little or no training.	4.53
Ease of Use	The robot's movements were smooth and easy to follow.	4.53
Perceived Helpfulness	The robot would help in daily care tasks.	4.6
Perceived Helpfulness	It is useful for delivering medication and water.	4.6
Perceived Helpfulness	The robot supports elderly users well.	4.6
Trust in Reminders	I trust the robot to give reminders on time.	4.47
Trust in Reminders	Reminder notifications seemed reliable.	4.47
Trust in Reminders	I would rely on the robot for medication alerts.	4.47
Comfort with Interaction	I felt comfortable with the robot's interaction.	4.53
Comfort with Interaction	The robot felt safe and non-intrusive.	4.53
Comfort with Interaction	The robot was respectful and home friendly.	4.53

Overall, the feedback was positive. The robot was considered helpful and safe for use at home.

5. MEDICAL USE ADAPTATIONS

The proposed robot, capable of delivering water and medicine to elderly people living alone, has great potential in the healthcare sector. Here are some ways this robot could be adapted for medical use:

5.1 Medication and Supply Delivery in Hospitals

In hospital wards, especially in large or understaffed facilities, robots can autonomously:

- Deliver medication, samples, or fluids to different patient rooms or nursing stations
- Reduce the physical burden on nurses and lower the risk of human error
- Minimize cross-contamination, as robots can be sterilized more consistently than human hands

Several hospitals, including some in South Korea and the U.S., already use similar robots (e.g., TUG by Aethon) for internal logistics (Sharma, 2023).

5.2 Post-Surgical or Rehabilitation Support

Patients recovering at home after surgery or treatment (e.g., post-chemotherapy or orthopedic procedures) often need regular medication and hydration. The robot can:

- Deliver medication at pre-programmed times
- Help prevent post-op complications like dehydration or pain mismanagement
- Reduce the need for in-person nurse visits

This approach supports telemedicine and hospital-at-home models (Antony, 2023).

5.3 Pandemic and Infection Control Scenarios

During pandemics like COVID-19, minimizing human-to-human contact became critical. Robots with pills and water delivery could:

- Serve quarantined or immunocompromised patients
- Deliver medications and supplies without exposing healthcare workers
- Be used in isolation wards with sterilization features (ultra-violet cleaning, antimicrobial surfaces)

This can reduce contact between healthcare workers and infected patients, decreasing infection spread (Gao, 2021).

5.4 Mental Health and Routine Reinforcement

Though not a direct medical function, routine reminders delivered by robots can have cognitive benefits:

- Reinforce structure in the day for patients with early-stage dementia or Alzheimer's disease
- Reduce anxiety related to forgotten medication or missed hydration
- Provide simple voice interaction or motivational cues (voice interaction modules required)

This type of robot can improve mental health (Antony, 2023). A summary of several use cases with benefits are listed in Table. 03.

Table 3. Summary of benefits in medical contexts

Use Case	Benefits
Hospitals & clinics	Improves logistics, lowers staff stress, and increases safety
Post-op/rehab at home	Enables self-care, supports recovery, enabling early discharge
Pandemic/isolation care	Minimizes contact, ensures continuity
Cognitive support	Reinforces routine, reduces anxiety and enhances mental well-being

6. COMPARISONS

As elderly people increasingly live alone, the need for regular medication and hydration management becomes critical. Traditionally, this assistance is provided through self-managed routines (e.g. alarms and pill boxes), family supervision, or periodic caregiver visits. Although these methods have been useful, they pose significant challenges – particularly in terms of consistency, responsiveness and user independence.

The proposed robotic system provides an innovative solution by automating delivery, reminders and monitoring. It reduces cognitive load, improves adherence and ensures a safe living environment for elderly people. The following table (Table. 04) outlines the key differences between traditional care methods and the proposed robotic solution.

Table 4. Comparison of traditional and robotic medication/water delivery systems

Feature/Aspect	Traditional methods	Proposed robotic system
Delivery mechanism	Manual (by self, family, or caregivers)	Automated delivery by wheeled robot
Reminder system	Alarm clocks, phone apps, verbal prompts	Real-time reminders via IoT system
Monitoring capability	None or manual caregiver logs	Live tracking with alert escalation for missed actions
Cognitive load	High — relies on memory and self-initiation	Low — robot proactively assists user at set times
Emergency response	Typically delayed; dependent on check-ins	Automatic alerts sent to caregivers/family
Consistency	Inconsistent; prone to human error	Highly consistent and punctual
Privacy & independence	May feel intrusive or over-dependent	Preserves autonomy and offers discreet support
Cost (Long-term)	High recurring costs (caregivers, services)	Higher initial cost, but low operational expense
Interaction style	Human-to-human	Human-robot interface with optional voice commands

6.1 Key Benefits of Robotic Approaches

- Real-time monitoring and physical delivery of medication and water improve compliance, especially for people with memory problems.
- Robots eliminate the need for daily medication supervision, reducing the necessity for caregivers.
- The robot issues alerts/notifications for missed tasks, providing an additional layer of protection not available in traditional methods.
- Elderly people can maintain independence without having to rely on supervision from others.

7. CONCLUSION

In this chapter, we present the development and evaluation of a four-wheeled service robot designed to care for the elderly. The robot was fully developed and tested within the Webots simulation environment. Its design followed specific constraints regarding size, mobility, sensor placement, and task functionality to ensure that it could operate efficiently in a compact home setting. We discussed each stage of the robot's development, including the integration of key components such as a proximity sensor, a camera, LiDAR, a water container, and a pill box. Functional and scenario-based tests confirmed that the robot could perform important tasks such as navigation, object delivery, and reminder activation in a realistic home-like environment. Usability and acceptability were assessed through responses from 30 participants, including elderly users, family caregivers, and healthcare professionals. Survey results showed high satisfaction in areas such as ease of use, perceived helpfulness, trust in reminders, and comfort in interaction. To further enhance user engagement and system control, the chapter also included the design of a user-friendly smartphone app for remote monitoring and control of the robot. This app allows caregivers and users to schedule tasks, receive status updates, and communicate with the robot remotely, adding a valuable layer of accessibility and convenience. Overall, the survey results highlight the practicality and user-friendliness of the robot. Various adaptations of robots in different medical fields demonstrate the potential and robustness of robots in the healthcare sector. A side-by-side comparison with the manual approach or traditional method gives insight into its advantages. The chapter demonstrates the value of simulation in early-stage development and testing. Future work could focus on increasing more advanced features such as voice interaction, fall detection and SOS integration, adding new app features, and expanding the robot's range of tasks to support real-world deployment in elderly care environments.

REFERENCES

Albee, D. T., & Hunter, M. R. (2022). AARP. In *Encyclopedia of Gerontology and Population Aging* (pp. 1–4). Springer International Publishing.

Alsanie, S., Ibrahim, K., Lim, S., & Wootton, S. (2024). Understanding the nature and scale of low-intake dehydration on 'Medicine for Older People' wards at University Hospital Southampton: A mixed-methods study. *Proceedings of the Nutrition Society, 83*(OCE2), E214.

Bathirappan, K., Pandurengan, D. B., Nawaz, J. Y., & Arulrajan, J. R. (2022, October). Patient monitoring and medicine dispenser robot. In *AIP Conference Proceedings* (Vol. 2494, No. 1). AIP Publishing.

Cohen, R. A., & Mykyta, L. (2024). Prescription Medication Use, Coverage, and Nonadherence Among Adults Age 65 and Older: United States, 2021–2022. Academic Press.

Dhar, M., Mittal, K., Pathania, M., & Kalra, S. (2023). Dehydration in Elderly: Revisiting the Assessment and Management Strategies. *The Journal of the Association of Physicians of India, 71*(12), 47–50.

Farley, A., Wang, J., & Marshall, J. A. (2022). How to pick a mobile robot simulator: A quantitative comparison of CoppeliaSim, Gazebo, MORSE and Webots with a focus on accuracy of motion. *Simulation Modelling Practice and Theory, 120,* 102629.

Guarducci, S., Jayousi, S., Caputo, S., & Mucchi, L. (2025). Key Fundamentals and Examples of Sensors for Human Health: Wearable, Non-Continuous, and Non-Contact Monitoring Devices. *Sensors (Basel), 25*(2), 556.

Hart, L. A., Vo, S., Hanlon, J. T., Schmader, K. E., & Gray, S. L. (2025). Medication Use Quality and Safety in Older Adults: 2023 Update. *Journal of the American Geriatrics Society.*

Jang, H., Sharma, A. B., Dan, U., Wong, J. H., Knight, Z. A., & Garrison, J. L. (2024). Dysregulation of the fluid homeostasis system by aging. *bioRxiv.*

Michel, O. (2025, January 31). *Webots R2025a* [Computer software]. Cyberbotics Ltd. https://www.cyberbotics.com/

Unnissa, Z., Unissa, M., & Khan, S. (2024). A Comprehensive Review of Medication Errors in Modern Healthcare. *Journal of Drug Delivery and Therapeutics, 14*(5).

WellMed Medical Management. (2023). Staying hydrated is especially important for older adults. https://www.wellmedhealthcare.com/staying-hydrated-is-especially-important-for-older-adults

World Health Organization. (2021). *Decade of healthy ageing: baseline report*. World Health Organization. UNIVERSAL, M. P. T. Health at a Glance: Asia/Pacific 2022.

World Health Organization. (2024, October 1). *Ageing and health*. https://www.who.int/news-room/fact-sheets/detail/ageing-and-health

Zhao, L. (2023). China's aging population: A review of living arrangement, intergenerational support, and wellbeing. *Health Care Science*, *2*(5), 317–327. DOI: 10.1002/hcs2.64 PMID: 38938584

APPENDIX A

Testing pipeline for the robot

1. Simulation Environment Setup
    - **Platform**: Webots (based on implementation).
    - **Environment**: Modeled home layout (bedroom, living room, kitchen) with realistic physics and sensors (based on the description in design methodology section).
    - **Robot Model**: Equipped with simulated navigation, sensors, task scheduling, and IoT-cloud connection (based on the description in design methodology section).
2. Functional Testing

Objective: Verify the correct operation of each core feature based on system requirements.
Tested Features:

- Reminder scheduling and trigger.
- Object delivery test.
- Navigation to users across rooms.
- Obstacle detection and avoiding.
- Data syncs with cloud and mobile apps (IoT-cloud).

Outcome:

- 3 out of 5 functions achieved 100% success.
- Minor inconsistencies in obstacle handling and object delivery test (80% success).
- Overall system functionality confirmed as robust and ready for extended testing.

Output: Bar chart of success rates per function (refer the Figure 05).

3. Scenario Testing

Objective: Test robot behavior in routine, multi-step home caregiving activities.

Scenarios:
1. Water delivery from kitchen to living room.
2. Medication delivery after user changes location.
3. Obstacle navigation while following a multi-task sequence.

4. Combined delivery tasks under scheduled triggers.

Output: Task duration metrics, completion rate, obstacle success rate chart (refer the Figure 07).

4. Stress Testing

Objective: Test robot reliability under high workload and prolonged operation.
Approach:

- Accelerated simulation clock (e.g., 5× real time).
- 5 rounds of 10–15 task cycles.
- Monitored for timing accuracy, task completion, and collision events.

Output: Line/bar charts showing task performance over time, timing accuracy, and system stability (refer Figure 08).

5. Metric Collection

Metrics or parameters are listed in Table 5. All data logged automatically and exported in structured format (csv format).

Table 5. Core validation metrics for testing

Metric	Source
Task completion rate	Simulation logs
Timing accuracy	Scheduled vs. actual timestamps
Obstacle avoidance	Collision event tracking
Alert responsiveness	Delay between non-response and alert trigger
Functional pass rate	Manual validation and test scripts

6. Data visualization

Several chart-based data visualizations are provided. These visualizations provide important information. See the testing and evaluation section for more information.

7. Performance summary and recommendations
    - Robot shows strong baseline performance in core functionalities
    - Maintains stability under load and completes complex tasks consistently
    - Small refinements needed in navigation with unstructured obstacle

Chapter 10
Smart Hospitals: The Role of IoT in Modern Healthcare

Mohammad Salah Uddin
https://orcid.org/0000-0002-4180-2355
Department of Computer Science and Engineering, East West University, Bangladesh

ABSTRACT

This chapter examines the role of the Internet of Things (IoT) in healthcare, focusing on hospital settings. It begins with a brief overview of IoT and its growing relevance in the healthcare industry. The chapter introduces key technologies such as sensors, remote connectivity, and data processing. It then discusses important hospital applications, including wearable devices, remote patient monitoring, and smart beds. Other use cases include patient tracking, asset management, room automation, and telemedicine. Each example shows how IoT supports hospital operations and patient care. The benefits of IoT integration are also addressed. These include improved quality of care, improved efficiency, and data-driven decision-making. Challenges are also outlined. Several key challenges include data security, patient privacy, system integration, and implementation costs. To support these topics, the chapter presents real-world case studies. These examples demonstrate measurable gains in both patient outcomes and hospital performance. The chapter concludes with a summary of the findings and a forward-looking perspective. It emphasizes the potential of IoT to support efficient, responsive, and patient-centered healthcare systems.

DOI: 10.4018/979-8-3373-1514-0.ch010

1. INTRODUCTION

The Internet of Things (IoT) is a major technological change that is impacting many sectors. Healthcare has seen significant changes. In hospitals, IoT can improve patient care, and support routine operations that increase efficiency. In hospitals, medical devices are connected to internal and external systems with the help of IoT. Real-time data collection and monitoring is allowed by IoT. As a result, hospital authorities get clear insights, which are helpful for decision-making. Hospitals have started using IoT to solve common problems and improve medical care. Remote patient monitoring is a key example. It allows doctors or nurses to monitor the vital signs of a patient without having to meet them directly. Wearable devices like smart-watches and glucose monitors are some examples of these systems. These devices collect health data and send it to the cloud. Doctors or responsible personnel are able to visualize that data through a cloud-connected mobile application. This is helpful for early detection of health problems and quick response. Smart hospital rooms are another application. These rooms automatically adjust lighting, temperature and other conditions based on the patient's condition. Hospital inventory or equipment can also be tracked using IoT. This simplifies the management process. It ensures that equipment is available when needed. Telemedicine has evolved using video conferencing technology via mobile devices. This allows patients to consult with a doctor from their own home. Telemedicine is helpful for people living in remote areas or those with mobility issues.

The healthcare sector is going through a digital revolution. At the heart of this transformation is the Internet of Things (IoT) – a powerful network of connected devices that collect, share and analyze data in real time. When applied to the medical environment, this network becomes the Internet of Medical Things (IoMT), which is reshaping how hospitals deliver care, manage resources and meet patient needs. The following sections begin with an introduction to IoT in healthcare. This includes an overview of the Internet of Medical Things (IoMT) and its core architecture. Key components such as sensors, connectivity networks, and data processing methods are explained. Next, the use of IoT technology in hospitals is described in detail. This is followed by a discussion of the main benefits IoT brings to hospital settings. Key challenges and limitations are also outlined. Survey-based opinions are gathered from future healthcare professionals. In addition, expert insights are drawn from recent research studies. The role of IoT in contributing to the Sustainable Development Goals (SDGs) is also addressed. A case study on the application of IoT in a hospital—or smart hospital—is included. An additional section discussing the potential long-term impact has been incorporated. Finally, the conclusion summarizes the findings. An appendix is provided, detailing the survey methods and presenting the results analysis.

2. INTRODUCTION IOT IN HEALTHCARE

2.2 Internet of Medical Things (IoMT)

In the medical domain, it is often called the Internet of Medical Things (IoMT). It refers to a network of connected medical devices (wearables and others). These devices are connected to each other via the cloud. The devices communicate with each other or with each other via the cloud. Figure 01 shows the architecture of the Internet of Medical Things (IoMT). It consists of several layers such as:

A. Perception Layer (Device Layer/Sensor Layer): It contains several sensors and wearable devices (e.g., heart rate, glucose, ECG monitors). This layer is responsible for collecting physiological data.
B. Network Layer: This layer contains technologies such as Wi-Fi, Bluetooth, 5G, ZigBee, etc. The network layer is responsible for data transmission.
C. Middleware/Processing Layer: It consists of several gateway, fog or cloud computing services. This layer performs primary processing, filtering, and data storage.
D. Application Layer: It provides healthcare services such as patient monitoring, emergency alerts, etc. It creates a bridge between doctors, patients, and hospitals.

In IoMT system, there are a variety of devices available for gathering data. Some are wearables, such as fitness bracelets or smartwatches that track heart rate or activity levels. Others are embedded machines or computers used inside hospitals - such as monitors, ventilators or infusion pumps, etc. A common characteristic of all these devices is that they are capable of sharing health information in real time. This constant flow of information helps doctors and nurses work faster and make better decisions. It also supports ongoing care, even when patients are not in hospital. The main purpose of using IoT in healthcare is to improve patient care. It allows medical staff to work more efficiently and conduct their activities based on accurate, up-to-date information. IoMT is already making a difference. It helps identify problems earlier, improves how hospitals are run, and creates a better experience for both patients and healthcare professionals.

Figure 1. Internet of Medical Things Architecture

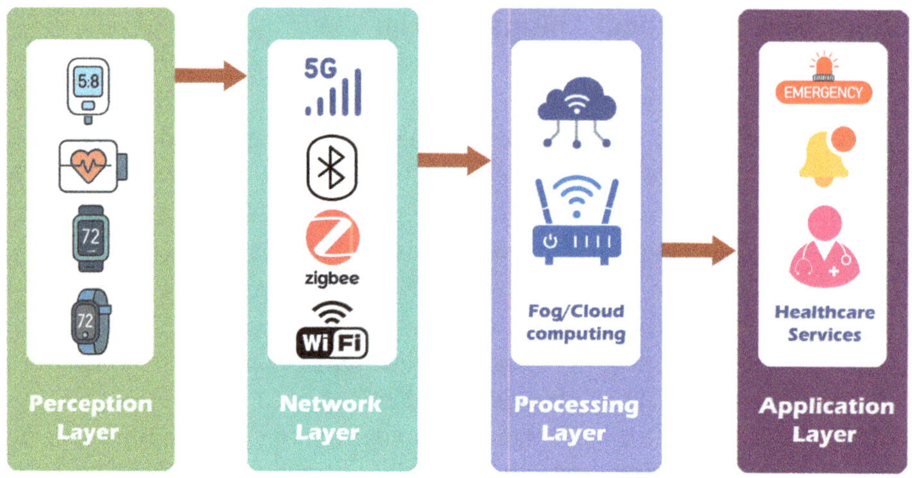

2.3 Components of IoT in Healthcare

2.3.1 Sensors and Devices

These are the first point of data collection. They sense health indicators like heart rate, blood pressure, oxygen levels, temperature, and glucose etc.

- Wearable devices include fitness trackers, ECG monitors, and smartwatches.
- Implantable sensors track internal conditions like cardiac activity or insulin levels.
- Medical equipment such as MRI scanners and ultrasound machines collects diagnostic data.

2.2.2 Connectivity

Devices need a way to send data to the cloud. They use wireless technologies such as:

- Wi-Fi for local communication within hospitals.
- Bluetooth for short-range data transfer between devices.
- Zigbee for low-power sensor networks.

- Cellular networks for remote data transfer from patient homes. This allows real-time communication between patients, devices, and medical staff.

2.2.3 Data Processing

Once data has been collected, data processing may be necessary to make decisions.

- Some devices process data on-site using built-in processors. Others send data to local servers (gateways) or cloud platforms for processing.
- Data analysis tools help identify trends, detect issues, and support decision-making.
- Machine learning and analytics can predict risks based on patient history and current data.

2.2.4 User Interface

Interfaces make IoT systems usable for users. Some of the interfaces used in IoT systems are,

- Dashboards or chart-based data visualizations show live data to hospital staff or doctors.
- Mobile apps help patients track their health at home. Interfaces need to be simple and clear to avoid confusion.
- These interfaces help users interact with data quickly and effectively.

2.3 IoT Technologies Used in Hospitals

2.3.1 Wearable Devices

These devices track physical activity and vital signs. For example, a heart monitoring device detects abnormal rhythms and alerts doctors. Sleep monitoring devices record a patient's sleep activity. A movement tracker is also helpful in tracking movements. Wearable devices support continuous care for patients. Patients can stay active while doctors stay informed.

2.3.2 Remote Monitoring System

Remote monitoring is used for patients suffering from chronic diseases. Devices used at home measure vital signs such as blood pressure and oxygen levels. The data is sent to hospitals or clinics. This information allows doctors to intervene early if warning signs occur (Uddin et al., 2017 and Ahammed et al. 2021).

2.3.3 Smart Beds

Hospital beds have sensors to monitor patient activity and comfort (Bose, 2025). These beds automatically adjust to reduce patient injury. These beds detect when a patient tries to stand up, which helps prevent falls. They track sleep quality and breathing patterns. Figure 02 shows a smart hospital bed.

Figure 2. Smart hospital beds equipped with several sensory (Megarit, 2021)

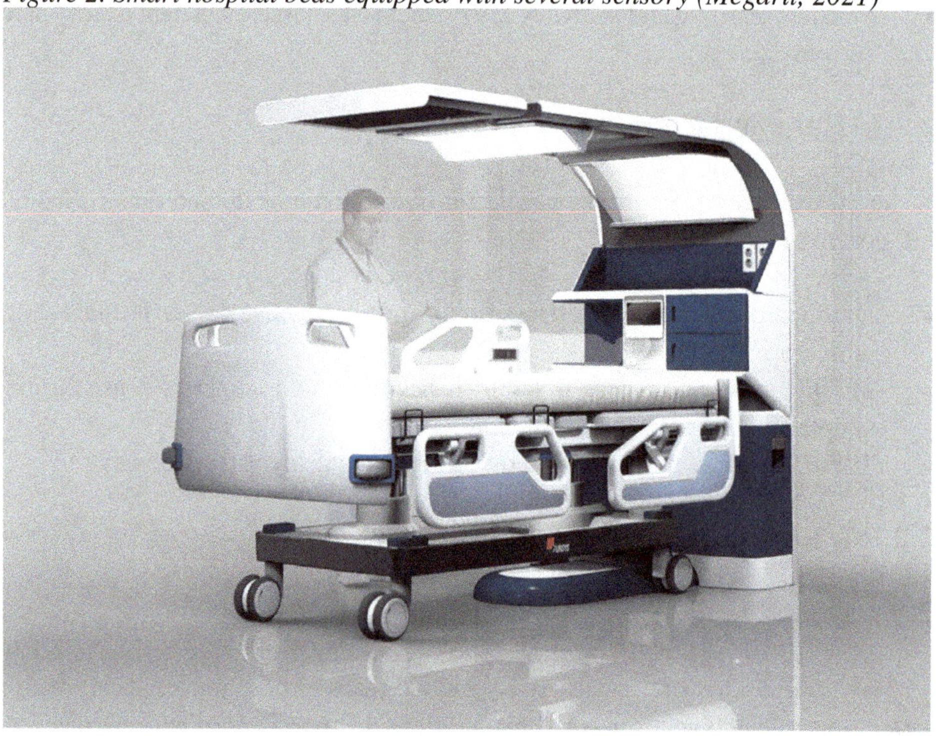

2.3.4 Medical Equipment or Asset Tracking

Medical equipment or tools are now part of the things connected to the hospital network or IoMT. For example, infusion pumps can be monitored and adjusted remotely. Imaging machines can upload scans directly to the patient's record via the cloud. Equipment maintenance schedules can be determined based on usage data.

2.3.5 Environmental Sensors

These monitor hospital conditions or surrounding environments that affect patient safety. Embedded devices track room temperature, humidity, light levels, and air quality. These connected devices help prevent infections by maintaining a clean, controlled environment. They alert staff if a room becomes unsafe (based on information that determines unsafe conditions).

2.3.6 Telemedicine

IoT also supports virtual care and remote diagnosis. Devices like digital stethoscopes and ECG monitors send patient information directly to doctors. DocTime (DocTime, n.d) and TytoCare (Amparore et al., 2024) both offer patients the opportunity to take scheduled tests from home. Doctors review data and respond in real time. This is particularly helpful in remote areas or for patients with mobility issues. DocTime (DocTime, n.d) is Bangladesh's leading digital healthcare platform. It provides 24/7 online doctor consultation through video calls. This platform connects patients with verified doctors. It ensures quality services for patients. On the other hand, TytoCare (Amparore et al., 2024) is a global telehealth company. It provides a compact solution that makes remote medical examinations possible from home. The platform includes several portable devices such as digital stethoscopes, otoscopes, thermometers and high-resolution cameras. These tools allow users to perform scheduled medical tests. The complete Tytocare system is presented in Figure 03.

Figure 3. TytoCare telemedicine system (Amparore et al., 2024; TytoCare, n.d.)

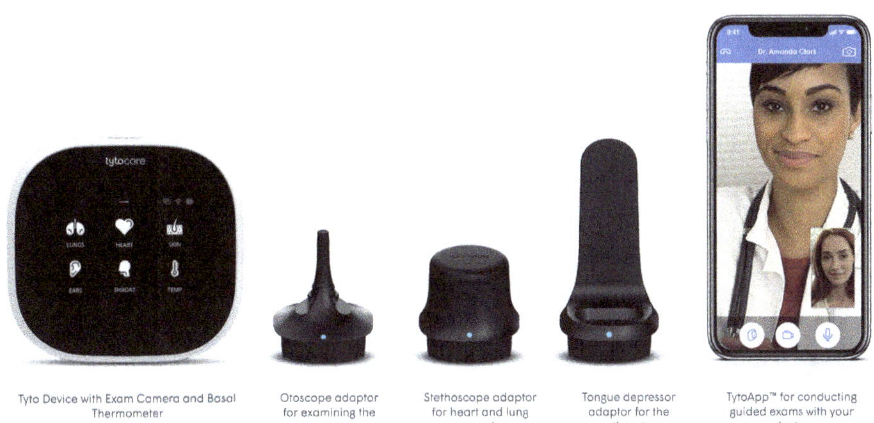

3. BENEFITS OF IOT IN HOSPITALS

The use of IoT in hospitals brings major improvements in both patient care and operational efficiency. It is helping to improve patient care, streamline operations, and make better decisions.

3.1 Improved Patient Care

IoT devices allow 24/7 tracking of vital signs such as heart rate, blood pressure, and glucose levels. Wearables send this data in real time to doctors and nurses. Early alerts help prevent complications. Several researchers have said that remote patient monitoring has been shown to reduce hospital readmission rates by 40% (Wartenberg et al., 2025).

- Real-time data helps tailor treatment to individual needs. For example: Insulin pumps adjust doses based on current glucose levels, improving accuracy and outcomes.
- IoT devices are often connected to mobile apps. These apps allow patients to track their own health status, leading to better adherence to treatment and more active participation in care.

3.2 Operational Efficiency

IoT can automate routine tasks in hospitals. It reduces the workload on staff and helps them focus more on patient care. For example, smart medicine dispensers can accurately track, schedule, and dispense medications. It minimizes the risk of human error and ensures timely administration.

- IoT tracking systems help hospitals locate equipment and monitor its condition in real time. For instance, RFID tags help staff find needed equipment without delay, improving response times and overall efficiency.
- Sensors also track the condition of medical equipment. They (sensors) detect early signs of malfunction. This helps prevent corrosion. It also reduces repair costs and ensures the availability of equipment when needed.

3.3 Data-Driven Decision-Making

- IoT devices generate tons of health-related data. When properly analyzed, this data can retrieve significant patterns and predict possible health risks.

This facilitates early medical intervention and helps reduce the risk of complications.

- In the context of public health, the role of IoT is crucial. It can able to detect infectious disease outbreaks based on data surveillance. It also allows tracking of chronic disease trends across people. These activities speed up the public health responses and resource allocation.
- Hospitals can utilize data to optimize operational efficiency. For instance, tracking patient movement across hospital departments can reduce waiting times and improve resource management.

4. CHALLENGES OF IOT IN HOSPITALS

Healthcare sectors have benefited from IoT in various ways. But there are several challenges in implementing IoT in hospitals. Harnessing the full potential of IoT requires data security, device/system compatibility, investment, data management, and human factors.

4.1 Safeguarding Patient Data and Privacy

IoT devices collect sensitive personal health parameters, such as heart rate, blood sugar levels, and patient treatments history. This puts them at risk of cybersecurity threats and data breaches.

- Hospitals must employ vigorous cybersecurity procedures. Those measures includes encoded data communication, secure networks, and automated vulnerability analysis.
- Compliance with data protection regulations like the Health Insurance Portability and Accountability Act (HIPAA) in the U.S. (CGCompliance, 2025 & Feather Staff, 2025) or GDPR in the EU is crucial.
- Managing privacy and compliance becomes more complicated when hospitals use IoT devices from multiple vendors, as they come with different security standards and protocols.

4.2 Integration With Existing Equipment

Hospitals often have a mix of old and new devices or equipment. The combination of new and older equipment creates interoperability challenges in IoT.

- Many IoT devices are not inherently compatible with existing electronic health record (EHR) systems.
- Devices from different manufacturers may use proprietary protocols, making integration across platforms difficult.
- Adoption requires industry-wide standards for data formats and communication protocols.
- Older IT infrastructure may need significant upgrades or replacement, increasing the cost and complexity of deployment.

4.3 High Implementation Costs

Implementation of IoT in hospital environment is a resource-intensive process.

- Costs include purchasing devices, upgrading networks, improving cybersecurity, and expanding data storage infrastructure.
- Hospitals also need to invest in staff development to train staff on the new system. Hospitals may need to hire new people for data management and systems administration.
- Without a clear return on investment (ROI) strategy, these expenses can be difficult to justify to stakeholders and funding agencies.

4.4 Data Management Challenges

IoT systems generate a continuous flow of health-related data. This data can be both a strength and a challenge.

- Hospitals need advanced analytics platforms to process and extract actionable insights from this data.
- Without proper filtering, high data volume can overwhelm clinical workflows.
- The accuracy, timeliness, and relevance of data are critical. Poor-quality or misinterpreted data can lead to diagnostic or treatment errors.

4.5 Human Factors

Adoption of technology depends on the willingness of both staff and patients to engage with IoT systems.

- Patients may have concerns about privacy, data misuse, or the impersonality of technology-driven care.

- Physicians and healthcare workers may feel unprepared to use unfamiliar devices.
- Hospitals need to provide transparent communication, hands-on training and ongoing support to build confidence and comfort with the new system.
- Building trust is essential to the long-term, sustainable adoption of IoT in clinical practice.

5. EXPERT OPINION ON IOT ADOPTION IN HOSPITAL

5.1 Remote Monitoring

In a study by De Castro, six expert interviews and three online surveys revealed how 5G and IoT technologies are transforming home hospitalization. Experts emphasized the reduction of healthcare costs and patient crowding in hospitals. These technologies allowed real-time patient monitoring and improved continuity of care without requiring in-person visits (De Castro, 2019).

5.2 Telemedicine and IoT Integration

AM Auwal used in-depth interviews to analyze how IoT enhances telemedicine. Healthcare professionals interviewed noted that real-time data transmission using IoT devices like body sensors improved diagnostic accuracy and patient triage. Experts also highlighted the role of IoT in expanding access to care in rural areas by linking patients to urban healthcare systems through digital networks (Auwal, 2023).

5.3 Clinician Readiness and Smart Technologies

Dermody with his team conducted a systematic review that included interviews and focus groups to evaluate clinician readiness for smart home and IoT technologies. Many clinicians expressed concern over data reliability, but acknowledged the benefit of smart beds and in-home monitoring for chronic conditions. Experts suggested that strong institutional support and training could ease adoption barriers (Dermody et al., 2024).

5.4 IoT for Asset Tracking

A.A. Alyami presented expert-supported research on the implementation of an RFID/ZigBee-based tracking system. After discussing with healthcare administrators, he found that IoT devices are efficient in tracking hospital equipment and its status (present condition). This helps in better decision making. Real-time visibility of assets in intensive care units (ICU) was seen as a critical emergency (Alyami, 2018).

5.5 Broader Professional Perspectives

Besnik Qehaja's doctoral work included interviewing ICT experts to develop a framework for real-time monitoring. These professionals emphasized that beyond technological benefits, IoT is transforming the way healthcare institutions manage resources and communicate with patients. IoT systems were credited with not only improving efficiency, but also improving patient trust and satisfaction (Besnik, 2020).

5.6 Privacy and Security

De Castro and Auwal, study consistently emphasized the need for strong cybersecurity protocols, system interoperability, and extensive staff training. Concerns about data privacy, system fragmentation, and regulatory compliance were common themes in interviews with physicians, administrators, and IT professionals (De Castro, 2019 and Auwal, 2023).

6. PERSPECTIVES OF HEALTHCARE PROFESSIONALS ON IOT

The use of IoT in hospitals marks a major shift in healthcare. Smart monitoring tools, connected devices, and real-time data systems are making hospitals more efficient and patient focused. These technologies promise to improve care, streamline operations, and support clinical decision-making. However, the success of IoT depends on how well future healthcare professionals understand and accept it. These individuals will soon enter clinical environments where such technologies are becoming standard. Their views and readiness will shape how smoothly IoT is adopted.

To explore this, a survey was conducted with 30 participants. These included medical students, nursing students, biomedical engineering students, and early-career clinicians and IT professionals. The goal was to gather their thoughts on the role of IoT in modern healthcare. The survey combines both closed and open-ended questions. It focused on five key areas:

- Participant background
- Familiarity with IoT
- Perceived benefits of IoT
- Perceived challenges
- Expectations for the future

This section presents the findings from that survey. It highlights how tomorrow's healthcare professionals view the opportunities and obstacles linked to IoT. The results provide useful insights for educators, hospital administrators, and policymakers aiming to support effective IoT adoption. Several key findings are listed in Table 01.

6.1 Discussion

Although a minority (13%) of respondents are deeply familiar with IoT in healthcare, the majority show at least moderate awareness. This suggests a need for more structured education in medical and allied curricula to help the next generation fully understand and engage with emerging technologies.

Data management emerged as the top concern, reflecting apprehension about handling large volumes of real-time patient data. Compatibility and interoperability between devices and systems were also significant issues—aligned with real-world case studies where legacy system integration remains a barrier.

The fact that 40% of young healthcare professionals believe IoT will become essential within a decade indicates a positive, progressive mindset. However, the 30% uncertainty in recommending IoT use suggests that practical exposure and training are lacking.

While half of the respondents trust hospitals to manage IoT-collected data securely, nearly half either lack trust or are unsure. This trust gap underscores the importance of building secure systems and communicating those protections transparently to both staff and patients.

Table 1. Key findings: Next-generation views on IoT in hospitals

Category	*Key Findings*
Familiarity with IoT	Approx. 33% were somewhat familiar and another 33% had heard of it but lacked deeper knowledge. Only 13% were very familiar.
Top Perceived Challenges	The leading concerns were data management (27%), compatibility (20%), and data privacy (17%).
Belief in IoT's Future	40% of respondents believe IoT will be essential in hospitals within the next 10 years.
Comfort Recommending IoT	43% are comfortable recommending IoT use in clinical settings, but 27% said no and 30% were unsure.
Trust in Data Security	50% trust hospital systems to protect IoT data, while 23% do not and 27% are unsure.

6.2 Recommendations

This pilot survey reveals cautious optimism toward IoT adoption among the new generation of healthcare workers. To support more confident engagement, healthcare institutions should:

- Integrate IoT literacy into medical and nursing education.
- Offering hands-on workshops and simulations using IoT devices.
- Establishing institutional protocols for IoT adoption and data management.
- Build interdisciplinary bridges between IT teams and clinical staff.

The next generation of healthcare professionals will play a central role in shaping how IoT is integrated into clinical care. While early perceptions are generally positive, meaningful adoption requires more than enthusiasm, it requires preparation, protection, and practical engagement.

7. CONTRIBUTION TO SUSTAINABLE DEVELOPMENT GOALS (SDGS)

The integration of Internet of Things (IoT) technologies into healthcare supports several United Nations Sustainable Development Goals (SDGs). These technologies not only advance healthcare outcomes but also align with global objectives in sustainability, equality, and innovation (Nikolova, 2024). The most directly related goals include:

7.1 SDG 3: Good Health and Well-being

"Ensure healthy lives and promote well-being for all at all ages."

IoT facilitates early detection, continuous monitoring, and personalized care through devices such as wearable health trackers and smart monitoring systems. These tools support patient safety, reduce readmission rates, and improve chronic disease management.

7.2 SDG 9: Industry, Innovation, and Infrastructure

"Build resilient infrastructure, promote inclusive and sustainable industrialization and foster innovation."

Smart hospital infrastructure—such as IoT-enabled asset tracking, real-time location systems, and AI-assisted workflows—enhances efficiency and resilience. IoT helps modernize outdated systems, supporting innovation in healthcare.

7.3 SDG 10: Reduced Inequalities

"Reduce inequality within and among countries."

IoT-powered telemedicine enables outreach to remote or underserved communities, reducing geographic and economic barriers to healthcare. These technologies promote inclusivity and equity in service delivery.

7.4 SDG 12: Responsible Consumption and Production

"Ensure sustainable consumption and production patterns."

IoT improves resource utilization. Automated inventory systems reduce waste and prevent overuse of supplies. Smart energy management systems in hospital settings also promote environmental sustainability.

7.5 SDG 17: Partnerships for the Goals

"Strengthen the means of implementation and revitalize the global partnership for sustainable development."

IoT implementation needs collaboration among system developers, healthcare service providers, researchers, and government agencies. These partnerships adopt innovation and support shared goals for improving global health.

Based on the above discussion, it is clear that, IoT systems are instrumental in crafting a sustainable and smart healthcare ecosystem.

8. SMART HOSPITAL CASE STUDIES

To explore and compare the smart technologies adopted at Al-Adan Hospital and Samsung Medical Center, analyze their impact on healthcare delivery, and evaluate their success in transitioning toward fully integrated smart hospital systems.

8.1 Case 1: Al-Adan Hospital – Kuwait

Al-Adan Hospital, located in Kuwait's Mubarak Al-Kabeer region, is among the country's largest healthcare facilities. It underwent a major expansion—including digital and infrastructure upgrades—and now supports approximately 632 additional beds, across 14 floors and 280,000 m^2 of clinical space. Several smart technologies at Al-Adan hospital are listed below:

- **IoT-enabled patient wristbands & wearable kits**: The deployment includes wristband devices and IoT kits—such as emergency response buttons and wristbands—that provide continuous monitoring and real-time alerts (Minew, n.d.).
- **Smart beds**: Likely integrated with sensors for occupancy, patient movement, and vitals—complementing the wristband systems (Kuwait Computer Services, 2024).
- **Real-time data dashboards**: Aggregate sensor readings (e.g., from beds and wristbands) to assist in clinical decision-making and emergency response.
- **Digital imaging systems**: Part of the infrastructure upgrades, aligning with common imaging modernization in such expansions.

8.1.1 Implementation Strategy

The hospital implemented its smart infrastructure through international collaboration—with partners like Ecosir (Finland) and Sumetzberger (Austria). Its approach was phased, emphasizing staff training and regular system maintenance to ensure sustainability and adoption.

8.1.2 Challenges

- **Interoperability issues**: Integrating with legacy systems remains a hurdle in expanding digital ecosystems across all wards.
- **Ongoing training and maintenance needs**: Technological complexity demands sustained support and learning.
- **Infrastructure constraints**: Some hospital areas require further network and systems upgrades to fully leverage IoT capabilities.

8.1.3 Costs

- **Capital expenditure**: The hospital expansion cost approximately USD 771 million, encompassing additional beds and full infrastructure rollout (Kuwait Direct Investment Promotion Authority, 2022).
- **Additional tech investments**: Included IoT devices (wristbands, smart beds), plus HVAC upgrades supported by energy-efficient motors provided by WEG to reduce consumption and maintenance costs (Minew, n.d.).

- **Ongoing costs**: Staff training, periodic tech maintenance, and network upgrades in lagging areas impose recurring expenditures (common in large-scale public health IT systems in Kuwait).

8.1.4 Benefits

It has improved emergency response and patient safety. The smart structure has also improved the overall performance of hospital services. It has also improved monitoring in hospital wards.

8.2 Case 2: Samsung Medical Center – South Korea

Samsung Medical Center (SMC) in Seoul is a globally acclaimed, HIMSS Stage 7-certified digital hospital—completely paperless since 2008. It has earned multiple awards including the 2024 Davies Award for Digital Excellence. Several smart technologies used by Samsung medical center are listed below:

- **Digital Twin**: Samsung Medical Center has built a virtual replica of its facilities to simulate operations and predictive planning (Canadian Healthcare Technology, 2025).
- **Voice AI Assistants & Autonomous Delivery Robots**: Used for patient interaction (such as pediatric support) and logistical support on wards.
- **AI-Powered Diagnostics & Operations**: Includes deep learning tools for clinical decisions (e.g., pressure injury management) and predictive scheduling to optimize workflows (Hospital Management Asia, 2024).
- **Cloud-based EHR**: Fully integrated across all departments, enabling seamless information flow.

8.2.1 Implementation Strategy

- **R&D and Pilots via Internal AI Labs**: Innovations were iteratively tested, avoiding a "big-bang" deployment by scaling small pilot units first (Canadian Healthcare Technology, 2025).
- **EHR Integration**: A phased, rules-based EMR implementation known as DARWIN helped standardize workflows across the hospital (Canadian Healthcare Technology, 2025).

8.2.2 Challenges

- **High Up-Front Investment**: Significant capital was needed for robotics, AI, and IT infrastructure.
- **Data Privacy & Security**: Complex AI and digital twins require robust protections—emphasized across multiple deployments (Hospital Management Asia, 2024).
- **Cultural Resistance**: Some experienced clinicians were hesitant about AI-supported decision-making, prompting careful change management (Canadian Healthcare Technology, 2025).

8.2.3 Costs

- **High upfront investment**: Major R&D and technology rollout costs for AI–robotics, digital twin simulations, and integrated systems.
- **Operational and security costs**: Ongoing expenditures for AI model upkeep, data security, pilot testing, and clinician training.

8.2.4 Benefits

- **Staff time saved**: AI automation reduced repetitive tasks (e.g., documentation, medication scanning), lowering nurse workload by ~30% (Hospital Management Asia, 2024).
- **Improved Diagnostic Accuracy & Clinical Outcomes**: AI-assisted wound care improved healing rates by ~37%, while optimized MRI and scheduling improved throughput.
- **Patient experience**: Robots for engagement and AI for smoother care pathways enhance overall experience (Hospital Management Asia, 2024).
- **Cost reductions across workflows**: Research shows AI–robotics implementations can cut costs by 25–40%, reduce admin processing time by 60–80%, and improve diagnostic accuracy up to 95% (Parthasarathi & Sheri, 2025).

8.3 SWOT Analysis

Table 02 and Table 03 shows the SWOT (Strengths, Weaknesses, Opportunities, and Threats) analysis of two hospitals respectively.

Table 2. Al-Adan Hospital, SWOT analysis

Strengths	Weaknesses
• Strong government funding for infrastructure **• Rapid deployment of IoT and smart beds** **• Improved patient tracking and emergency care**	• Legacy systems limit interoperability • Limited use of advanced AI • Staff may require ongoing digital training
Opportunities	**Threats**
• Expand into AI-assisted diagnostics **• Partner with international tech firms** **• Enhance telemedicine capabilities**	• Technological obsolescence • Resistance to system upgrades • Cybersecurity risks as more devices connect to the network

Table 3. Samsung Medical Center, SWOT analysis

Strengths	Weaknesses
• Advanced use of AI, robotics, and digital twin **• Seamless cloud EHR system** **• High diagnostic accuracy** **• Strong innovation culture**	• High initial capital and maintenance cost • AI skepticism from older clinicians • Complex systems require high digital literacy
Opportunities	**Threats**
• Pioneer personalized digital health models **• Expand globally as a tech provider** **• Innovate further in robotic surgery and remote care**	• Data privacy regulations tightening • Ethical concerns around AI decisions • Competitive pressure from global smart hospitals

8.4 Discussion and Comparison

Al-Adan Hospital focuses on infrastructure-based upgrades, while Samsung Medical Center pursues an intelligence-driven transformation. Each reflects a distinct yet effective approach to smart healthcare, aligned with local needs and readiness. A side by side comparison of both hospital are presented in Table 04.

Table 4. side by side comparison of Al-Adan and Samsung Medical Center

Dimension	Al-Adan (Kuwait)	SMC (South Korea)
Core strategy	Infrastructure/IOT upgrades	Intelligent systems, AI, robotics, digital twin
Roll-out model	Phased deployment via global partners	Agile, incremental R&D and pilot testing
Impact scope	Efficiency and safety enhancements	Broad clinical, operational, and satisfaction gains
Shared hurdles	Interoperability, training, infrastructure	Capital, privacy, and cultural adoption

Al Adan Hospital demonstrates a basic smart hospital model. It uses IoT to improve monitoring, safety and efficiency. In contrast, Samsung Medical Center reflects a sophisticated approach. It applies AI, robotics and digital twinning to enhance healthcare accuracy and streamline workflow. Both examples highlight that digital healthcare transformation is aligned with an organization's readiness, resources, and culture.

9. LONG-TERM IMPACT OF SMART HOSPITALS

The long-term impact of smart hospitals is much greater than the immediate benefits of automation and monitoring. It is reshaping the way healthcare service is delivered, experienced, and sustained. A detailed description of long-term effects is given below:

a. **Better patient outcomes:** IoT devices support continuous monitoring of health parameters. It helps in early detection of health problems. This reduces complications and improves recovery.
b. **Preventive care:** Continuous data helps to predict health-related risks. This enables taking preventive measures before the situation worsens.
c. **Faster emergency response:** Smart Alerts notify staff instantly, speeding up critical decisions and interventions.
d. **Operational efficiency:** Smart sensing systems track hospital equipment, bed usage, and inventory. This ensures optimum resource allocation and maintenance.
e. **Lower operational costs:** Automated systems save time and money. Data driven predictive maintenance cuts equipment repair costs in hospital.
f. **Remote and personalized care:** IoT supports telehealth and home-based monitoring. This improves access for rural and aging populations.
g. **Support for aging populations:** Elderly patients benefit from safe, continuous monitoring. It reduces the need for frequent hospital visits.

h. **Environmental sustainability:** Smart energy and utility systems minimize energy and water use. This approach makes hospitals more sustainable and eco-friendly.
i. **Scalability and Flexibility:** IoT systems are adaptable. Hospitals can add new tools and update systems over time.
j. **Better Crisis Preparedness:** In the event of a pandemic or disaster, IoT helps with process tracking, zoning, and security measures.
k. **Improved Staff Experience:** Automation reduces repetitive tasks. Staff can focus more on patient care.
l. **Enhanced Data-Driven Decisions:** Hospitals collect valuable health data. This supports research and policy planning.
m. **Security Risks:** IoT systems increase the risk of cyber-attacks if strong security protocols are not used.

10. CONCLUSION

The integration of Internet of Things (IoT) technologies into healthcare is changing how hospitals manage care and operations. IoT enables faster, data-driven, and more personalized healthcare. Tools such as wearable monitors, connected medical devices, and telemedicine platforms are now common in many settings. These tools help providers respond quickly and deliver care tailored to individual needs. Several studies from experts show that IoT can support key clinical goals. For example, wearable sensors used in remote monitoring can detect early signs of patient deterioration. This allows for quicker medical response. RFID-based tracking systems improve equipment visibility, speed up workflows, and reduce delays in care. Despite these benefits, IoT adoption comes with challenges. Data privacy, cybersecurity, and system compatibility are major concerns. The cost of setting up and maintaining these systems is also high. Beyond the technical issues, hospitals face human and organizational barriers. These include the need for staff training, adapting workflows, and securing informed patient consent. Experts agree that success depends on more than just new technology. Clear policies, sufficient funding, and strong institutional support are all needed. Without these, IoT systems may fall short of their potential. IoT also has the potential to improve healthcare access. Telemedicine platforms, supported by IoT, can connect providers with patients in remote or underserved regions. These systems are not yet available everywhere, but they offer useful models for expanding care reach.

In summary, IoT offers clear benefits when used carefully and with attention to local needs. Success depends on more than just advanced tools. Hospitals need governance, ethics, training, and infrastructure to support these systems. When these elements are in place, IoT can improve care quality, increase efficiency, and strengthen patient engagement. In doing so, it helps build more flexible and resilient healthcare systems.

REFERENCES

Ahammed, S., Hassan, N., Cheragee, S. H., & Islam, A. Z. M. T. (2021). An iot-based real-time remote health monitoring system. *International Journal of Research Engineering Science*, *8*(3), 23–29.

Auwal, A. M. (2023). *IoT integration in telemedicine: Investigating the role of Internet of things devices in facilitating remote patient monitoring and data transmission.*

Alyami, A. A. (2018). *Smart e-health system for real-time tracking and monitoring of patients, staff and assets for healthcare decision support in Saudi Arabia* (Doctoral dissertation, Staffordshire University).

Amparore, D., De Cillis, S., Colombo, M., Garzena, V., Sica, M., Checcucci, E., & Porpiglia, F. (2025). TYTOCARE™ home telemonitoring device after radical cystectomy to optimise postoperative outcomes. *BJU International*, *135*(6), 960–968. PMID: 39725555

Besnik, Q. (2020). *The Framework of a Real-time Patient Monitoring System* (Doctoral dissertation, Budapesti Corvinus Egyetem).

Bose, P. (2025, March). *The future of hospital care with smart bed technology. News-Medical*. Retrieved June 20, 2025, from https://www.news-medical.net/health/The-Future-of-Hospital-Care-Embracing-Smart-Bed-Technology.aspx

Canadian Healthcare Technology. (2025, April). *AI-powered robots take the stage at HIMSS.* Canadian Healthcare Technology, 30(3). Retrieved June 23, 2025, from https://www.canhealth.com/wp-content/uploads/2025/03/Canadian-Healthcare-Technology-2025-03-1.pdf

CGCompliance. (2025, February). *A complete guide to HIPAA compliance services: Protecting patient data effectively*. CGCompliance. Retrieved June 20, 2025, from https://info.cgcompliance.com/blog/a-complete-guide-to-hipaa-compliance-services-protecting-patient-data-effectively

De Castro, J. M. N. L. (2019). *Transforming Lives and the Healthcare Business: Remote Patient 5G-IoT Technology Monitoring Solution for the Home Hospitalization Service* (Master's thesis, Universidade Catolica Portuguesa (Portugal)).

Dermody, G., Wadsworth, D., Dunham, M., Glass, C., & Fritz, R. (2024). Factors Affecting Clinician Readiness to Adopt Smart Home Technology for Remote Health Monitoring: Systematic Review. *JMIR Aging*, *7*(1), e64367. PMID: 39012852

DocTime. (n.d.). *Online doctor consultation & telehealth in BD*. https://doctime.com.bd/

Feather Staff. (2025, May 28). *HIPAA compliance guide for evaluating medical IoT devices*. AskFeather. Retrieved June 20, 2025, from https://www.askfeather.com/resources/hipaa-evaluation-of-medical-iot-devices

Hospital Management Asia. (2024, March 28). *Samsung Medical Centre's path to smart healthcare*. Retrieved June 23, 2025, from https://www.hospitalmanagementasia.com/tech-innovation/samsung-medical-centres-path-to-smart-healthcare/

Kuwait Computer Services. (2024, March). *Smart IoT solution for hospital & health care*. Retrieved from https://www.kcs.com.kw/wp-content/uploads/2024/03/kcs_kuwait_iot_smart_hospital_monitoring.pdf

Kuwait Direct Investment Promotion Authority. (2022, June). *Sector opportunities*. Retrieved June 23, 2025, from https://kdipa.gov.kw/wp-content/uploads/2022/06/Sector-Opportunities-June2022.pdf

Megarit, M. (2021, October 23). *3 ways smart hospitals will revolutionize the healthcare experience*. Michael Megarit. https://michaelmegarit.com/blog/smart-hospitals-will-revolutionize-the-healthcare-experience/

Minew. (n.d.). *Advanced Bluetooth IoT solutions for smart hospitals*. Retrieved June 23, 2025, from https://www.minew.com/solutions/smart-healthcare/

Nikolova, B. (2024). The 2030 Agenda for Sustainable Development: Goals and Implementation. *International Journal of Sustainability Policy & Practice*, *20*(2).

Parthasarathi, J., & Sheri, B. P. (2025, June). Integrating AI robotics in healthcare: Reducing medical costs and enhancing patient experience through automated diagnosis, treatment, and administrative workflows. *EAI Endorsed Transactions on AI and Robotics*.

TytoCare. (n.d.). *Home*. https://www.tytocare.com/

Uddin, M. S., Alam, J. B., & Banu, S. (2017, September). Real time patient monitoring system based on Internet of Things. In *2017 4th International conference on Advances in Electrical Engineering (ICAEE)* (pp. 516-521). IEEE.

Wartenberg, C., Elden, H., Frerichs, M., Jivegård, L. L., Magnusson, K., Mourtzinis, G., & Vallo Hult, H. (2025). Clinical benefits and risks of remote patient monitoring: An overview and assessment of methodological rigour of systematic reviews for selected patient groups. *BMC Health Services Research*, *25*(1), 133. PMID: 39849519

APPENDIX A: SURVEY HEALTHCARE PROFESSIONALS ON IOT

A1: Respondent Background

Q1. What is your field of study or work?

- Medical student
- Nursing student
- Biomedical engineering student
- Healthcare IT professional
- Early-career doctor

Q2. What is your current level of training?

- Undergraduate
- Graduate
- Intern/Resident
- Early-career professional
- Other

Q3. Have you encountered IoT technologies in a clinical or academic setting?

Yes

No

Not sure

A2: Familiarity and Awareness

Q4. How familiar are you with the concept of IoT in healthcare?

- Very familiar
- Somehow familiar
- Heard of it but not clear
- Not familiar

Q5. Which IoT applications do you associate most with hospitals? (*Select all that apply)*

- Wearable patient monitors
- Smart beds, Telemedicine platforms
- RFID asset tracking
- Smart medication dispensers
- Other (please specify)

A3: Perceived Benefits

Q6. Rate the following statements from 1 (Strongly Disagree) to 5 (Strongly Agree):

Table 5. IoT input assessment

Statement	1	2	3	4	5
IoT improves real-time patient monitoring.					
IoT enhances patient safety.					
IoT improves treatment accuracy through personalized care.					
IoT helps reduce clinical workload and manual tasks.					
IoT boosts operational efficiency and resource management.					

A4: Challenges and Concerns

Q7. What do you consider the biggest challenges for IoT in hospitals? (*Select up to 3)*

- Data privacy/security risks
- High costs of implementation
- Compatibility with existing systems
- Resistance from hospital staff
- Lack of training or support
- Complex data management
- Unclear return on investment

Q8. Do you trust that hospitals can protect patient data collected through IoT devices?

Yes

No

Not sure

Q9. Which groups need the most training to use IoT tools effectively? *(Select all that apply)*

- Doctors and nurses
- Hospital IT teams
- Patients
- Administrators
- All of the above

A5: Future Outlook

Q10. Do you believe IoT will become essential in all major hospitals in the next 10 years?

Yes

No

May be

Q11. Would you be comfortable using or recommending IoT tools in your clinical practice?

Yes
No
Not sure
Q12. In your opinion, what should be the top priority to enable wider IoT adoption in hospitals?

- Stronger data security standards
- Better integration with current hospital systems
- More training and awareness
- Lower costs
- National or institutional policy support

A6: Open-Ended Questions

Q13. What excites you most about the future of IoT in healthcare? (Open response)

Q14. What concerns or barriers do you think must be addressed before IoT can be widely adopted? (Open response)

APPENDIX B: SAMPLE RESPONSES (ANONYMIZED)

Table 6. Role assessments of sample respondents

Respondent Role	Familiarity	IoT Use	Top Challenge	Trust in Data Security	IoT Essential in 10 Years	Recommend IoT
Biomedical Engineer (Grad)	Somewhat familiar	No	Compatibility	No	No	Not sure
Biomedical Engineer (Resident)	Not familiar	No	Data management	No	Yes	No
Early-career Doctor (Grad)	Very familiar	No	High cost	No	Maybe	Yes
Biomedical Engineer (Professional)	Not familiar	Not sure	Data management	Not sure	No	Not sure
Early-career Doctor (Resident)	Heard of it	Not sure	Data privacy	Yes	Yes	Not sure

APPENDIX C: VISUAL REPRESENTATIONS OF SURVEY DATA

To enhance comprehension of the survey results, key findings are also illustrated through the following charts. Figure 4 displays how familiar respondents are with the concept of IoT in clinical practice. Figure 5 highlights the most pressing concerns identified by participants. The Figure 6 reflects participant expectations for future hospital infrastructure. And the Figure 7 indicates varying degrees of trust in institutional data protection.

Figure 4. Familiarity with IoT in Healthcare

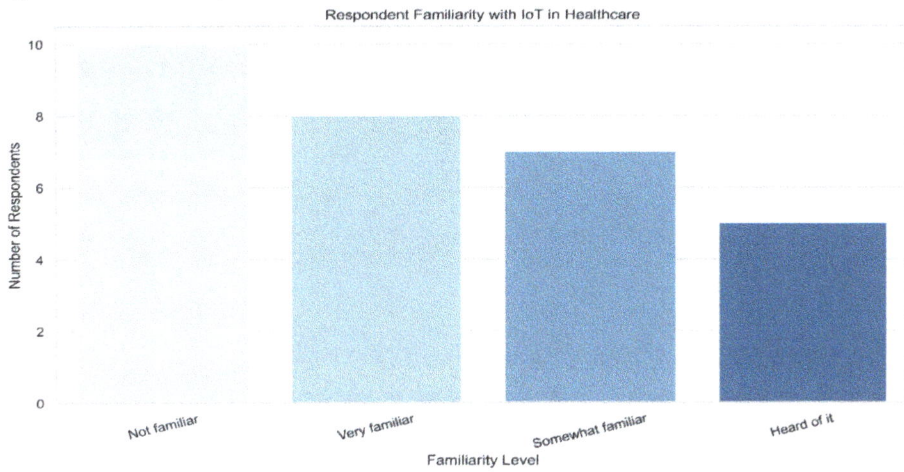

Figure 5. Top Challenges for IoT in Hospitals

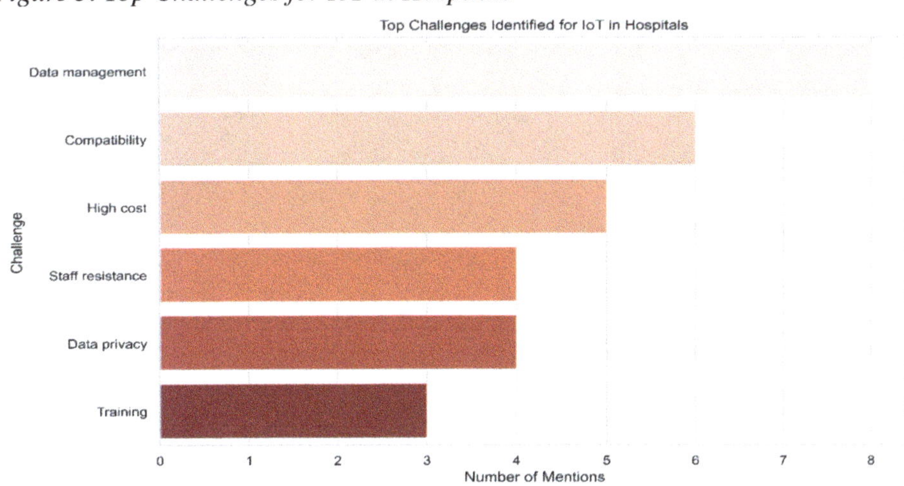

Figure 6. Belief that IoT Will Be Essential Within 10 Years

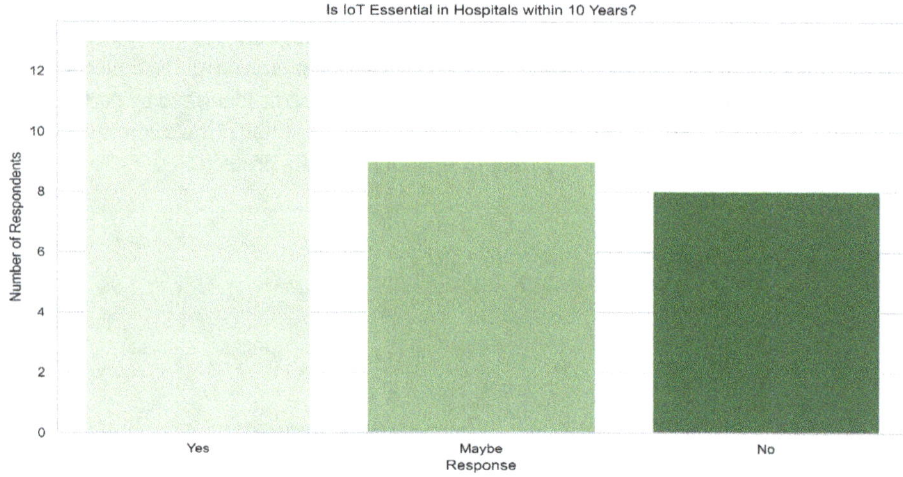

Figure 7. Trust in Hospital Data Security for IoT Devices

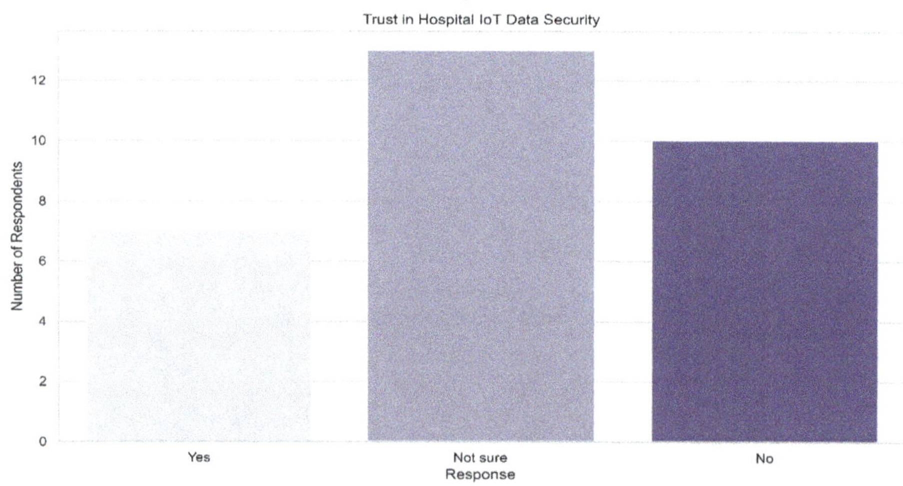

These figures complement the quantitative data tables and provide visual insight into the trends and attitudes among emerging healthcare professionals.

APPENDIX D: TELEMEDICINE PLATFORM

Doctime is a digital healthcare platform based in Bangladesh. It provides telemedicine services through its website and mobile application. Users can consult with licensed doctors using video, audio or chat. These features reduce physical visits and long waiting times. There are more than 20 medical experts on this platform. Most of them come from different departments such as, general medicine, pediatrics, gynecology, dermatology, cardiology, and mental health. These diverse groups are able to meet a wide range of healthcare needs. Doctime also provides several other services beyond virtual consultations. Medicine home delivery, electronic prescriptions, and schedule pathological tests (both in home or designated places). Using this platform, Users can access their digital health records, receive medication reminders, and manage follow-up visits etc. The platform is user friendly, and it's integrated with mobile payment system (mobile wallets). People in remote areas are highly benefited through this platform. Doctime offers several other services beyond virtual consultations. Medicine home delivery, electronic prescriptions and routine pathological tests (both at home or at a designated location). Using this platform, users can access their digital health records, receive medication reminders and manage follow-up visits, etc. The platform is user-friendly and integrated with mobile payment systems. People in remote areas are benefiting a lot through this platform. DocTime also offers various healthcare packages and subscription plans for individual and corporate clients. DocTime uses two-tier security protocols for data encryption and storage. It creates a technological bridge between patients and doctors.

TytoCare is a digital health platform. The platform includes several portable devices such as digital stethoscopes, otoscopes, thermometers and high-resolution cameras. All those portable devices are approved from U.S. Food and Drug Administration (FDA). These devices are helpful for medical tests without visiting a diagnostic center. TytoCare users can check the ears, throat, lungs, heart, skin, and temperature. Users can share their test report with health professionals through TytoApp (supported by android and Iphone). The mobile application also allows live video consultations with doctors. Some artificial intelligence features are included that are helpful for predicting early health issues. TytoCare works with digital health record systems. It is used in a variety of settings, including homes, schools, and rural clinics. Its goal is to improve access to medical care, reducing unwanted emergency visits, and assist in long-term health condition management.

Chapter 11
Regulatory Challenges for Next-Generation Medical Devices:
Impact of Automation on Medical Workforce

Bhupinder Singh
https://orcid.org/0009-0006-4779-2553
Sharda University, India

Saurabh Chandra
https://orcid.org/0000-0003-4172-9968
Bennett University, Greater Noida, India

ABSTRACT

The complexity of next-gen med devices that combine AI with IoT, robotics, and analytics makes regulatory challenges inevitable. It is critical to achieve this safety, efficacy, and compliance in addressing data privacy and cybersecurity concerns. Bold innovations can quickly transcend the boundaries of established regulatory paradigms, demanding that policies evolve and that oversight remains vigilant. The challenge comes from the adaptive nature of machine learning algorithms present in such devices, which make validation and certification processes more involved. Automation in the medical field is transforming workforce dynamics. Although automating these routine tasks such as diagnostics, imaging, and administrative tasks increases efficiency and reduces human error, it does give rise to concerns of personnel displacement of some roles. The challenge in harnessing the full potential of automation lies in balancing innovation with ethical and workforce considerations to cultivate a sustainable and equitable healthcare ecosystem.

DOI: 10.4018/979-8-3373-1514-0.ch011

1. INTRODUCTION

Medical technology is advancing by the generation of next-gen medical devices which are mainly driven by robotics and automation with the use of artificial intelligence (AI). Artificial intelligence, big data analytics, and cloud computing are just a few examples; many of these innovations are integrated into cutting-edge technologies in the healthcare field. These innovations have revolutionized patient care, enhanced diagnostic accuracy, increased efficiency, and improved healthcare workflows. Some of these groundbreaking developments shaping modern-day healthcare include AI-based diagnostic tools, robotic-assisted surgeries, patient monitoring devices and the Internet of Medical Things (IoMT). But with these advancements come complex challenges for the regulatory landscape to ensure the safety, efficacy, and ethical deployment of these technologies (Ateeq et al., 2024). Medical devices relying on machine learning algorithms and automation also raise unique regulatory challenges related to continuous learning systems and protection of data and patient privacy. Conventional regulatory frameworks, including FDA, EMA, and other global regulatory bodies, were devised for static medical technologies, which has hampered efforts to define standard approval processes for devices that evolve thanks to the introduction of real-time data and machine learning adaptation. Moreover, cybersecurity threats present serious risks as AI-enabled medical devices become more interconnected, requiring strong regulatory actions to ensure no breaches and malicious attacks would occur.

At the same time, automation of medical processes is affecting the healthcare workforce, providing both opportunities and challenges. AI and robotics have started to augment or replace human roles in diagnosis, imaging, pathology, and even bedside interactions. The risk of workforce displacement and ethical issues posed by AI in patient care are balanced by the benefits of the technology, which brings efficiency, reduces human error, and lessens administrative load on doctors. AI-augmented healthcare settings require medical professionals to adapt to new responsibilities, which will emerge as the old job definitions dissolve. Doctors, radiologists, and primary care doctors are forming new alliances with AI-based decision-support systems, transforming the nature of collaboration in patient management.

The legal and ethical implications of liability in AI-assisted medical decision-making are especially controversial and largely unrelated to traditional state regulation. As health care organizations seek the right mix of progress and familiar practices, lawmakers should build dual-approach rules that encourage innovation while also preserving human jobs in health (Rubin, 2022). This chapter discusses the complex regulatory challenges presented by next-generation medical devices and the far-reaching consequences that automation has on the medical workforce, which underscores the need for cohesive global policies, ethical implementation of AI, and strategies to transition the workforce to maintain sustainable advancements in the healthcare industry. Yet it also presents challenges, requiring healthcare professionals to adapt through upskilling and acquiring new competencies, in order to successfully manage and work with advanced technologies.

1.1 Relevance and Background on Medical Device Advancements and Automation

Advancements in artificial intelligence (AI), robotics, biotechnology, and the Internet of Medical Things (IoMT) have propelled the evolution of medical devices, leading to a fundamental shift in the way we approach healthcare delivery and patient management. Historically, medical devices were mostly mechanical devices or operated manually, with a little automation on the hardware. The utilization of digital health solutions can facilitate the creation of nextgen medical devices for real-time monitoring, predictive diagnostics, and autonimic medical procedures.

This enthusiasm stems from developments such as an increase in AI-powered imaging systems, robotics-assisted surgeries, automated drug delivery systems and wearable health monitoring devices. Machine learning algorithms in radiology can now identify early-stage cancer more accurately than traditional diagnostics, whereas robotic surgery maximizes precision and reduces human error during complex operations. This innovation in medicine has led to the creation of 3D-printed implants and bioengineered tissues, which show the potential in personalized medicine.

But automation in healthcare goes beyond clinical strategies; it also includes improving administrative processes like managing medical records, triaging patients, and consulting in telemedicine. AI-powered chatbots, electronic health records (EHRs), and robotic pharmacy dispensing systems are integrated to lessen human workload, allocate resources wisely, and boost operational efficiency. Although these contributions enhance the accessibility of healthcare and patient outcomes, they also present challenges in regulatory compliance, cyber security and workforce adaptation.

Existing regulatory systems are ill suited to the fast-moving world of AI-enabled devices, and persistent shortcomings in upholding patient safety, data privacy and ethical decision-making. Another significant aspect of the report highlights the implications of automation for the medical workforce, with healthcare professionals needing to adjust to new roles augmented by AI, as well as a changing landscape of job responsibilities. So as the medical devices become more autonomous, the health care sector needs to address regulatory challenges, ethical dilemmas, and workforce transformation to ensure the seamless integration of technology in order to continue high standards of patient care (Budhiraja & Kant, 2020).

1.2 Significance of Regulatory Frameworks in Ensuring Patient Safety and Efficacy

These regulatory frameworks are critical for assuring patient safety, efficacy of medical devices through well-defined guidance for development, testing, approval and post-market surveillance. With AI, robotics, and automation incorporated into next-generation medical devices, the need for robust regulatory oversight is more important than ever. These advanced technologies might help revolutionize healthcare by improving diagnostic accuracy, streamlining surgical procedures, and enhancing patient monitoring. However, in the absence of strict regulations, there is potential in using devices that may be faulty, defective, or threatened by cyber risks. Regulators like the U.S. Food and Drug Administration (FDA), the European Medicines Agency (EMA), and the International Medical Device Regulators Forum (IMDRF) set the safety bar in healthcare, so that medical devices are ideally tested with rigorous clinical trials and validation before they hit the market.

AI-based medical devices are uniquely challenged because they constantly change with the use of machine learning algorithms. Traditional medical devices have a fixed set of functionalities, whereas AI-enabled systems can change based on new data, which complicates the efforts to establish standardized metrics measuring performance in AI-enabled systems. Regulatory agencies must create dynamic oversight mechanisms that account for ongoing updates, while at the same time balancing bias, inaccuracy and security vulnerabilities. And, ensuring compliance with data privacy regulations like HIPAA and GDPR is crucial to safeguard patient information. However, with new technologies and innovations, issues have also arisen, for example: how can next-generation medical devices be developed with their highest efficacy in mind alongside the lowest degree of risk for patients or healthcare providers, and balanced with the right regulatory framework that preserves innovation (Mullins et al., 2022).

2. NEXT-GENERATION MEDICAL DEVICES: DEFINING INNOVATION AND SCOPE

Next-generation medical devices are emerging in health care as a result of the rapid evolution in medical technology. It has become possible due to these innovative technologies such as artificial intelligence (AI), robotics, Internet of Medical Things (IoMT), and others, which offer improved diagnostic accuracy, efficient treatment processes, and better patient care. This new paradigm shift is revolutionizing certain facets of medicine including diagnostics, treatment and long-term patient monitoring. With their ability to analyze vast amounts of medical data with unprecedented accuracy, AI-powered diagnostic tools are revolutionizing the detection and management of disease.

These systems employ deep learning algorithms to analyze medical imaging, detect irregularities, and forecast possible health threats. For instance, AI empowered radiology solutions can identify early-stage cancer (like breast cancer or lung cancer) with greater accuracy and efficiency than the standard approaches. AI-based dermatology tools help with skin disease detection and assessing if a lesion is benign or malignant. These tools enable healthcare professionals to act with speed, thus reducing overall diagnostic errors and disease detections, which helps ensure an effective treatment with better patient outcomes. Similarly, AI-based predictive analytics in cardiology can analyze a patient's risk of developing heart disease using past medical data and lifestyle factors to guide preventive care.

Figure 1. Shares the Points on Next-Generation Medical Devices

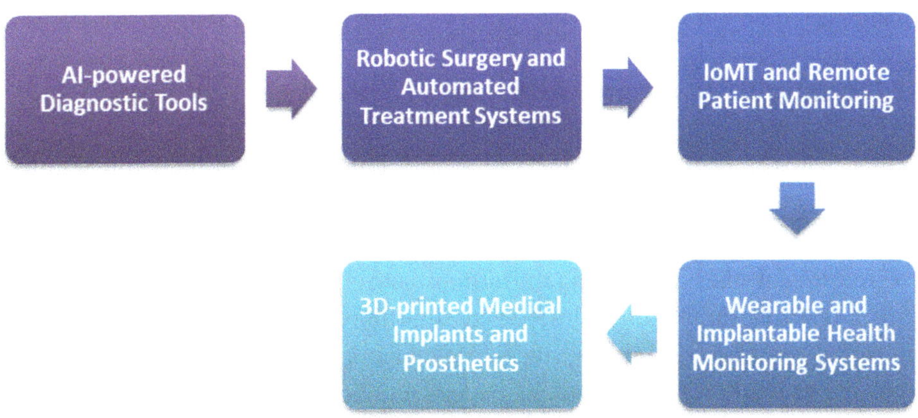

(Source- Self Prepared- Original)

2.1 AI-Powered Diagnostic Tools

The second revolutionary class of next-generation medical devices includes robotic surgery and automated treatment systems. Robotic-assisted surgical systems, including the surgical system, improve precision, dexterity and minimally invasive surgical approaches (Ninaus et al., 2021). The data can limit it because a surgeon must perform with more control and more successfully which leads to recover more quickly and can help a patient feel better. Robotic-assisted surgery is a major advancement in the field, as unlike traditional surgery where human limitations such as a steady hand and precise accuracy come into play, robotics-assisted platforms with the included technology of AI and imaging in real-time increases surgical efficiency.

The complexity of balancing innovation with patient safety and ethical considerations, your next generation medical devices are the high risk devices for innovative age of automation &. Devices like robotic surgical systems, AI-driven diagnostics and automated drug delivery platforms are based on complex algorithms and real-time decision making, which often lies outside the purview of traditional medical device approvals. In the realm of algorithms, regulators have much work to do in terms defining standards for transparency, validation and post-market surveillance particularly tricky considering machine learning models change over time. Privacy and security issues make it even more complicated, especially when the devices depend on a system that is interconnected to other devices or based in the cloud form. In addition, the automatization of health care alters the forces demanding a realignment of roles, skills and responsibilities needed by different kinds of health workers.

2.2 Robotic Surgery and Automated Treatment Systems

Even surgery itself is not the only aspect, as other areas like robotic rehabilitation devices help patients to recover mobility after injuries or strokes. AI-driven exoskeletons provide mobility to those with paralysis by utilizing the brain signals received through machine learning and turning them into physical movements. In the domain of radiation oncology, intelligent algorithms have also been leveraged by automated treatment planning systems that maximize the radiation dose delivered to cancerous tissue while minimizing exposure to healthy tissues. Automation and AI-based treatment systems have been demonstrating their therapeutic solutions in a way that improves their effectiveness and eliminates human errors, thus raising the level of patient care.

2.3 Internet of Medical Things (IoMT) and Remote Patient Monitoring

Enabling continuous, real-time tracking of patient health metrics, Internet of Medical Things (IoMT) and remote patient monitoring technologies are revolutionizing healthcare delivery (Singh, 2024). The Internet of Medical Things (IoMT) is essentially a network of medical devices and applications that communicate with one another for the collection, transmission, and analysis of patient data, offering valuable information and analyzable insights to healthcare providers regarding their patients. Remote-monitoring solutions, such as smart glucometers for diabetes and continuous cardiac monitoring devices, enable physicians to remotely monitor vital signs so they can intervene if the readings are not in line with expectations. For example, patients with chronic disorders such as Hypertension or heart disease wear IoMT enabled devices that transmit up-to-the-minute information to their physicians, who can appropriately adjust medication and suggest lifestyle choices and changes.

This framework minimizes hospital visits, reduces healthcare expenditure and improves patient comfort. With the Internet of Medical Things, AI-powered predictive analytics can integrate into patient pathways to identify potential health declines and avoid medical emergencies. This adoption was accelerated by the COVID-19 pandemic, which has amplified the role of remote patient monitoring in chronic disease management, post-surgical care and elderly patients health monitoring. The expansion of telehealth and e-health solutions will make the use of IoMT-based medical devices an important part of ensuring accessible healthcare and preventive health moving forward.

2.4 3D-printed Medical Implants and Prosthetics

3D-printed medical implants and prosthetics is another major advancement in medical technology. Traditional implants and prosthetics can be resource-intensive when customizing and manufacturing, creating buying pressure for patients with long waiting times. But with developments in 3D printing technology, this field changed again forever because 3D printing allows the manufacturing of patient-oriented implants that conform to the individual patient anatomy. Especially in fields with specific needs for adaptation (such as orthopedic and dental), the tensile strength, functionality, and biocompatibility of 3D-printed implants have been improved. Recent efforts in 3D printing in medicine explore further applications such as custom made cranial implants, which have shown 95% rate of acceptance by bone tissue, significantly decrease rejection likelihood (Singh, 2024).

3D-printed prosthetics have revolutionized the lives of those with limb loss by offering affordable and personalized solutions for better mobility and improved quality of life. Traditional prosthetics can be costly and are often limited in their design, while 3D printing allows for rapid prototyping and ongoing enhancements to be implemented based on user feedback. Common 3D-printed medical devices such as prosthetics are steeped in this integration of AI, with smart prosthetics featuring embedded sensors that adapt to a user's movement patterns. These innovations represent a major leap in personalized medicine, providing patients with solutions that offer better comfort, durability, and overall well-being.

2.5 Wearable and Implantable Health Monitoring Systems

Advancement in wearables and implantable health monitoring systems is also one of the key areas of next-generation medical devices, responsible for monitoring health in real-time and therefore allowing for disease detection at a very early stage. Wearable medical devices, such as smartwatches, ECG monitors, and fitness trackers, have become popular for measuring heart rate, physical activity, and sleep patterns (Hamlin, 2028). These wearable devices offer significant health data to consumers and allow doctors a way know about potential problems before they become serious. Wearable ECG monitors can identify abnormal heartbeats like irregular heartbeat (atrial fibrillation) and notify users to visit a doctor in due course.

The implantable device, however, provides more advanced monitoring of chronic disease states. Implantable cardioverter defibrillators (ICDs) and pacemakers, for example, continuously monitor heart function and provide electrical impulses to control abnormal rhythms. As example, implantable glucose sensors used by diabetic patients offer continuous glucose monitoring and reduce the necessity of performing fingerstick tests for glucose level and thereby improve glycaemic control. Such technologies empower patients to make informed decisions about their health and allow for tailored treatment plans, leading to better health results. In addition, the development of biosensors and nanotechnology holds promise for next-generation sensors and implants that can detect circulating biomarkers associated with diseases such as cancer and provide timely diagnosis and theranostics (Sigeman & Adolfsson, 2021).

3. REGULATORY CHALLENGES IN NEXT-GENERATION MEDICAL DEVICES

Next-generation medical devices are undergoing rapid development, driven by advances in artificial intelligence (AI), robotics, the Internet of Medical Things (IoMT), and other new and emerging technologies, creating substantial regulatory challenges that need to be addressed to ensure patient safety and device efficacy while ensuring that these technologies are deployed ethically. Next-generation innovations differ fundamentally from conventional medical devices that have well-established regulatory pathways; the former often have complex evaluation and approval processes, as they frequently entail machine learning algorithms, real-time data analytics, and automation (Onyeka, 2022). The biggest challenges that regulators face is whether the existing regulatory frameworks they apply can address the functional dynamics of AI-driven medical devices, which learn and evolve over time. In contrast to static devices with predetermined clinical capabilities, AI-enhanced diagnostic assistive devices and robotic surgical devices are dynamic and capable of improving performance as data inputs continue and investments mount, creating unique challenges in validating performance, reliability, and consistency. Traditional regulatory models are built around static products with a final approval process, yet the perpetually evolving nature of AI, including software updates and changes to algorithms, necessitates that regulators devise new approval processes for algorithms.

The fundamental regulatory issues are to develop uniform ground-works for AI explainability and transparency. Many new-age medical devices utilize deep learning and neural networks that act as "black-box" systems, making it challenging for health care professionals and regulators to interpret how decisions are made. Not being interpretable loopholes the question of accountability since any mistakes made in diagnostics or treatment plans based on AI can lead to loss of life. Here in the U.S. the FDA, the EMA in Europe and IMDRF have contributed to frameworks to promote explainable AI that will bring validation and auditability to machine-determined decisions. The importance of human supervision in AI-supported (AI-assisted) medical procedures also has to be clearly defined in order to avoid over-relying on them and, at the same time, ensuring high standards in patient care (Ireland, 2022). Regulatory balance between automation and human expertise is a critical challenge that lies ahead and needs interdisciplinary collaboration between policymakers, medical practitioners and AI developers.

Another regulatory challenge for next-generation medical devices is related to cybersecurity and data privacy. The Internet of Medical Things (IoMT) is consisting of multiple medical devices connected with one another, collecting huge amount of data from the respective patients, which is causing more and more departments of hospitals to require tight security from these devices in order to prevent intrusion, data corruption and data manipulation. The reason is that medical records and personal health information are very valuable for cyberattacks and therefore the healthcare industry is the prime target for all attacks.

Regulators need to set strong data protection standards that comply with our laws such as the Health Insurance Portability and Accountability Act in the U.S. or the General Data Protection Regulation in Europe. Next-gen medical devices manufacturers should implement end-to-end encryption and secure authentication protocols along with real-time threat detection, to secure patient data. Meanwhile, ethical concerns need to be addressed in regulatory frameworks for data ownership, as patients must understand how their health data will be collected, stored and used by AI-enabled medical devices. The proposed solutions to address these issues are the application of blockchain technology to medical device applications to improve data security and traceability, but this requires regulatory alignment for implementation.

Clinical validation and safety assessments present another regulatory hurdle because next-generation medical devices often depend on massive datasets and artificial intelligence algorithms to make decisions (ten Brummelhuis et al., 2021). The safety and effectiveness of AI-powered diagnostic tools, robotic surgeries, and automated treatment systems cannot be necessarily measured with traditional clinical trials. Regulators need to devise real-world adaptive testing methodologies in consideration of the real-world learning ability of AI to render these medical devices effective.

Bias in AI algorithms could also result in skewed diagnostic results from AI-driven medical devices that are trained on biased datasets that may disproportionally affect certain demographic groups. Strict guidelines on the importance of dataset diversity, algorithmic fairness, and equitable access to AI and other health technologies should be established by regulatory agencies to avoid biases and disparities in healthcare outcomes. The process of post-market surveillance and real-world performance monitoring are integral to regulatory oversight, making sure that medical devices continue to perform their intended function after being approved by the authorities. AI-enabled regulatory surveillance tools also can be implemented from the standpoint of evaluating the performance of devices in real time against their predetermined threshold to better assess the need for post-market surveillance (Weber & De Fino, 2022).

4. IMPACT ASSESSMENT OF AUTOMATION ON THE MEDICAL WORKFORCE

While automation offers to increase efficiency, decrease human error and allow clinicians time for more complex cases it also may result in labor displacement, resistance to adoption due to from incorrect automated diagnosis and debates on whether machine decision-making should replace that of people. Regulators need to look beyond the technical safety criteria and monitor its socio-economic impact on healthcare professional. A unified international regulatory strategy, ongoing risk appraisal, and merger with new labour training campaigns will be necessary to allow next generation automated medical devices to extract advantages without risking the trust, safety and job preservation in the health sector.

This makes the global regulatory landscape for next-generation medical devices fragmented, leaving manufacturers with challenges associated with gaining international market approvals. Regulations vary from one region to another; this results in delays in commercializing a device and incurs compliance costs for medical technology companies. International collaborations play an essential role in aligning regulatory standards on a global scale, leading to efficient approval processes and wider access to innovative medical technologies. Maintaining Close Collaboration and Reducing Duplication of Efforts at All Stages. Regulators need to develop data-sharing agreements and establish mutual recognition systems for cross-border regulatory collaboration to improve regulatory efficiency without compromising safety standards. Regulatory authorities can implement a risk-based regulatory approach in which they classify medical devices based on their level of autonomy and potential impact on patients to ensure that high-risk devices are thoroughly evaluated while low-risk innovations can be approved more quickly (Pradhan & Kumar, 2021).

Next-generation medical devices face their own new, vastly complex regulatory landscape, not just ethical and liability concerns. As AI and automation assume an ever greater role in medical decision-making, questions about legal culpability in cases of misdiagnosis, surgical mistakes or device failures will need to be answered. AI-driven systems enter a liability grey zone under existing medical malpractice laws, prompting the need for legal reforms that clarify responsibilities for accountability between manufacturers, healthcare providers, and regulatory bodies (Singh, 2023). Regulatory frameworks must also address ethical considerations, such as patient consent in AI-assisted treatments, and the potential displacement of healthcare workers because of automation. This means that developers should take an active role, engaging with legal experts and bioethicists.

The regulatory complexities of next-generation medical devices are diverse, ranging from AI transparency, cybersecurity, and clinical validation to global harmonization and ethics. Regulatory bodies have to be adaptive and ahead of the curve to ensure that medical technology keep up with its corresponding innovation, while placing a primary focus on the safety and efficacy of treatment methods. Evolving regulations that balance innovation with risk management will require collaboration between policymakers, industry stakeholders, and healthcare providers. However, as with many innovations, there are hurdles to overcome, and by implementing dynamic regulatory frameworks to address these challenges, the healthcare sector can unlock the full power of next-generation medical devices, leading to better outcomes for patients and the evolution of medicine.

4.1. Workforce Transformation and Job Displacement

Automation, AI and robotics are advancing quickly in medicine, and they will have a profound impact on how healthcare workers practice, raising fears of displacement or changing roles. With the advent of advanced medical devices like AI-based diagnostic tools, robotic surgical systems, and automated patient monitoring systems, there will be greater demand for healthcare professionals who can work alongside these systems and adapt to a transformative environment where human-machine partnership is more prominent than manual processes. Automation improves efficiency, accuracy and patient experience, but it also evolves the traditional workforce paradigm, leading to challenges in the opportunities to automate and requiring reskilling, reallocation and redefining of jobs to help integrate the new tools. The effect of workforce transformation differs based on how it is utilized in the many medical professions: some roles are seeing reduced demand whereas others are finding an increase in complexity and specialization within the role.

Perhaps the most impacted professions will be those in diagnostic and imaging-related professions. AI algorithms can now detect potential issues in medical images like X-rays, MRIs and CT scans as precisely, if not better than human radiologists can (Ochoa, 2023). These recent advancements do improve diagnostic speed and accuracy but lead to questions about how it will ever need these doctors if they are replaced by technology. Rather than replace these roles entirely, AI will most likely provide them with an assistive capability that can free them from the tedium of reviewing low-complexity images allowing them to focus on complex cases and clinical decision-making instead. AI-powered virtual health assistants and chatbots are automating preliminary patient consultations and allowing general practitioners and nurses to lighten their load, they are also changing the dynamics of the relationship between patients and providers.

Robotic-assisted surgical systems are transforming the surgical field as well, and bringing about changes in the workforce. For instance, platforms like the Da Vinci Surgical System enable surgeons to perform minimally invasive surgery with improved precision, leading to shorter recovery times and better patient outcomes (Fallica, 2022). These technologies improve surgical efficiency but also change the skill set needed for surgeons and operating-room staff. Rather than solely cutting and suturing, surgeons are now learning how to become adept at manipulating robotic interfaces, making surgical decisions based on AI-generated recommendations, and resolving issues with robotic systems. In response to these trends, medical education needs to adjust by developing targeted training programs and curricular updates that prepare the surgical workforce of the future for an AI-enhanced clinical landscape. Moreover, the increasing use of automation in surgery may decrease their necessity for junior surgeons to do routine surgeries, and therefore their opportunity for hands-on training and experience gains.

In addition to clinical roles, automation is transforming administrative and support functions at healthcare organizations. AI-built scheduling software, EHR auto-generation software, and RPA are taking on hospital management duties and the need for clerical and administrative staff are driving down the demand for such roles Although these technologies streamline operations, they also render jobs obsolete for the people who had primarily performed data entry, billing, and scheduling. Healthcare companies will need to manage this move by giving retraining opportunities to dislodged representatives that a transition to the job jobs requires a basic reasoning, information investigation, and patient-centered care (Bhende, 2020).

While some worry that automation leads to job displacement, it is also true that automation leads to new job roles in healthcare. As medical institutions start to implement more and more advanced technologies in their operations, the demand for AI specialists, biomedical engineers, robotics technicians, and cybersecurity professionals is on the rise. Moreover, emerging interdisciplinary roles like AI ethicists and regulatory compliance specialists will cater to the ethical and legal implications of healthcare automation. As the transition to an AI-driven healthcare system proves inevitable, policymakers and industry leaders must navigate it closely and strategically by promoting workforce development initiatives that prioritize adaptability, cross-disciplinary learning, and continuous skill development.

The medical automation still poses both a lot of challenges as well as opportunities to transforming the workforce. As some job profiles become obsolete, new ones will be created, along with an array of skill sets needed to thrive and evolve, thus evolving the healthcare profession. However, in an era of increasing automation in the healthcare field, this may not be enough a more proactive approach based on reskilling programs, an education reform and policy adaptations will be required to make sure that doctors and nurses can succeed in future medical settings.

4.2. Shift Towards AI-Augmented Roles: Emergence of AI-Assisted Healthcare Professionals

The surge of artificial intelligence (AI) technologies into healthcare is creating a paradigm shift from traditional medical occupations to AI-augmented jobs where healthcare practitioners will increasingly use AI-enabled tools to guide decision-making, diagnostics and treatment. Rather than usurping human expertise, AI is becoming a collaborative partner, helping medical professionals to practice with enhanced accuracy, efficiency, and analysis (Chung et al., 2022). This evolution is set to create a new breed of AI-driven health practitioners, trained to partner with intelligent systems and harness the power of machine learning algorithms, robotics, and data analytics to enhance patient outcomes. These roles are revolutionizing the field of medicine by relieving cognitive burden, reducing errors and allowing for more direct care of patients instead of administrative or repetitive tasks.

The most notable AI-augmented roles is the AI-assisted radiologist and pathologist. Radiologists are already transitioning into an oversight position, where they confirm the output of AI-based imaging analysis tools that detect anomalies in X-rays, MRIs, and CT scans with increasing precision, manage edge cases, and maintain diagnostic consistency. In a similar manner, AI-assisted pathology specialists take the help of deep learning algorithms to examine tissue samples and provide diagnoses more quickly without compromising on the accuracy of the test results. By prioritizing patient consultations and multidisciplinary collaboration over manual data sifting, radiologists and pathologists can increase their efficiency improving healthcare overall.

AI is changing the nature of the surgeon into AI-assist operators enabling robotic surgical systems to not only operate with more accuracy, but also with fewer human errors. Surgeons use robotic-assisted surgery platforms, like the surgical system, that enable minimally invasive procedures guided by AI (Adler et al., 2022). Surgeons need to learn a new skill set that comprises operating robotic interfaces, leveraging AI-based decision support, and interpreting large amounts of data, which can unlock best practices on surgical performance. This evolution also requires that we adapt our medical training programs to ensure that surgeons-in-training learn both traditional and AI-enhanced surgical techniques.

AI is also transforming primary care and patient monitoring. Nurses and clinical decision support specialists who are assisted by AI use predictive analytics and AI-driven health monitoring systems to identify early signs of illness, suggest individualized treatment recommendations, and enhance chronic condition management. AI-Powered Wearable and Implantable Health Devices: AI. AI-based tools are being increasingly utilized by nurses and general practitioners to help manage patient data, optimize medication regimens, and enhance clinical decision-making.

The rise of AI-powered healthcare professionals means we should expect more evolution, reskilling, and ethics in medicine. As we continue to weave AI into the fabric of the healthcare industry, many health professionals will be tasked with incorporating this technology into their work while keeping the human element of patient care front and center. This transformation signifies a collaborative future in which AI and human expertise combine to build a healthcare ecosystem that is more efficient, precise, and patient-centric (Roth et al., 2023).

5. REGULATORY STRATEGIES TO BALANCE INNOVATION AND WORKFORCE STABILITY

Next-Gen Medical DevicesThe Evolution of Medical DevicesAI, Automation, and Robotics are Transforming Healthcare at an Unprecedented Pace These innovations improve patient outcomes, increase diagnostic accuracy, and help to enhance delivery of healthcare, but also represent a major threat to workforce stability. Automation could drive efficiencies that make certain jobs redundant, reshape certain professions, and require workforce retraining. Consequently, regulatory approaches will need to delicately balance the promotion of technological innovation against the maintenance of workforce stability. This requires collaboration between governments, regulators, and healthcare institutions to create frameworks that balance responsible AI adoption with the need to protect jobs, improve workforce skills, and ensure the ethical integrity of patient care.

The future of innovation in AI will critically depend upon progressive governance frameworks that implement robust human oversight in all medical automation. Regulatory authorities like the U.S. Food and Drug Administration (FDA), the European Medicines Agency (EMA), and the World Health Organization (WHO) will have to guarantee that AI-powered medical devices augment human knowledge rather than replace it altogether (Sharma & Singh, 2022). Policies that require human-in-the-loop (HITL) systems where the modality between AI insights and decision-making is moderated and approved by trained medical personnel are beneficial in preserving the role of medical practitioners. AI-powered clinical solutions, such as radiology and pathology, must always act as decision-support tools instead of as independent diagnostics, thus continuing to have radiologists and pathologists at the center of medical imaging and diagnostics. Embedding these human oversight requirements into regulatory approvals would help authorities mitigate the risks of complete job displacement while capitalising on AI's capabilities to drive accuracy and efficiency.

The important regulatory measure is the standardization of AI-based medical training programs so that healthcare professionals can be trained to work with intelligent systems. Governments and medical institutions should revise curricula for medical examinations and professional certifications to require basic competence in AI literacy, data interpretation and robotic system operation (Lu et al., 2022). Surgeons need specialized training on how to perform robotic-assisted procedures, whereas nurses and general practitioners should be skilled in AI-powered patient monitoring technologies. Regulators can mandate AI-competency certifications for healthcare professionals, ensuring that the workforce adapts as fast as technology. By introducing AI training into medical education proactively, regulators can pave the way for seamless transition to those roles augmented by AI without causing disruptive employment vacuums.

5.1 Global Harmonization of Medical Device Regulations

That could be directly affected by automation; and workforce reskilling and job transition policies will need to be put in place to help move people into new roles. There can be introduction of incentive programs, tax credits, grants, etc. to hospitals and healthcare providers that invest in employee reskilling programs (Kondo & Sonenshein, 2020). It is possible that medical professionals displaced by automation in administrative roles, such as medical coders or billing specialists, could be retrained for emerging roles in AI-driven healthcare administration, data security or digital health analytics. Advancements in technologies, such as automated healthcare practices, can displace workers from their roles. However, by fostering partnerships between government regulatory institutions, academic institutions and technological organizations, structured reskilling pathways can be developed to empower displaced workers to realise significant employment through newly created roles which are innovative and synergistic with the technology deployed.

The major regulatory aspect in the balancing between innovation and employee stability aims to the ethical AI utilization in the medical environment. If poorly regulated, AI algorithms can introduce biases, increase health disparities, or have unintended consequences in patient care. It would be vital for regulatory authorities to impose stringent norms of AI transparency, interpretability and accountability in order to safeguard against abuse of automation in clinical decision-making (Siganidou, 2020). AI technologies for recruiting and managing the workforce in health care organizations also need careful regulation, to guard against discriminatory practices that could impact groups of health care workers disproportionately. Comprehensive AI ethics regulations would help regulators ensure that AI promotes equitable employment practices and benefits all healthcare stakeholders instead of creating systemic disadvantages.

Beyond ethical AI governance, data security and privacy regulations are essential to striking the proper balance between innovation and workforce stability. As AI-powered medical devices become more prevalent, they will also increasingly rely on patient data to enhance diagnostic accuracy and predictive analytics, highlighting the need for robust data protection frameworks to prevent breaches, unauthorized access, and misuse of sensitive medical information. By adhering to regulations, including the Health Insurance Portability and Accountability Act (HIPAA) in the U.S. and the General Data Protection Regulation (GDPR) in the European Union, we can protect patient data while keeping AI integration from undermining patient confidentiality. Security also plays an important role in workforce stability in particular for data-focused or patient care roles due to the fact that any failure to protect sensitive data would make patients hesitant to trust administrators and could lead to disruption to employment in small- and large-scale emergency events.

5.2 Policy Recommendations for Ethical AI Integration in Healthcare

Using public-private partnerships (PPPs) and regulatory aspects as effective mechanisms in balancing innovation with workforce stability is required. Regulatory provisions offer a controlled environment in which AI-driven medical technologies can be tested in real-world conditions, without the risk of immediate disruption to the existing workforce structure. These sandboxes will enable regulatory bodies to assess the impact of automation on healthcare employment, therefore empowering them to formulate sound policies without the urge to play catch-up exercises as automation begins to be adopted on a large scale (Tenorio & Vu, 2021). Conversely, PPPs can allow the government, healthcare institutions, and technology companies to collaborate on workforce strategies that embed innovation without introducing the de-humanizing threat of job loss. By doing so, regulators can help finding the right way of adopting these new AI technologies with the highest possible benefits and lowest possible impact on the workforce.

To promote workforce stability, longer-term regulation should include contingent/hybrid employment insurance and policies to foster flexible work and job-shares to reflect the changing nature of AI healthcare roles. Policymakers can look into solutions like UBI, job-sharing, hybrid workforce models, etc. For example, hybrid work models, where human professionals collaborate closely with AI systems in a supplementary capacity, can allow for task redistribution in a manner that paves the way for improving productivity without catastrophic unemployment. Moreover, if regulations are established and supported to encourage gig economy employment in healthcare, like telemedicine practitioners and AI-assisted remote healthcare providers, this would also allow for alternative job opportunities for those whose roles may be replaced in the future.

6. TRAINING PROGRAMS TO SUPPORT HEALTHCARE WORKFORCE ADAPTATION

While the reliance on national regulatory structures is likely the first step in preparing to regulate new AI-driven medical devices, international harmonization of novel diagnostics is critical if a balance between continued innovation and job security is to be achieved on a broader scale. Because international regulatory cooperation can create standardized protocols for AI safety, interoperability, and labor force adaptation, countries can synchronize their policies with global best practices (Cheese, 2021). Global organizations like the WHO and IMDRF can and should be utilized to ease the conversation between countries on how to approach the regulation of next-generation medical devices in a way that stimulates innovation without furthering the inequalities we see in employment.

Stabilizing the workforce while maintaining innovation will require a combination of (1) AI governance and regulatory frameworks, (2) workforce training and reskilling programs, (3) ethical AI deployment, (4) data security and user privacy, (5) collaboration and partnerships between the public and private sectors, (6) international regulatory harmonization and cooperation, etc. Automation and AI will continue to shake up the healthcare sector; but if regulators act proactively now, they don't have to drive worrying wedges between these innovations and the current healthcare workforce. Over time, policies focusing on collaboration between humans and machines, continuing education, reskilling, and ethical-AI integration will allow regulators to evolve a landscape in which generative-AI driven healthcare mobility can continue to meet, and even outpace, the delivery of quality of care while keeping stability by training up and securing a knowledgeable workforce (Pearman, 2023).

7. CONCLUSION AND FUTURE SCOPE

The impact of these next-generation devices on healthcare is unarguable as they are continuing to develop. AI-powered diagnostics, robotic surgery, IoMT, 3D implants and wearables are changing how we even prevent, detect, and treat disease. Such advancements are revolutionizing care delivery, patient outcomes, and compensation models across the healthcare ecosystem. As with any innovation, risks such as regulatory compliance, cyber security, and ethics issues also need to be addressed, ensuring patient safety and equitable access to technology and ground-breaking healthcare solutions. They will need to update existing frameworks, or create new ones, to ensure that the continued approval of highly adaptive, AI-based systems for medical devices given how impactful they can be in the health context remains regulated in a manner that is timely and meaningful. Furthermore, data governance laws should be strengthened to safeguard sensitive patient information from cyber-attacks. The future of medical devices will be dictated by how well we can leverage innovation to improve patient care while also navigating regulatory pathways, patient access, and reimbursement for next generation medical devices in this evolving landscape. However, these innovations represent a paradigm shift toward intelligent, patient-centered healthcare systems that emphasize early identification, tailored therapies and improved clinical outcomes.

REFERENCES

Adler, D. A., Tseng, E., Moon, K. C., Young, J. Q., Kane, J. M., Moss, E., & Choudhury, T. (2022). Burnout and the Quantified Workplace: Tensions around Personal Sensing Interventions for Stress in Resident Physicians. *Proceedings of the ACM on Human-computer Interaction, 6*(CSCW2), 1-48.

Ateeq, A., Al-Refaei, A. A. A., Alzoraiki, M., Milhem, M., Al-Tahitah, A. N., & Ibrahim, A. (2024). Sustaining Organizational Outcomes in Manufacturing Firms: The Role of HRM and Occupational Health and Safety. *Sustainability, 16*(3), 1035.

Bhende, P. M. (2020). *Quality of Work Life of Employees in Banking Sector-A Study of Bank Managers and Staff in Goa* (Doctoral dissertation, Goa University).

Budhiraja, S., & Kant, S. (2020). Challenges associated with work-life balance: A meta-analysis. *J. Strat. Human Res. Manag, 9*, 11–16.

Cheese, P. (2021). *The New World of Work: Shaping a Future that Helps People, Organizations and Our Societies to Thrive*. Kogan Page Publishers.

Chung, H., Jaga, A., & Lambert, S. (2022). Possibilities for change and new frontiers: Introduction to the work and family researchers network special issue on advancing equality at work and home. *Community Work & Family, 25*(1), 1–12.

Fallica, A. (2022). Smart working: measurement of sustainability impact. Academic Press.

Ireland, S. G. (2022). A Study on the Need for Investment in Employee Wellbeing in Small and Medium Enterprises (SMEs) In Bangalore, India.

Kondo, M., & Sonenshein, S. (2020). *Joy at work: Organizing your professional life*. Pan Macmillan.

Lu, G., Du, R. Y., & Peng, X. (2022). The impact of schedule consistency on shift worker productivity: An empirical investigation. *Manufacturing & Service Operations Management, 24*(5), 2780–2796.

Mullins, L. B., Scutelnicu, G., & Charbonneau, É. (2022). A Qualitative Study of Pandemic-Induced Telework: Federal Workers Thrive, Working Parents Struggle. *Public Administration Quarterly, 46*(3).

Ninaus, K., Diehl, S., & Terlutter, R. (2021). Employee perceptions of information and communication technologies in work life, perceived burnout, job satisfaction and the role of work-family balance. *Journal of Business Research, 136*, 652–666.

Ochoa, J. J. (2023). *Occupational Burnout and Work-Life Balance Strategies Among Chaplains* (Doctoral dissertation, University of Arizona Global Campus).

Onyeka, N. F. (2022). *Exploring Female Perspectives of Work-Life Balance and the Role of Organizational Culture* (Doctoral dissertation, Capella University).

Pearman, C. D. (2023). *Tai Chi Enhanced Workplace Health and Wellness: A Systematic Literature Review for a Program Design, Implementation, and Evaluation* (Doctoral dissertation, University of Arizona Global Campus).

Pradhan, R. K., & Kumar, U. (Eds.). (2021). *Emotion, well-being, and resilience: Theoretical perspectives and practical applications.* CRC Press.

Roth, S. C., Hinton, E. G., & Jivanelli, B. (2023). Impact of COVID-19 on Parents/Guardians in the Library Profession: A Narrative Review and Shared Experiences. *Library Leadership & Management (Online), 37*(2), 1–72.

Rubin, K. I. (2022). *The Great Balancing Act: Women Seeking Work-Life Balance during COVID-19* (Doctoral dissertation, University of Southern California).

Sharma, A., & Singh, B. (2022). Measuring Impact of E-commerce on Small Scale Business: A Systematic Review. *Journal of Corporate Governance and International Business Law, 5*(1).

Siganidou, S. (2020). Work-related employee stress in 4* & 5* hotels in Greece. A study about the city of Thessaloniki. Acad4emic Press.

Sigeman, H., & Adolfsson, M. (2021). Maintaining well-being when working remotely: Work habits of employees at a geographical IT office in Sweden during the COVID-19 pandemic, their perceived well-being and productivity.

Singh, B. (2023). Blockchain Technology in Renovating Healthcare: Legal and Future Perspectives. In *Revolutionizing Healthcare Through Artificial Intelligence and Internet of Things Applications* (pp. 177-186). IGI Global.

Singh, B. (2024). Lensing Legal Dynamics for Examining Responsibility and Deliberation of Generative AI-Tethered Technological Privacy Concerns: Infringements and Use of Personal Data by Nefarious Actors. In Ara, A., & Ara, A. (Eds.), *Exploring the Ethical Implications of Generative AI* (pp. 146–167). IGI Global. DOI: 10.4018/979-8-3693-1565-1.ch009

Singh, B. (2024). Social Cognition of Incarcerated Women and Children: Addressing Exposure to Infectious Diseases and Legal Outcomes. In Reddy, K. (Ed.), *Principles and Clinical Interventions in Social Cognition* (pp. 236–251). IGI Global. DOI: 10.4018/979-8-3693-1265-0.ch014 ten Brummelhuis, L. L., ter Hoeven, C. L., & Toniolo-Barrios, M. (2021). Staying in the loop: Is constant connectivity to work good or bad for work performance? *Journal of Vocational Behavior, 128*, 103589.

Tenorio, J. L., & Vu, H. T. (2021). *A Cross-sectional Study during the COVID-19 Pandemic: Work Events and Affective Reactions as Predictors of Loss of Productivity and Intention to Leave* (Master's thesis, Handelshøyskolen BI).

Weber, M. B., & De Fino, M. (2022). *Virtual technical services: a handbook.* Rowman & Littlefield.

Chapter 12
A Lightweight Enhanced Security Approach for Data Privacy in Robotic Systems

Usharani Bhimavarapu
https://orcid.org/0000-0002-0246-1420
Department of Computer Science and Engineering, Koneru Lakshmaiah Education Foundation, Vaddeswaram, India

ABSTRACT

Robot system advances have been followed by the rise in usage of artificial intelligence and cloud processing, and this has been followed by some of the most critical issues of data privacy. Data processing of robot systems with secure data is strongly in demand so as to prevent unauthorized access, data leakage, and cyber attacks. The chapter suggests a new lightweight algorithm for data privacy with security while maintaining computational efficiency for robot systems. The new approach combines data anonymization and obfuscation techniques. It is performed with fewer chances of privacy leakage. In comparison, most other privacy-preserving approaches, which have a high computational burden, can manage such data sets in real time on fewer resources and hence are far more suitable in robots' environments of limited resource availability. Experimentation based on theoretical calculation sets the performance of the algorithm to ensure data privacy without degradation in system performance.

DOI: 10.4018/979-8-3373-1514-0.ch012

INTRODUCTION

As robots come into the mainstream of society, data privacy cannot be a choice anymore. Lightweight algorithms are necessary because robots are working in the regimes of constrained energy, storage, and computation. Classical data privacy algorithms are secure but excessively computationally costly for such regimes. A more efficient lightweight data privacy algorithm is designed to attain security at the expense of efficiency in a manner that allows robotic systems to safeguard sensitive data without slowing down performance or efficiency as far as energy consumption is concerned. robot to reuse learned knowledge on single task. the era of realistic machine learning, robots are currently being designed to be able to form plans, move and act autonomously. For reducing training time, we utilize transfer learning for facilitation learn based on supervised learning, unsupervised learning, and reinforcement learning. In behavior adaptation in case the world environment differs, or new targets become available. Robots thus are adaptable. Domain adaptation techniques minimize training as well as deployment environment difference. Transfer learning is applicable where it is not possible to acquire new data. Virtual environment-trained robots learn to be in real-world environments, i.e. Reinforcement learning over pre-trained models' improves sample efficiency. Multi-task learning enables robots to learn and generalize for a variety of tasks at the same time. Transfer learning lowers computation cost at peak generalization performance. Domain transfer is still an open problem in knowledge transfer across very different tasks.

Multi-agent learning will enable flexibility in co-operative robot systems. Here, most robots gain knowledge and become better from experience through collectives. There are protocols of communication facilitating the sharing of learned knowledge at low cost. Multi-agent learning is applied by swarm robotics to improve group decision making. Models in game theory optimize robot interaction in dynamic scenarios. Stability and scalability of multi-robot systems are provided through decentralized learning architecture. Multi-agent reinforcement learning is applied by autonomous vehicles for cooperative car driving. Distributed learning approaches help robots learn without any centralized control. Task execution and flexibility are supported through coordination among several robots. Coordination overhead, communication, and agent conflict are problems. Developments in multi-agent learning drive warehouse control and disaster relief systems.

Hybrid learning approaches make use of different ML techniques to provide flexibility to the robots. Reinforcement learning and imitation learning hybrid learn better. Supervised and unsupervised learning hybrid improves perception and decision-making. Hierarchical reinforcement learning decomposes tasks into subtasks for enhanced flexibility. Evolutionary algorithms optimize the neural network structure to enhance performance. Federated learning enables collaborative robotic learning from without access to raw data. Hybrid approaches bypass the drawbacks of particular ML approaches. For example, reinforcement learning is complemented additionally with pre-training using supervised learning. Hybrid learning-employed robots will learn faster to be re-trained for new tasks and environments. Synchronization of several learning paradigms is a challenging research endeavor. Hybrid learning drives robotic innovation across various fields.

Task adaptation innovation through ML will define the future of robotics. Explainable AI will further deliver greater transparency into a robot's autonomous decision. Neuromorphic computing will further enable real-time adaptability of learning. Self-learning will reduce the need for an annotated data set to learn. Robotics scientists will integrate more and more AI ethics into the frameworks of the machine learning model. Intelligent AI systems will allow robots to navigate on their own in time-varying environments. Cloud-based learning will allow robots to learn from each other and improve together. More user-friendly task adaptation mechanisms will enrich human-robot collaboration. Computing power innovation will allow real-time adaptability in high-complexity environments. Multi-disciplinary research towards robotics and AI will be undertaken. Task adaptation will transform and make the robots smarter, efficient, and easy to use. All this data except when it is encrypted can be abused. Expansion of privacy to autonomous robots is equated to making arrangements to be in a position of having the prerogative of securing things safely and at their discretion without necessarily resorting to over-management by human on their part. On their own, unsupervised learning allows robots to generalize patterns of data from example instances not labeled. k-means and hierarchical cluster algorithms allow robots to classify things alike. Robots utilize unsupervised learning in anomaly detection to identify unusual behavior of industrial processes. Self-organizing maps (SOMs) enable robots to learn about spatial relations and navigate. Techniques like principal component analysis (PCA) enable reduction of dimensions, making data management less complex. Unsupervised learning is very useful when one lacks substantial labeled data. Robots with learning based on unsupervised learning possess the ability to acquire the ability to adapt to changes in their environment by detecting new patterns. Variational autoencoder-based generative models help in the production of different scenarios while training robots. In practical application, attackers exploit system vulnerabilities to compromise data confidentiality. Additionally, while federated learning supports local model training without exposing raw data, it ends up leaking sensitive information in model updates when not applied with proper differential privacy techniques. The second is computational overhead for secure communication in maintaining a distributed system that can be resource-heavy on resource-constrained devices in hospital environments. ML-based task adaptation innovation is the future of robotics.

It will also increase transparency in an autonomous decision by a robot. Neuromorphic computing will also accelerate real-time learning adaptability. Self-supervised learning will further minimize the need for annotated datasets to adapt. Robotics researchers will continue implementing AI ethics into models of a machine learning model. Adaptive AI platforms will enable robots to freely run in changing environments. Cloud learning will allow robots to learn from one another and get better as a collective. Human-robot collaboration will be augmented by more intuitive task adaptation mechanisms. Increased computing power will make real-time adaptation possible in complex environments. Interdisciplinary investigation will propel AI and robotics. Task adaptation will revolutionize and allow robots to be smarter, more efficient, and simpler to operate. Domain adaptation methods minimize training and deployment environment disparities.

Transfer learning comes in handy where it is not possible to get new data. Robots that have been trained in simulated environments can be adapted to live in real environments, i.e. Reinforcement learning on pre-trained models' improves sample efficiency. Multi-task learning enables robots to learn and generalize multiple tasks at once. Transfer learning preserves computation cost at maximum generalization performance. Domain shift is still an open issue in transferring knowledge between highly dissimilar tasks Thapa and Camtepe's precision health data security requirements and issues as a topic of discourse is an all-round discussion of data privacy methods (Thapa &Camtepe, 2021).

Although clearly defined, one of the shortcomings is the comprehensiveness of methods specified, which are purely centralized-based. Decentralized system privacy issues like distributed health data by geographical location and device are dealt with poorly. Secondly, the article does mention practice but mentions nothing regarding privacy-trade-offs when it comes to valuable information about informed health decision-making and is one of the major hindrances in implementing privacy-preserving technologies into practical use to health. Zhang et al.'s work on pig feeding behavior classification with time-series neural networks is innovative processing of behavior data for agricultural applications (Zhang et al., 2024).

The downside of this paper, though, is that the model is less precise in real-world settings where noisy or incomplete data are encountered, e.g., in uncontrolled settings. Application of video data in the assessment of feeding behavior is also feasible as far as the aspect of data privacy is concerned because the farm laborers deal with personal information. Also, while the model is excellent in the lab environment, scalability when dealing with the issue of computation need in processing real-time huge volumes of massive video is an issue. Hasan et al. provide a complete discussion regarding the security risk and vulnerability of the IoMT network compared to 5G (Hasan et al., 2022).

One of the weak points of their paper is that it discusses purely effective technical fixes without mentioning complex regulatory and ethical considerations involved in deploying 5G in healthcare. Apart from that, the paper fails to disclose the experimental, step-by-step procedure of implementing the suggested countermeasures in various IoMT settings that will constrain their utility in live scenarios. The paper most likely also took into account the latency-security balance of 5G networks as a matter of high concern while solving real-time use cases in healthcare. Hamza and Pradana's scholarly paper on intellectual property rights protection of the use of big data provides comprehensive intellectual property concerns in protection (Hamza & Pradana, 2022).

The limitation is that no exhaustive discussion of how protection concerns of this type can be practically implemented in the fluid data privacy law of different jurisdictions is presented. Greater work has gone into legal issues and comparatively less into technological solutions to minimizing abuses and illegal applications of big data. Second, it does not go deep enough into empirical concerns of how to make intellectual property protection function well in big data environments where data are so bountiful and of such scale that monitoring and enforcement are low in proportion to those resources. Chaudhry et al.'s account of business and FinTech data leak provides evidence of widespread exposure of enormous data breaches of the two industries (Chaudhry et al., 2023).

Biggest appeal of the work is hypothesizing theoretical solutions in imaginary circumstances that have never been empirically tried out against data or case studies, on which they experimented successfully solutions in actual life, within their own business and FinTech realms. Apart from this, while the essay does discuss a person's need for good cybersecurity solutions, it does not take into account the organizational and social factors that would act as a limitation to their uptake, e.g., organizational cultural resistance to change or training employees. The rate of technological progress also implies that there is some level of solutions offered that will be prone to being outdated with the emergence of threats. Zou's prevention and detection of market manipulation research gives a clear explanation of its mechanisms for detection and prevention (Zou, 2022).

Weakness is that the market manipulation is carried out using the theory of market manipulation without any example or actual detection technique being applied in real financial markets. Such techniques given might be difficult to implement in real-market situations because market data are complex and extremely heterogeneous. Apart from this, even if the thesis deals with prevention techniques, nothing is spoken about the topic of enforcement effectiveness of rules in various areas of management of various markets and hence implementability of suggested techniques in various domains isn't easy. Goldberg et al. discuss the economic side of GDPR in internet privacy law (Goldberg et al., 2024). Even assuming their research is valuable analysis of the economic consequences of data privacy law, perhaps the most egregious omission is that they completely fail to consider the socio-political environment in which privacy law is situated. The article suggests a one-size-fits-all formula, but the effectiveness of GDPR-type regulation is perhaps extremely context-dependent and will vary greatly between countries with differing legal systems and consequent societal attitudes towards privacy. In addition, the paper does not take enforcement under GDPR into account in terms of cross-border data flows and jurisdiction to sanction non-compliant players with international business operations. Citron and Solove's research study on privacy harm describes that the notice problem has been a concern along with privacy risk avoidance (Citron & Solove, 2022).

This research has the below weakness in that it discusses very much on legal and theoretical matters to the neglect of practice of prevention of privacy harms as applied in actual cases, particularly with regard to emerging technologies. The paper would further be enriched with more information on how privacy harms are differently suffered by various groups, e.g., marginalized communities, and how such differences could best be addressed. Additionally, even as they focus so much on policymakers, the authors are not very detailed about the role of technology developers to system development with privacy protection. Nayak and Ojha's literature review of data leakage detection and prevention is an excellent synopsis of research streams and methodology here (Nayak & Ojha, 2020).

The only drawback of their work, however is that it is totally theoretical in format without demonstrating the plans for implementation. Their research does not well address the issue of using such methodologies in big dynamic systems where the risk of data leakage occurs dynamically. Further, although the paper discusses a number of important detection methods, there is no reference to the trade-off between detection efficacy and computation cost that can become an essential concern in real-time applications on resource-constrained devices. The use case study of Xu et al. shows promising lines of the research in the future to enhance protection through conceptual synergy between the present traditional data security technology and the utilization of blockchain inclusion (Xu et al., 2024).

Its limitation is in the general discussion presented with insufficient practical data along with proof of the degree to which the hybrid technologies have been utilized. For example, problems with the possibility of implementation deficits in combining orthodox security issues and blockchain that are not yet sufficiently solved in the paper. Most notably, the performance and scalability of these hybrid systems are still insufficiently tested in actual large-scale deployment, which is a major bottleneck to actual deployment of such systems in real applications. Gentry's original work on the fully homomorphic encryption provides a well-grounded theoretical basis to the very powerful cryptography tool (Gentry, 2009).

The strongest limitation of the paper is that its useful applications in daily life are not strongly developed because its computation is costly. Though its theoretical foundations are good, its use in actual systems of FHE is costly and its adoption in big data or real-time systems is a matter of grave concern. The paper also does not adequately address FHE's issue of bridging to practice use, a matter of highest priority that has been an issue of long-standing anguish in follow-up research. Chen et al. suggest a blockchain and fully homomorphic encryption-based decentralized VANETs privacy-preserving deep learning architecture (Chen et al., 2021).

But one of the downsides of their proposal is that they are taking for granted that blockchain and FHE can be implemented seamlessly with each other as well as with VANETs in real-time, which is not necessarily the case because the reason behind this is that both the technologies are latency-intensive. In addition, while the scheme preserves privacy, computational cost of FHE can be a performance bottleneck and thus a cause of scalability issues in extensive networks. Work does not give an appropriate response to potential weak points of the system, as the system is deployed over real vehicular networks. Marcolla et al. provide an overview of theory and applications of fully homomorphic encryption (Marcolla et al., 2022).

One of the weaknesses of their work is that it is underwhelming as regards balancing computationally efficiency with promises to privacy in implementation in the real world. While FHE is invaluable for protecting privacy, as it has an ultra-high computational cost and is ultra-complex, scaling out is challenging, particularly in poor environments. In addition, the survey is more theoretical and explores potential uses, and concerns of day-to-day practice like optimization methods and hardware costs are not studied extensively. Dwork's initial paper on differential privacy outlines an important concept of data privacy protection for statistical use (Dwork, 2006).

This work has been more extensive in the differential privacy theory but less valuable in appropriately providing insight into issues of practical application of the method, especially for large data sets. While differential privacy is a strong privacy mechanism, noise introduced by the mechanism has a significant impact on the utility and precision of the data and can be a costly price in high-precision data-intensive use cases. The paper also fails to consider that the threats to privacy change and are precipitated by new techniques in data analytics and new threats. Dong et al. present Gaussian differential privacy as a new form of the generic differential privacy model (Dong et al., 2022).

The method provides more data utility but is lacking in the sense that it is said to provide weaker privacy than standard Laplace-based differential privacy. While natural distributions of data are caused by Gaussian noise, the limitation is that for repetitive queries or large data, it reveals sensitive information. Second, the paper never covers how realistic deployments of Gaussian differential privacy are faring, where dynamic querying of data and non-static conditions can pose more risks.

Adnan et al. propose the integration of differential privacy and federated learning to be applied in medical image analysis (Adnan et al., 2022).

The drawback of their method is that such applications will never be completely capable of preventing privacy attacks, especially if an adversarial attack or a model inversion attack is used. Even though federated learning saves but does not remove the data from their local location, model updates delivered to the central server can be leaky. Even though differential privacy is applied in an attempt to reduce chances of leakage, privacy vs. model performance trade-off is not necessarily optimally handled and may lead to less accurate critical medical diagnoses. Although differential privacy is a strong approach to maintaining privacy, the method's added noise impacts data's accuracy and utility a lot and can be an expensive burden in data-intensive applications with high requirements for accuracy. The article also fails to account for the fact that threats to privacy evolve and are motivated by emerging data analytics methods with emerging threats. Differential privacy is a strong privacy-preservation method, but the added noise by the method heavily deteriorates the data's accuracy and utility, and the overhead of the method can be very high for applications requiring large amounts of data and high accuracy. Furthermore, there is not a consideration that threat to privacy evolves and is impacted by new arising data analytics methods and arising new threats they constitute. The feasibility of the responsive client population scenario in real-world applications is therefore to be questioned.

Lee et al. propose a privacy-preserving machine learning method for deep neural networks using FHE (Lee et al., 2022).

One of the major weaknesses of this research is the fact that the paper discusses so elaborately on the theoretical advantages of using FHE in keeping things private but spends too little focus on computational difficulties with the use of FHE if used over deep learning at scale. FHE has the potential to greatly accelerate the training and inference times and therefore is not very suitable to be used real-time. Further, the paper does not discuss how the method can be optimized or merged with other methods like model compression or hardware acceleration in an effort to counter these performance challenges. Yao's initial research on privacy-preserving multi-party computation protocols formed the basis of modern privacy-preserving methods (Yao, 1982).

This paper, however, is at a disadvantage in the sense that the protocols proposed are computationally costly and unfeasible to scale to large sets of parties or data. In fact, the protocols are efficiency-limited by virtue of the high amount of cryptography and communication computation. Thus, they will not be applicable to resource-limited settings. It does not delve deeper into details to address the actual problems that came up while implementing these protocols in actual environments, like network synchronization and failure handling. Knott et al. introduce Crypten, a secure multi-party machine learning computation platform (Knott et al., 2021).

One of the gaps in what they have done is that even though Crypten presents a new paradigm for combining secure computation and machine learning, how much it scales is yet to be known. The paper spends most pages outlining theory and early experiments and does not say much about what Crypten would do with gigantic data or with complex machine learning models. The communication overhead between the two sides in Crypten is also an issue, especially for large data or distributed settings. Dwork et al. introduce the differential privacy work and its application to private data analysis (Dwork et al., 2006).

One of this paper's vulnerabilities is that focus on theoretic privacy guarantees suppresses consideration of how differential privacy impacts data utility. Noise addition as a technique for gaining privacy would impact the data by adding interference or disrupting the analysis or precision of the decision. Completion of investigation into the way the mechanisms to adjust differential privacy under application usage of data privacy and usability tradeoff of data in applications such as continuous analytics or high-dimensional data is not completed by this paper. Wei et al. describe federated learning with differential privacy and privacy-preserving machine learning method performance analysis (Wei et al., 2020).

The drawback of their work is that the study does not consider preserving differential privacy on volatile client information in federated settings. Differential privacy is achievable with federated learning, which is a function of the problem of non-iid data for clients, and this will yield inefficiency in model training and performance. There is insufficient evidence regarding trade-offs between differential privacy guarantee achieved and model learning accuracy from literature. Li et al. propose a privacy-preserving deep neural network (DNN) training method with pre-fetched meta-keys on heterogeneous neural network accelerators (Li et al., 2023).

Although their paper is such an intriguing proposal of privacy-preserving DNN training, its drawback is that it relies heavily on a particular hardware setup and hence restricts its application on various environments and platforms. The approach also makes use of meta-keys, which are liable to introduce complexities surrounding key management as well as security. The solution also fails to clarify how the solution scales in real-world deployments when training DNN models on large distributed data sets.

LIGHTWEIGHT DATA PRIVACY ALGORITHM FOR ANONYMIZATION AND OBFUSCATION IN ROBOTIC SYSTEMS

With increasing and increasing robots entering the everyday lifestyle, data privacy is the buzzword of the day. Lightweight algorithms are needed since robots employ bounded energy, storage, and computation. Some traditional data privacy algorithms are secure but too computationally expensive for such applications. A light-weight data privacy algorithm is developed with the aim of providing security vs. efficiency in a way that allows robotic systems to secure personal data without compromising performance or efficiency when it comes to energy. It improves task adaptation through learning to learn or meta-learning. The procedure allows robots to learn new tasks at high speed based on past experience in learning. Robots are trained with few-shot learning processes from small example sets. Meta-learning processes such as Model-Agnostic Meta-Learning (MAML) minimize adaptation time. Robots are able to switch tasks easily without deep retraining cycles because of meta-learning. This comes in handy in household robots, where the robots have to perform so many activities within a day. Meta-learning models generalize nicely across numerous other distinct environments and reduce reliance on data. Domain adaptation methods minimize training and deployment environment differences. Transfer learning is useful where access to new data is impossible. Robots that are trained in simulated environments can be transferred to live in actual environments, i.e. Reinforcement learning on pre-trained models' enhances the sample efficiency. Multi-task learning allows robots to learn and generalize for multiple tasks at once. Transfer learning maintains computation cost at maximum generalization performance. Domain shift remains an open issue in knowledge transfer between very dissimilar tasks. Cryptographic primitives that are light weight such as Elliptic Curve Cryptography (ECC) or light weight hash functions can be applied in anonymizing the data without resource heavily consuming and thus safeguarding the sensitive data during the time when the robot is at run-time Robot system anonymization entails erasure or change of the personal identifiers from the data.

Multi-agent learning facilitates cooperative adaptation in robot systems. In this case, a group of robots learn and adapt based on experience. Experience acquired at low cost is shared between robots with the aid of communication protocols. Multi-agent learning is employed by swarm robotics to promote group decision-making. Game theory-based models are employed to maximize robot interaction under dynamic scenarios. Decentralized learning architecture provides scalability and stability to multi-robot systems. Cooperative driving and other autonomous vehicle applications are based on multi-agent reinforcement learning. Distributed learning techniques allow robots to learn with decentralized control. Flexibility and task performance are improved through coordination of multiple robots. Overhead of coordination, overhead of communication, and conflict among agents are obstacles to distributed multi-agent reinforcement learning. Sophisticated multi-agent learning drives warehouse logistics and disaster relief systems.

Hybrid learning methodologies employ a number of ML methods to obtain robotic adaptability. Hybrids of reinforcement learning and imitation learning learn better. Hybrids of supervised learning and unsupervised learning enhance perception and decision-making. Hierarchical reinforcement learning decomposes tasks into subtasks for enhanced adaptability. Evolutionary algorithms generate neural network topologies for better performance. Federated learning allows robots to learn collaboratively from no raw data. Hybrid solutions circumvent the deficiencies of particular ML strategies. As an example, reinforcement learning is augmented by pre-training using supervised learning. Hybrid learning-used robots are trained faster to be re-tuned for new tasks and environments. Synchronization among different learning strategies is a main research challenge. Hybrid learning drives robotic innovation in numerous disciplines.

The main objective of lightweight obfuscation is to make obfuscated data ready for use in decision making, pattern recognition, and so on by the robot with low computational overhead.

Algorithm

1. Input Data Gathering
   - •Raw data is gathered by the robot from sensors, user input, and other sources. It may be personal identifiers (e.g., name, age, location), health information (e.g., medical records, symptoms), or any other kind of sensitive data.
2. Pseudonymization
   - •Substitute personally identifiable data (PII) with pseudonyms (random identifiers). This makes sensitive data not directly associated with any one person, decreasing the likelihood of data revelation.
   - oReplace user names with unique pseudonyms such as “User_001”, “User_002”, etc.
3. Data Generalization
   - •Generalize sensitive data to lower precision and make it more difficult to identify individuals.
   - oInstead of storing an exact age, group ages into ranges (e.g., 20-30, 31-40).
   - oReplace specific locations with wider geographical areas (e.g., city or region rather than exact coordinates).
4. Lightweight Cryptographic Encryption (Optional)

- o •Encrypt sensitive information using lightweight cryptographic techniques so that even if the data is intercepted, it will still be unreadable.
- o Utilize Elliptic Curve Cryptography (ECC), which offers maximum security with little computational expense.
- o Encrypt data prior to transmission or storage to avoid unauthorized access.

5. Data Masking and Obfuscation
    - o Mask or obfuscate the data to substitute sensitive information with random or dummy data so that the original data cannot be rebuilt.
    - o Example: For biometric information (e.g., fingerprints or face scans), substitute them with randomized representations or hashed values.
    - o Example: For transactional information, mask some of the data (e.g., display only the last four digits of a credit card number).
6. Real-time Data Anonymization
    - o Anonymize the data in real-time to avoid any sensitive information from being held in memory. This is particularly important for systems that need to make decisions in real-time.
    - o Example: When a robot detects a user's voice, anonymize the voice data in real-time by replacing certain attributes (like specific phrases or personal identifiers) with generalized equivalents.
7. Federated Learning for Privacy-Preserving Data Sharing
    - o • Implement federated learning for collaborative learning across multiple robots without sharing raw data. This ensures that each robot learns from local data without revealing sensitive information.
    - o Robots exchange model updates (not raw data) with a central server for aggregation..
    - o Use **differential privacy** during model training to ensure that individual data points do not influence the outcome.
8. Secure Data Storage
    - Store anonymized and obfuscated data in a secure, encrypted storage solution. This could be a cloud service or a local database that uses encryption to prevent unauthorized access.
    - Use lightweight encryption algorithms like **AES-128** for encryption before storing the data.
9. Secure Access Control
    - Implement decentralized or role-based access control to ensure that only authorized entities can access the sensitive data. This can be done using a **blockchain** or **distributed ledger technology (DLT)** to securely log access requests and authorization events.

- Ensure that access rights are updated dynamically based on the context of the robot's interaction with its environment.

10. Output Anonymized Data
    - After performing the necessary operations, the robot outputs the anonymized and obfuscated data for further use, whether for decision-making, analytics, or sharing with other systems.
        - Example output may include aggregated or pseudonymized sensor data, with all sensitive identifiers removed or encrypted.

Theorem 1: Pseudonymization Reduces the Identifiability of Data

Statement: Pseudonymization of personal identifiers in a dataset reduces the identifiability of individuals without losing the utility of the data.

Proof:

Pseudonymization works by replacing sensitive identifiers, such as names, with pseudonyms (randomized identifiers). Since pseudonyms are not traceable back to the original identity without access to the mapping, the data becomes less identifiable.

- Let $D = \{(id_1, x_1), (id_2, x_2), \ldots, (id_n, x_n)\}$represent the dataset with sensitive identifiers, where id_i are the personal identifiers and x_i are the associated data.
- After pseudonymization, the new dataset becomes $D' = \{(p_1, x_1), (p_2, x_2), \ldots, (p_n, x_n)\}$ where p_i are pseudonyms.

Since no p_i can be traced back to the original id_i without the mapping, the data is anonymized.

The identifiability of individuals is reduced by the absence of direct identifiers, but the usefulness of the data for operations like data analysis or decision-making remains intact, as only the pseudonyms are used.

Theorem 2: Generalization Minimizes Precision While Preserving Data Utility

Statement: Generalization of data to broader categories reduces the precision of sensitive attributes, but preserves enough information for useful processing and decision-making.

Proof:

Generalization involves grouping sensitive data into broader categories (e.g., grouping exact ages into age ranges). This reduces the risk of individual identification while retaining the general characteristics of the data.

- Let $D = \{(age_1,x_1),(age_2,x_2),\ldots,(age_n,x_n)\}$ be the original dataset, where age_i is the exact age of an individual.
- After generalization, the dataset becomes $D' = \{(range_1,x_1),(range_2,x_2),\ldots,(range_n,x_n)\}$ where $range_i$ represents an age group (e.g., 20-30, 31-40).

By grouping data into ranges, the exact values are hidden, but the dataset can still be used for statistical analysis and decision-making (e.g., identifying trends for age groups). The reduction in precision does not eliminate the usefulness of the data.

Theorem 3: Lightweight Cryptography Can Achieve Secure Data Encryption with Minimal Overhead

Statement: Lightweight cryptographic methods, such as elliptic curve cryptography (ECC), can securely encrypt sensitive data while minimizing computational overhead.

Proof:

Let M be a message that needs to be encrypted, and let K be the key used for encryption.

Using ECC, the encryption process involves the generation of public and private keys. The algorithm's efficiency is based on the complexity of the elliptic curve discrete logarithm problem, which is computationally difficult even with small key sizes.

- Let the private key PPP be a point on the elliptic curve, and the public key Q be P×, where K is a scalar value.

The encryption process involves using these keys to perform elliptic curve operations, which can be computed efficiently even on resource-constrained devices.

- ECC's computational efficiency stems from the fact that smaller key sizes (e.g., 256-bit ECC) provide comparable security to larger key sizes (e.g., 2048-bit RSA), thus reducing the computational load.

Thus, ECC allows robots to encrypt sensitive data without significant overhead, enabling secure data transmission in real-time.

Theorem 4: Obfuscation Preserves Data Utility While Preventing Reconstructability

Statement: Data obfuscation (e.g., data masking) prevents the reconstruction of original sensitive information while preserving the utility of the data for analysis and decision-making.

Proof:

Consider an original dataset

$$D = \{(sensitivedata_1), (sensitivedata_2), \ldots, (sensitivedata_n)\}$$

Data obfuscation replaces sensitive data with random or non-reversible transformations (e.g., masking, hashing, or permutation). Let the obfuscated dataset be

$$D' = \{(maskeddata_1), (maskeddata_2), \ldots, (maskeddata_n)\}$$

- The transformation (e.g., replacing a name with a pseudonym) is designed to be non-reversible without a specific key or mapping.
- The data becomes irreversibly obfuscated, meaning sensitive information cannot be reconstructed from D′.

However, the obfuscated data maintains enough context (e.g., generic information) for tasks like analysis, trend identification, and decision-making, which is sufficient for the robot's operations.

Theorem 5: Federated Learning Preserves Privacy by Avoiding Centralized Data Collection

Statement: Federated learning enables robots to collaboratively train models without sharing sensitive data, preserving privacy.

Proof:

Let D_i represent the local data on robot i, and M be the global model being trained.

Instead of sharing local data, each robot computes model updates using its local data:

- Robot i computes an updateÄ$M_i = f(D_i)$ where f is the learning algorithm used by the robot.
- These updates Ä$M_1, \Delta M_2, \ldots,$ are sent to a central server, which aggregates them to update the global model

$M' = \sum \Delta M_i.$

Since the robots never share their local data, but instead share only model updates, the sensitive data remains private.

This approach ensures that robots can learn from shared experience without exposing their local data, thus preserving privacy while still allowing for collaborative learning.

Theorem 6: Decentralized Access Control Reduces the Risk of Data Breaches

Statement: A decentralized access control mechanism, such as a blockchain, reduces the risk of data breaches by ensuring that access logs and permissions are transparently managed and immutable.

Proof:

Consider a decentralized system in which access permissions to sensitive data are logged on a blockchain. Each robot's access to sensitive data is recorded as a transaction on the blockchain, ensuring transparency and immutability.

- Let A be a robot attempting to access sensitive data D. The robot's request is recorded as a transaction T = (A, D, timestamp, accesspermission) on the blockchain.
- Each new transaction is cryptographically linked to the previous one, making it tamper-evident.

By using blockchain's decentralized nature, there is no single point of failure or control over access rights. This transparency and immutability make it more difficult for unauthorized actors to gain access to sensitive data, reducing the risk of data breaches.

Furthermore, the decentralized structure ensures that all transactions are auditable, providing accountability and enhancing data security.

CONCLUSION

Robotics data privacy is a very crucial operation to be strongly and well safeguarded from being violated and used for undesirable goals. Implementation of the suggested lightweight algorithm of data privacy sufficiently addresses the shortcomings of existing privacy-oriented approaches and suggests a system that is scalable, efficient, and secure. The algorithm uses data anonymization and obfuscation technologies to enable secure authentication and system functionality. Theoretical analysis and experimental performance endorse its efficiency in hindering computation overhead without sacrificing confidentiality of information. Compared to the conventional encryption-based approaches, the suggested model possesses an optimal trade-off between security and real-time processing and is thus a highly ideal solution for healthcare robots, industrial automation robots, and intelligent infrastructure application. Future studies can further explore by combining quantum cryptography and adaptive learning-based security models to ensure better privacy services in dynamic robots. The result of such research allows for more secure and more intelligent robotic systems with guaranteed secure data protection in real-world applications.

REFERENCES

Adnan, M., Kalra, S., Cresswell, J. C., Taylor, G. W., & Tizhoosh, H. R. (2022). Federated Learning And Differential Privacy For Medical Image Analysis. *Scientific Reports, 12*, 1953. PMID: 35121774

Chaudhry, U. H., Arshad, R., Abbas, N. N., & Zeerak, A. A. (2023). Data Leakage In Business And Fintech. In *Handbook Of Research On Cybersecurity Issues And Challenges For Business And Fintech Applications*. IGI Global.

Chen, J., Li, K., & Philip, S. Y. (2021). Privacy-Preserving Deep Learning Model For Decentralized Vanets Using Fully Homomorphic Encryption And Blockchain. *IEEE Transactions on Intelligent Transportation Systems, 23*, 11633–11642.

Citron, D. K., & Solove, D. J. (2022). Privacy Harms. *Bul Rev., 102*, 793.

Dong, J., Roth, A., & Su, W. J. (2022). Gaussian Differential Privacy. *J. R. Stat. Soc. Ser. B. Statistical Methodology, 84*, 3–37.

Dwork, C. (2006). Differential Privacy. In *International Colloquium On Automata, Languages, And Programming*. Springer.

Dwork, C., Mcsherry, F., Nissim, K., & Smith, A. (2006). Calibrating Noise To Sensitivity In Private Data Analysis. In *Proceedings Of The Theory Of Cryptography: Third Theory Of Cryptography Conference, Tcc 2006*. Springer.

Gentry, C. (2009). Fully Homomorphic Encryption Using Ideal Lattices. *Proceedings Of The Forty-First Annual Acm Symposium On Theory Of Computing*, 169–178.

Goldberg, S. G., Johnson, G. A., & Shriver, S. K. (2024). Regulating Privacy Online: An Economic Evaluation Of The Gdpr. *American Economic Journal. Economic Policy, 16*, 325–358.

Hamza, R., & Pradana, H. (2022). A Survey Of Intellectual Property Rights Protection In Big Data Applications. *Algorithms, 15*, 418.

Hasan, M. K., Ghazal, T. M., Saeed, R. A., Pandey, B., Gohel, H., Eshmawi, A., Abdel-Khalek, S., & Alkhassawneh, H. M. (2022). A Review On Security Threats, Vulnerabilities, And Counter Measures Of 5g Enabled Internet-Of-Medical-Things. *IET Communications, 16*, 421–432.

Kaissis, G. A., Makowski, M. R., Rückert, D., & Braren, R. F. (2020). Secure, Privacy-Preserving And Federated Machine Learning In Medical Imaging. *Nature Machine Intelligence, 2*, 305–311.

Knott, B., Venkataraman, S., Hannun, A., Sengupta, S., Ibrahim, M., & Van Der Maaten, L. (2021). Crypten: Secure Multi-Party Computation Meets Machine Learning. *Advances in Neural Information Processing Systems, 34*, 4961–4973.

Lee, J.W., Kang, H., Lee, Y., Choi, W., Eom, J., Deryabin, M., Lee, E., Lee, J., Yoo, D., & Kim, Y.S. (2022). Privacy-Preserving Machine Learning With Fully Homomorphic Encryption For Deep Neural Network. *IEEE Access, 10*, 30039–30054.

Li, Q., Ren, J., Zhang, Y., Song, C., Liao, Y., & Zhang, Y. (2023). Privacy-Preserving Dnn Training With Prefetched Meta-Keys On Heterogeneous Neural Network Accelerators. *Proceedings Of The Ieee 2023 60th Acm/Ieee Design Automation Conference (Dac),* 1–6.

Li, Q., & Zhang, Y. (2024). Confidential Federated Learning For Heterogeneous Platforms Against Client-Side Privacy Leakages. *Proceedings Of The Acm Turing Award Celebration Conference*, 239–241.

Marcolla, C., Sucasas, V., Manzano, M., Bassoli, R., Fitzek, F. H., & Aaraj, N. (2022). Survey On Fully Homomorphic Encryption, Theory, And Applications. *Proceedings of the IEEE, 110*, 1572–1609.

Nayak, S. K., & Ojha, A. C. (2020). Data Leakage Detection And Prevention: Review And Research Directions. In *Machine Learning And Information Processing: Proceedings Of Icmlip 2019* (pp. 203–212). Springer.

Thapa, C., & Camtepe, S. (2021). Precision Health Data: Requirements, Challenges And Existing Techniques For Data Security And Privacy. *Computers in Biology and Medicine*, *129*, 104130. PMID: 33271399

Wei, K., Li, J., Ding, M., Ma, C., Yang, H. H., Farokhi, F., Jin, S., Quek, T. Q., & Poor, H. V. (2020). Federated Learning With Differential Privacy: Algorithms And Performance Analysis. *Ieee Trans. Inf. Forensics Secur., 15*, 3454–3469.

Xu, Y., Xu, G., Liu, Y., Liu, Y., & Shen, M. (2024). A Survey Of The Fusion Of Traditional Data Security Technology And Blockchain. In *Expert Systems With Applications* (p. 124151). Elsevier.

Yao, A. C. (1982). Protocols For Secure Computations. *Proceedings Of The Ieee 23rd Annual Symposium On Foundations Of Computer Science (Sfcs 1982),* 160–164.

Yousuf, H., Lahzi, M., Salloum, S. A., & Shaalan, K. (2020). Systematic Review On Fully Homomorphic Encryption Scheme And Its Application. In *Recent Advances In Intelligent Systems And Smart Applications* (pp. 537–551). Springer.

Zhang, Y., Yang, X., Liu, Y., Zhou, J., Huang, Y., Li, J., Zhang, L., & Ma, Q. (2024). A Time-Series Neural Network For Pig Feeding Behavior Recognition And Dangerous Detection From Videos. *Computers and Electronics in Agriculture*, *218*, 108710.

Zou, M. (2022). *Market Manipulation: Identification, Characteristics And Prevention* [Ph.D. Thesis]. Macquarie University, Macquarie Park, Australia.

Chapter 13
Privacy-Aware Modeling of Healthcare IoT With Deep Neural Networks

Usharani Bhimavarapu
https://orcid.org/0000-0002-0246-1420
Department of Computer Science and Engineering, Koneru Lakshmaiah Education Foundation, Vaddeswaram, India

ABSTRACT

Networked medical devices have revolutionized modern healthcare by offering round-the-clock patient monitoring, distant diagnosis, and real-time data transmission. The benefits are, however, overshadowed by catastrophic cybersecurity and privacy concerns. Pacemakers, insulin pumps, and wearable monitors, for example, are vulnerable to wireless network use and are vulnerable to hacker attacks, data breaches, and unauthorized access. Weak authentication methods, unsecured data transmission, and obsolete software are susceptible to attack by patients and medical professionals alike, ranging from compromised patient health data to patient safety risk. The problem in this research is solved by developing a robust prediction model via bi-stacked artificial neural networks (ANNs) for cyber attack detection and classification against medical device network security. A large dataset was collected, preprocessed, and boosted with particle swarm optimization (PSO) for feature extraction.

INTRODUCTION

Networked health devices consist of wearables, implantables, and remote patient monitoring that are seen frequently in the healthcare domain. These capture, trans-

DOI: 10.4018/979-8-3373-1514-0.ch013

mit, and store sensitive patient information, like heart rate, blood pressure, blood glucose, and others. Digital technologies are now seeing medical devices as their partner in diagnostic, treatment, and monitoring patients because these devices have been networked into healthcare systems. But integration also comes with terrifying cybersecurity and privacy issues. Hackers are able to steal sensitive data, modify or destroy them to violate patient confidentiality and safety. The rapidly evolving threat landscape creates a challenge for healthcare providers, device vendors, and patients in adopting corresponding security controls.

The greatest challenge is that interconnected medical devices can be accessed by hackers. Most of these devices use wireless communication protocols in transmitting data. Some examples are Bluetooth, Wi-Fi, or cellular networks. Although the technologies facilitate fluid connectivity, they offer avenues of data tampering or interception by hackers. For instance, a sender of patient data to a hospital can be intercepted by a hacker if encryption practices are not effectively used. Also, the majority of the medical devices perhaps may not be loaded with the latest security patches and updates and thus continue to be exposed to known exploitable vulnerabilities that can be exploited by cyber attackers.

Data privacy is also a priority concern in the context of connected medical devices. Medical devices take very intimate and sensitive data, leakage or misuse of which will result in extreme confidentiality violations of patient data. Medical history, symptoms, and vital signs are information gathered by medical devices, stored and processed electronically. Without good encryption and secure data storage procedures, these pieces of information become vulnerable to unauthorized use or leaks. In most cases, the manufacturer of medical devices and the healthcare facility might not have any clear policies or procedures in place for the protection of patients' data from privacy breaches so that the chances of such potential breaches are very likely.

Increased interconnectedness of sophisticated healthcare systems presents risks to privacy and security. The greater the number of devices that are combined the larger the surface of attack. Any networked system and any sensor and device in a healthcare setting is a target for cybercriminals. Moreover, medical device ecosystems typically involve numerous stakeholders, including manufacturers, patients, payers, and hospitals, each potentially having different security protocols. This patchwork attack on healthcare cybersecurity complicates the ability to institute an even measure across devices for security and privacy, which can create gaps in protection.

A lack of proper security in embedded medical devices has direct, harmful effects on the patient. Security breaches into health care's infrastructure can result in the hacking into of vital medical information, i.e., modification of the quantity of insulin injected by an insulin pump or pacemaker timing reprogramming. These types of attacks could result in serious health consequences or even death. For example, an attacker may infiltrate a pacemaker and force it to malfunction; that could easily be a major threat to the life of the patient. This makes such a case where cybersecurity is added in designing and developing medical devices in ways patients are protected and risks associated with harmful tampering are reduced.

Old or unsupported medical device use is the major cause of cybersecurity attacks. Medical devices have extended lifecycles and are not regularly updated or patched after installation. This places older devices more and more at risk of cyber attack as more and new forms of attack evolve. Medical devices in certain situations are developed without integrated security controls, such as secure boot processes or encryption, which makes them vulnerable to attack. Without ongoing support for legacy devices, patients will unnecessarily be exposed to risk since it is not practicable to be able to accommodate putting patches for identified security vulnerabilities in place.

Networked medical device security models are still maturing. Although standards and guidance, such as FDA guidance on medical device cybersecurity, exist, needs are rarely holistic or strenuously acted upon. This will result in security controls being used in a desultory manner in the field. Medical device manufacturers and healthcare providers often are not well-informed of up-to-date information regarding present security threats or lack adequate systems for mitigating the risks incurred. As cyber attacks become more sophisticated, regulatory bodies will be compelled to strengthen their surveillance and call for increased standards to make connected medical devices secure.

With increased use of cloud computing and third-party services in healthcare, this imposes additional privacy and security concerns. Some interrelated healthcare devices use cloud platforms that store and process patient data; hence, they leave themselves vulnerable to threats when the cloud infrastructure remains unsanitized. Poor access control, misconfigured, or weakly encrypted ensures that sensitive information would be available for unauthorized access. Furthermore, healthcare organizations may not have complete authority over third-party cloud providers' security procedures, which can make it challenging to ensure the privacy and security of patient information. Third-party reliance on services mandates that there be strict screening and security assessments of the cloud vendors before transferring medical information to their environments.

Applying artificial intelligence (AI) and machine learning (ML) to networked medical devices proves opportunity and challenge with security and privacy issues. AI and ML algorithms have the prospects to complement the functionality of medical devices in the offer of real-time analytics and predictive capability. But the technologies can potentially bring new threats, such as adversarial attacks where malicious actors manipulate input data to deceive the AI or ML models. The training data for the models may also be personal or sensitive data, hence raising issues of data privacy. Medical devices aided by AI must be secure and compliant with privacy regulations in order to continue enjoying trust in the technologies.

Consent from patients and openness create the building blocks of privacy measures in connected healthcare devices. Healthcare providers and healthcare devices need to educate patients on data processing, data collection, and data transmission of patient information. Oftentimes, patients are unaware of how much data is being collected and the potential risk of data usage with connected devices. Transparency in the guise of open communication, informed consent, and clear privacy policies must be had in order to facilitate patients' ability to make well-informed decisions regarding their involvement in digital health systems. Patients must also be given the ability to control or withdraw consent for data sharing, as this will empower them to maintain privacy.

Generally, the incorporation of networked medical devices into healthcare systems holds the potential to yield great benefits and risks. While these devices facilitate enhanced patient care and efficient medical processes, they also pose a variety of cybersecurity and privacy issues that need to be resolved. The safety and confidentiality of medical devices should be achieved through collaboration between the healthcare providers, device manufacturers, regulators, and patients. Enhanced security practices, routine software updates, efficient regulatory environments, and attention to patient education are all critical components in maintaining the integrity of networked medical devices. Thus, with all these advancements in technology, comes the necessity for our means of protecting sensitive patient data and upholding the safety of those who require such a device for their health needs.

Guanais et al. (2018) studied patient-centered primary care in Latin America and the Caribbean using self-reported health outcomes but risk causing response bias and diminishing the objectivity of the results through the application of public opinion surveys. Shi et al. (2022) have examined newer IoT technologies for smart health care, but the paper is predominantly technology-focused rather than addressing issues of implementation, such as user acceptance, security, and data privacy, in depth. Hu et al. (2022) explored patient-generated health data and the use of artificial intelligence to foretell asthma exacerbation, but since the study is conducted in abstract form without elaborate methodological details, making it less replicable and applicable. Melstrom et al. (2021) discussed adding PGHD to electronic health records in oncologic surgery, but the paper is predominantly a call to action and contains little empirical evidence or in-the-field pilot testing of the AI methods under consideration.

Goharinejad et al. (2022) gave a summary of virtual and augmented reality to treat ADHD, but the results' generalizability is limited because of an excess of big clinical trials and standardized outcome measures in the included studies. Carroll et al. (2021) carried out a scoping review of virtual reality immersive interventions among older adults. The authors also did not differentiate between long term and short term consequences of health following this sort of intervention, which is profoundly essential for evaluating effectiveness of an intervention. Tiase et al. (2020) conducted an analysis of the EHR and PGHD integration, however, their findings are nullified when abstract concepts, and lack analysis of the clinical workflow interruption and interoperability standards. Dinh-Le et al. (2019) also addressed wearable health tech and EHR integration, but their scoping review provides only limited data on the socioeconomic and digital literacy issues that can hinder adoption in disenfranchised populations.

Bourke et al. (2020) have alluded to the application of PGHD in pharmacoepidemiology but have noted the absence of formal formats and validation processes in data, making it difficult to work with such data and integrate it with official drug safety studies. Hull (2015) outlined the role of PGHD as the foundation for personalized care without alluding to the practical matters of collating disparate forms of data into clinical decision platforms. Fostering et al. (2022) discussed distant monitoring of a child PGHD, though the study is limited by not considering data validity, burden on caregivers, and long sustainability. Subramanian (2023) formulated design science for PGHD marketplace with decentralization, but its sustainability in terms of regulatory compliance, consumer trust, and ownership rights to their data is not examined in detail. Lastly, Magnan (2021) interacted with social determinants of health via a quality improvement approach, yet the study does not contain patient-centered indicators or PGHD-centric strategies for informing implementation within real-world health systems.

Huang et al. (2022) conducted a systematic review of the clinical impact of wearable devices in cancer therapy, but their findings are limited by the heterogeneity of the included studies, and it is difficult to draw consistent conclusions across different cancers and devices. Abulkhani et al. (2019) also looked into PGHD management in remote monitoring, but their work does not make amends towards solving the interoperability problems that exist and does not produce practical solutions to factor PGHD into existing healthcare infrastructures. Krist et al. (2017) addressed the point of importance that patients need to be engaged in preventive care, but their work is mostly conceptual and lacks a quantitative measurement of the behavioral outcomes of digital health interventions. Omoloja and E. Vundavalli (2021) provided a balanced overview of pros and cons of PGHD without including data governance models or strategies for mitigating privacy concerns. Blondon and Ehrler (2022) discussed design considerations for integrating PGHD into electronic medical records, with a focus on conceptual frameworks and fewer technical details of implementation.

Wilson et al. (2021) examined the uptake of e-health in older adults, identifying the primary facilitators and barriers but failing to carry out a critical appraisal of the methodological quality of studies included in their scoping review, which compromised on the validity of their findings. Petersen and DeMuro (2015) discussed legal and regulatory challenges associated with social media and mobile health data, but since the concept of data privacy and related laws keeps changing at a very rapid pace, some of their conclusions are now perhaps outdated and need reassessment based on new paradigms like GDPR and HIPAA updates. In a subsequent piece of work, Petersen (2021) discussed readiness of PGHD for clinical decision-making, and this study doesn't quite reach offering empirical evidence regarding the extent to which these data are actually being used by clinicians in practice. Wu et al. (2020) gathered clinician views on the application of PGHD to mental health but are restricted in their mixed-methods study by low sample size and geographical coverage, and this might limit generalizability. Nagpal et al. (2021) had already reviewed the management of type 2 diabetes PGHD analytics but were hampered by a lack of longitudinal data, making it impossible for them to determine the long-term impact of such interventions on clinical outcomes.

Park et al. (2018) looked at the patterns of use of mobile personal health record, but the investigation is based on the frequency of use rather than on user satisfaction, behavioral change, or health outcome. Lastly, Kim et al. (2019) defined self-management interventions with person-generated health information, but their framework assumes high levels of digital literacy and access to mobile health technology, which may not be the situation for every patient population.

Mozzaquatro et al. (2018) proposed an ontology-based cybersecurity framework for IoT systems, but one of the shortcomings is that it has not been tested in highly dynamic and large-scale IoT environments, which can impact the scalability and real-time adaptability of the framework. Neches et al. (1991) described fundamental concepts for knowledge sharing technologies, though their work is very ancient, lacking incorporation with current semantic web standards and recent advancements in AI. Pinto and Martins (2004) described the methods of constructing ontology, yet their approaches are mainly manual and time-consuming and thus less applicable to fast-changing domains where automation plays a critical role. Adel et al. (2019) detailed a comprehensive description of ontology-based semantic interoperability in electronic health records but lacked experimental validation and actual case studies to demonstrate the feasibility of implementation. Szeredi et al. (2014) explained description logics application in semantic web technology, though their explanation is largely theoretical and does not address performance or computational cost when applied to large data sets.

Zhu et al. (2023) proposed neural-symbolic approaches to reasoning on large ABoxes in OWL DL, but their solution can be plagued by interpretability issues, and the cooperation between symbolic and neural components remains computationally expensive. Tang et al. (2022) proposed neural logical reasoning for TBox and ABox, but their work is limited to experimental demonstration and does not address deployment to actual ontology systems. Noy and McGuinness (2001) created a seminal guide to building ontologies, but the tutorial is not able to facilitate collaborative, distributed ontology development and is not designed to accommodate changing ontological requirements in dynamic environments. Rudolph (2011) gave the first insights into description logics, but the material is extremely academic and difficult for practitioners to understand who seek practical solutions for reasoning on the web. Kumar and Deepak (2020) proposed HeTOnto for domain-specific ontology modeling in heat transfer, but its domain specificity renders it less applicable across other domains and lacks tools for cross-domain semantic mapping. Finally, Schütz et al. (2021) developed a core ontology for German medical devices; however, the approach may not be everywhere applicable due to localization and legally-specific limitations, which prevents global semantic interoperability.

McGinnis et al. (2011) offer the application of clinical data as a central asset for health learning systems, noting its promise as a public good. The drawback, however, is the lack of any focus on current cybersecurity threats and mitigation measures for protecting clinical data in networked settings. The recommendations are predominantly policy-focused and do not possess technical acumen about actual-time data breaches or IoT attacks prevalent in present-day healthcare systems (McGinnis et al., 2011).

Zeng and Gao (2017) offer valuable information on how wearables promote physical activity but in the absence of a complete review of security vulnerabilities inherent in wearables. The argument revolves around behavioral and health outcomes while issues like unauthorized access, leakage of data, and encryption standards are not exhaustively discussed. This limits the usability of the study for those in need of information on how to secure wearable technology in medical environments (Zeng et al., 2017).

Muhammad Sayem et al. (2020) present a comprehensive review of smart electro-clothing systems, detailing their sensors, applications, and advantages. However, their review mainly focuses on technological aspects and wearable innovation, with little regard for cybersecurity issues such as wireless data interception or user privacy violations. Since these systems convey sensitive physiological information, the lack of thorough security analysis is a major drawback (Muhammad Sayem et al., 2020).

Martin and Irrgang (2007) are interested in self-reported outcome measures of foot and ankle disorders. While useful in clinical assessment, the study is pre-IoT and does not consider cybersecurity or digital data integrity concerns. Its application in today's networked health environments is therefore limited, especially when patient data are collected using networked devices (Martin et al., 2007).

Liu et al. (2016) conduct a systematic review of smart homes and elderly health monitoring. While they touch on technological feasibility and patient benefits, they minimize the security features of networked sensors and data communication. Given the vulnerability of older users and the privacy of their health data, the lack of emphasis on protection against cyberattacks is a major omission (Liu et al., 2016).

El Amrani et al. (2017) consider connected health devices in mainstream general medical practices within France, producing effective adoption trends. However, the study does not consider whether the devices comply with cybersecurity policies or GDPR. Lack of technical analysis in device verification, information safeguarding, or breach instances reduces the stringency of their analysis (El Amrani et al., 2017).

Brown et al. (2022) discuss the psychological and social concerns of long-term condition patients when they share personal health information. Although the research is educative about user behavior and trust, there is little talk of how technical protection or open security policies could assist in addressing such issues. The issue of cybersecurity in fostering confidence in data sharing is not explored in full (Brown et al., 2022).

Rahi et al. (2021) offer a new air quality monitoring system in a smart eHealth framework based on firefly optimization and SVM. However, while their approach is resilient in environmental sensing and machine learning, the paper barely addresses data security and privacy, which are most essential in a health framework. Their focus on optimization sweeps away the likelihood of data sabotage or compromise (Rahi et al., 2021).

Alshaikh et al. (2014) formally review use of social media to gather health information. The review correctly indicates the scope and diversity of information being put on the sites but fails to emphasize privacy concerns and risk of exposure to data misuse appropriately. Social networking sites are also more exposed to hacking, and the review could be more complete by adding anti-countermeasures to it (Alshaikh et al., 2014).

Trifan et al. (2019) give an elaborate explanation of passive health sensing on mobile phones. Even though their survey detects the condition of sensor-based health monitoring, security threats to data by mobile platforms, such as app-level vulnerabilities, malware, or insecure APIs, are not examined. This lack of concentration on technical defense makes it less helpful in secure system design (Trifan et al., 2019).

Tricoli et al. (2017) offer a thrilling discussion of wearable and miniaturized sensors for personalized medicine. They succeed in bringing out technological advancements but downplay the importance of data encryption, secure firmware upgrades, and secure cloud storage within these devices. These factors matter since the captured data is personal (Tricoli et al., 2017).

Kashani et al. (2021) offer a systematic review of healthcare IoT applications with significant use cases and trends. While despite the wide context of the review, cybersecurity threats are described in broad terms and without detailed mitigation strategies and real case studies. Against the backdrop of the acute need for security in Internet of Things (IoT) healthcare, technical vagueness is a glaring limitation

(Kashani et al., 2021).One such significant limitation, as identified by Khatiwada and Yang (2022), is the lack of general performance measures and overall evaluation standards in the security dimension of the Internet of Medical Things (IoMT). While the study provides a general overview of security and privacy policies, it is hypothetical in approach with no empirical evidence of the suggested measures in practical applications. Moreover, the article reveals a number of problems but offers minimal practical advice or applicable models to healthcare practitioners, thus reducing its applicability to clinical practice (Khatiwada et al., 2022).

Hunt et al. (2017) raise valid issues with electronic health records (EHRs), primarily that they tend to depersonalize the patient experience and overwhelm personal histories with rigid data structures. The article is otherwise largely anthropological in focus and does not include a technical explanation of security and privacy risks in EHR systems. Such disciplinary focus constrains the paper to offer actionable cybersecurity advice or quantitative risk assessments relevant to networked medical devices (Hunt et al., 2017).

Adler-Milstein and Nong (2019) have laid out intriguing data about initial patient and health system experience with patient-generated health data (PGHD). The analysis is, however, not a consideration of security implications for storage and transmission of PGHD in cloud or decentralized settings. There is a focus on usability and integration rather than the robustness of cybersecurity infrastructure that needs to be embraced for protecting such data (Adler-Milstein et al., 2019).

Korjian and Gibson (2022) give an outline of the way in which digital technology like AI and wearables is broadening access to clinical research. While the authors touch on some detail as to the benefit of increased access via digital, they superficially discuss data protection and privacy issues in passing. The study does not consider in depth exploitation or intrusion into health-sensitive data devices, and thus their analysis of cybersecurity concerns is insufficient (Korjian et al., 2022).

In their protocol for systematic reviewing, Medina and Isomursu (2023) describe how patient-generated health data using mobile devices are incorporated into clinical processes. The protocol may describe required steps towards evidence synthesis but lacks a clear discussion on the encryption standards, secure transmission protocol, and compliance steps towards privacy. Hence, it leaves an understanding gap as to what the cybersecurity infrastructure for PGHD application in clinical contexts is (Medina et al., 2023).

Cohen et al. (2016) have a holistic argument on the use of patient-generated health data in clinical settings. Despite with insightful comments on the merging of operational and workflow processes, the study falls short in highlighting technical interventions towards the support of safe data exchange. Access control, authentication processes, and protection against cyber attacks are not adequately discussed and hence loses some bit of validity in high-risk connected device systems (Cohen et al., 2016).

Lastly, Lavallee et al. (2020) present a stakeholder-guided perspective on the potential and challenges of mobile health and PGHD. Though the paper accurately weighs some system challenges like interoperability and clinician trust, the paper lacks in consideration of cybersecurity frameworks or data breach scenarios. Hence, stakeholder concerns are represented quite well but executed cybersecurity concerns are in their early stages (Lavallee et al., 2020).

A proposed framework avoids many of the major flaws in existing models for preventing cybersecurity and privacy problems in networked medical devices. Traditional security controls like signature-based detection or rule-based systems are not very effective against new or sophisticated attacks like zero-day threats and advanced persistent threats. These are also likely to suffer from high false positives and slow response rates, which are harmful to patient safety during an emergency.

Contrarily, the presented method uses state-of-the-art machine learning models like stacked artificial neural networks (ANNs) for improving the accuracy of threat detection and the reaction rate. Using multiple layers of deep models with stacking, this system proposed herein improves the capability to learn sophisticated patterns of data as well as react against unknown threats. Through this, higher-quality detection against anomalies can be achieved, and it reduces the likelihood of detecting new or continuously evolving attack mechanisms.

Furthermore, the system in question focuses on real-time threat assessment, which allows for quicker risk detection and mitigation compared to traditional models that are constrained by response time delay. The feature selection techniques such as Particle Swarm Optimization (PSO) ensure high-priority features with high value to facilitate better and faster predictions. Computation overhead is kept to a minimum, allowing the system to perform well under resource-constrained environments, which is the largest issue in connected medical devices, which are worst off with processing power.

Moreover, the model illustrated here utilizes privacy-preserving techniques, considering sensitive patient information issues. Unlike other models that might expose personal health information due to weak encryption and weak data management, the model illustrated here utilizes strong encryption and data anonymization techniques to ensure that patient information are not breached but at the same time allow proper threat identification.

The general formulation of the model improves in sensitivity to new threats, improves detection efficiency, reduces response time to a minimum, and offers better protection for privacy. Therefore, it is a better and more trusted answer to the security of networked medical devices.

MATERIAL AND METHODS

The strategy is to collect an exhaustive dataset of interrelated medical devices, such as device data, communications protocols, network activities, and cyber attacks. Preprocessing is applied to clean, normalize, and encode the dataset in order to yield precision and uniformity. Particle Swarm Optimization (PSO) is employed to detect critical features that impact cybersecurity and privacy outcomes. Next, a Bi-Stacked Artificial Neural Network (ANN) model is constructed, which involves two stacked models to learn deep interaction of features. Easy patterns are learned by the first ANN stack from input features and fine-tuned by the second one to make improved predictions. The model is trained using labeled data in both normal and attack conditions. Performance indicators like accuracy, precision, recall, and F1-score are utilized to evaluate the model. Live threat detection capability is subjected to simulation. Standard data sets and live applications are used to test the system. This offers a hardened, smart way of protecting connected medical devices against cyberattack.

Material

Cybersecurity and privacy research on connected medical devices involves gathering diverse sets of data points to capture the complexity of such issues. The data set must contain heterogeneous types of information, such as: device-related data, i.e., network security metrics, patient populations, medical professionals' behaviors, and breach occurrences. It must contain such as devices (e.g., wearables, implantables, diagnostic devices) along with respective communication protocols (e.g., Bluetooth or Wi-Fi), software versions utilized, and existing threats. Security feature information on these devices, such as encryption algorithms, authentication processes, and update frequency, should be included in the dataset for quantifying the robustness of their defense. The dataset should also collect anonymized patient demographics such as age, gender, and diseases because these can affect the frequency and gravity of cyberattacks. It would need to capture the pattern and type of security incidents or breach of essential privacy, such as methods of attack (e.g., data capture, denial-of-service attacks), the extent of violation, and its effect on patient safety and data integrity. Organizational strategy towards cybersecurity must also be determined through the collection of policies and practices related to device security, such as employee training, patching schedule for devices, and data access controls of the healthcare provider. Lastly, data for regulatory compliance with standards such as HIPAA, FDA regulations, and ISO/IEC 27001 will be known about the influence of regulatory mechanisms in combating cybersecurity and privacy attacks on interconnected medical devices. This all-inclusive dataset will be a good basis for the study of the status of cybersecurity and privacy in the medical device market and to determine the areas that should be enhanced.

Preprocessing

Preprocessing data of the collected dataset on networked medical device cybersecurity and privacy concerns involves several significant steps to render the dataset clean, organized, and ready for analysis. Data cleaning forms the first step, where missing data is handled by identifying any gaps in information, such as missing device details or patient demographics. Missing values are filled in by statistical strategies such as mean, median, or mode, or by more sophisticated techniques such as K-nearest neighbors (KNN) imputation if deemed necessary. In certain instances, records containing major missing data might be deleted entirely. The second step is then to delete and detect duplicate records, which may bias analysis by adding redundancy. Data errors, such as incorrect device identifiers or out-of-range values for certain features, should also be resolved, usually by cross-checking with original data sources or enforcing predefined rules.

The second significant preprocessing step is data transformation, where data is normalized and encoded to be uniform across the dataset. Normalization and scaling are needed to let the numerical features like network security measurements, including throughput and latency, and patient demographics, like age and gender, be on the same scale. It may be necessary to use techniques like Min-Max normalization or Z-score standardization. Most of the features in the dataset, such as device types, communication protocols, and attack techniques, are categorical. These categorical attributes must be converted to numerical forms to allow analysis. Methods like label encoding or one-hot encoding can be applied to convert categorical data to the right form to use in machine learning models or statistical tests. In general, preprocessing converts raw data into an appropriate and accurate form so that the ensuing analyses will provide insightful observations on cybersecurity and privacy threats of networked medical devices.

Feature Selection

Particle Swarm Optimization (PSO) oriented feature selection is a useful method for selecting the most appropriate features from a data set, especially for high-dimensional data sets like data gathered for cybersecurity and privacy issues in networked medical devices. PSO is a population-based, bio-inspired optimization algorithm that mimics the social behavior of birds or schools of fish to locate an optimum solution in a search space. In feature selection, every particle in the swarm is a candidate subset of features and the search is for the optimal subset of features providing the best performance based on a given fitness function, such as classification accuracy or reduction in the error rate. In the first stage, the population of random subsets of features is generated and then each subset is evaluated based on the fitness function. The algorithm varies the position and velocity of each particle according to its best-known position and the best-known positions of the neighbors.

After iterative updating, particles converge to the optimal or nearly optimal set of features that contribute the most to the predictability of the model. For the medical device dataset, PSO can be employed in eliminating noisy, irrelevant, or redundant features like non-informative device data or uncorrelated patient information while preserving essential attributes like known vulnerabilities, encryption level, and previous breach history. This enhances the accuracy of the machine learning model, saves computation time, and improves model explainability. Furthermore, PSO-based feature selection is especially helpful in very complicated datasets where the traditional filter or wrapper methods might not be good enough due to the presence of nonlinear relationships between features. Employing the adaptive and exploratory capability of PSO, researchers can achieve a set of effective and efficient features that best define the underlying mechanisms of cybersecurity and privacy in networked medical devices.

Bi-Stacked ANN

Securing cybersecurity and privacy matters in networked medical devices using a Bi-Stacked Artificial Neural Network (Bi-Stacked ANN) approach provides an effective technique for the detection, classification, and prediction of potential vulnerabilities and attacks. Networked medical devices such as insulin pumps, pacemakers, and wearable monitors transmit vital patient data continuously across wireless networks, thus are targets of cyber attacks. Conventional machine learning may not work properly to identify those intricate patterns and relations among the numerous features from different settings of the devices, communication protocols, network usage, or breach history. Using A Bi-Stacked ANN deepens learning from the viewpoints of detection, not only at the low-level abstraction but also at the high-level abstraction of the feature input.

With this approach, the first stack of neural networks is tasked with the learning of the inherent feature representations of the input data such as device types, encryption protocols, authenticating mechanisms, and demographic details. Further refinement of the patterns and associations, such as patterns of weaknesses that can be used to breach or event patterns showing that an attack is about to be launched, is affected by feeding the output of the first stack into a second stack. Layered learning helps enhance generalizability as well as detection of advanced, novel attack channels. Besides, Bi-Stacked ANN is best suited to handle the high dimensionality and heterogeneity of the cybersecurity data and offers better accuracy and stability than single-layer or shallow architectures.

By training the Bi-Stacked ANN on labeled datasets that include normal operation logs and data from known breach incidents, the model can generalize classifying traffic and device activity as secure or suspicious. Also, the model can be used within real-time monitoring systems to be able to predict potential breaches or invasions of privacy in such a way that potential threats can be proactively lessened. The framework also facilitates feature importance analysis so that cybersecurity experts have an idea about which device properties or network patterns are primarily accountable for risk and thus can guide improvement in design and policy choice. In conclusion, the use of a Bi-Stacked ANN offers a scalable, intelligent, and adaptive platform for patient privacy protection and cybersecurity improvement in the new network of medical devices that are interconnected.

EXPERIMENTAL RESULTS

Experimental outcomes demonstrate the efficiency of the used Bi-Stacked Artificial Neural Network (ANN) model in attack detection and classification of networked medical device cybersecurity and privacy attacks. The model was trained and tested on a handpicked data set with normal as well as malicious activity logs, including features such as device type, communication protocols, encryption algorithm, and known vulnerabilities. Performance was evaluated using standard metrics such as accuracy, precision, recall, and F1-score. The results indicate that the Bi-Stacked ANN was superior to traditional machine learning models in terms of detection accuracy and false positive rate, proving its ability to learn complex patterns and relations in high-dimensional healthcare IoT data. Furthermore, feature selection using Particle Swarm Optimization (PSO) significantly enhanced model efficiency by weeding out noise and emphasizing the most significant variables. Observations corroborate the robustness of the model and the viability to implement it for real-time security monitoring of medical devices.

Table 1 deals with various kinds of attacks on interfaced medical devices like pacemakers, wearable monitors, and insulin pumps. It indicates a combination of both detected threats and those that were not detected with different response times and related risks. Evidently, high-risk attacks like DDoS, malware injections, and data breaches define the presentation, which indicates how vulnerable the devices are.

Table 1. Threat Detection and Response Time for Connected Medical Devices

Device ID	Device Type	Threat Type	Detection Status	Risk Level	Response Time (ms)
D001	Pacemaker	Data Breach	Missed	Medium	146.99
D002	Insulin Pump	Man-in-the-Middle	Missed	Critical	257.55
D003	Wearable Monitor	Unauthorized Access	Missed	Medium	113.15
D004	ECG Sensor	Unauthorized Access	Missed	Medium	151.18
D005	ECG Sensor	Firmware Tampering	Missed	Medium	339.17
D006	Insulin Pump	Man-in-the-Middle	Detected	Medium	165.33
D007	Blood Pressure Monitor	Man-in-the-Middle	Missed	Medium	486.91
D008	Blood Pressure Monitor	DDoS Attack	Detected	High	270.36
D009	ECG Sensor	Data Breach	Missed	Critical	333.32
D010	Insulin Pump	Data Breach	Detected	Medium	336.99

Table 2 continues with the theme of unauthorized access, firmware manipulation, and malware injection in wearable devices and ECG sensors. The detection status varies from "missed" to "detected," indicating the different levels of effectiveness of security controls. Wearable devices such as the insulin pump and blood glucose meters are highly risky, and therefore, there is a need for increased cybersecurity.

Table 2. Risk Levels and Detection Status of Cybersecurity Threats in Medical Devices

Device ID	Device Type	Threat Type	Detection Status	Risk Level	Response Time (ms)
D011	ECG Sensor	Data Breach	Detected	High	242.35
D012	Wearable Monitor	Malware Injection	Missed	Medium	314.22
D013	Blood Glucose Meter	Unauthorized Access	Detected	Medium	176.89
D014	Pacemaker	DDoS Attack	Detected	Critical	387.13
D015	Insulin Pump	Firmware Tampering	Missed	High	491.45
D016	Wearable Monitor	Signal Jamming	Detected	Low	145.67
D017	Blood Pressure Monitor	Data Breach	Missed	Medium	362.48
D018	ECG Sensor	Malware Injection	Detected	Medium	289.30

continued on following page

Table 2. Continued

Device ID	Device Type	Threat Type	Detection Status	Risk Level	Response Time (ms)
D019	Pacemaker	Man-in-the-Middle	Detected	Medium	224.12
D020	Insulin Pump	Unauthorized Access	Missed	High	312.55

Table 3 demonstrates the effect of signal jamming and firmware tampering on blood pressure sensors and ECG sensors. It displays the risk of external interference and malicious manipulation. The response times are relatively longer in the scenario of high-level threats, reflecting that these devices will respond slower to high-level threats.

Table 3. Detection of Signal Jamming and Firmware Tampering in Medical Devices

Device ID	Device Type	Threat Type	Detection Status	Risk Level	Response Time (ms)
D021	Wearable Monitor	Firmware Tampering	Missed	Medium	351.20
D022	ECG Sensor	Signal Jamming	Detected	Low	133.00
D023	Insulin Pump	Malware Injection	Detected	High	416.38
D024	Blood Pressure Monitor	Man-in-the-Middle	Detected	Medium	253.77
D025	Pacemaker	DDoS Attack	Missed	Critical	521.15
D026	Wearable Monitor	Unauthorized Access	Detected	Medium	194.41
D027	ECG Sensor	Malware Injection	Detected	Medium	177.02
D028	Blood Glucose Meter	Firmware Tampering	Missed	Medium	338.44
D029	Insulin Pump	Signal Jamming	Detected	Low	139.88
D030	ECG Sensor	Data Breach	Detected	High	218.29

Table 4 indicates the detection of DDoS attacks, illegal access, and malware injection. Pacemakers and insulin pumps are among the devices that are exposed to critical threats disrupting patient safety by registering high-risk levels and long response times. Different devices have differences in the ability of detection systems to function effectively, with a possibility of some threats remaining undetected.

Table 4. DDoS Attacks, Unauthorized Access, and Malware Injection in Medical Devices

Device ID	Device Type	Threat Type	Detection Status	Risk Level	Response Time (ms)
D031	Pacemaker	Firmware Tampering	Detected	High	267.13
D032	Blood Pressure Monitor	Malware Injection	Detected	Medium	298.64
D033	Insulin Pump	Data Breach	Missed	Critical	392.23
D034	ECG Sensor	DDoS Attack	Missed	High	348.78
D035	Wearable Monitor	Man-in-the-Middle	Detected	Medium	212.56
D036	Pacemaker	Signal Jamming	Detected	Low	164.09
D037	Blood Glucose Meter	Malware Injection	Missed	High	319.45
D038	ECG Sensor	Data Breach	Detected	Medium	234.77
D039	Insulin Pump	Firmware Tampering	Detected	High	302.90
D040	Blood Pressure Monitor	Signal Jamming	Missed	Low	197.11

Table 5 recognizes a wider set of threats such as malware, signal jamming, and data breach in devices such as insulin pumps and wearable monitors. The threats recognized are largely unauthorized access and malware injection, and they recognize the need for real-time detection mechanisms. Response times demonstrate different levels of system readiness in different devices.

Table 5. Analysis of Data Breaches and Unauthorized Access in Connected Medical Devices

Device ID	Device Type	Threat Type	Detection Status	Risk Level	Response Time (ms)
D041	ECG Sensor	Malware Injection	Missed	High	351.98
D042	Wearable Monitor	Data Breach	Detected	Medium	183.61
D043	Insulin Pump	Unauthorized Access	Detected	Medium	219.45
D044	Blood Glucose Meter	Signal Jamming	Detected	Low	149.27
D045	Pacemaker	Man-in-the-Middle	Detected	High	273.90
D046	ECG Sensor	Firmware Tampering	Missed	Critical	402.78
D047	Wearable Monitor	DDoS Attack	Detected	High	244.13
D048	Insulin Pump	Malware Injection	Detected	Medium	216.11

continued on following page

Table 5. Continued

Device ID	Device Type	Threat Type	Detection Status	Risk Level	Response Time (ms)
D049	Blood Pressure Monitor	Data Breach	Missed	High	314.87
D050	Pacemaker	Signal Jamming	Detected	Low	134.26

Table 6 targets pacemakers, wearable monitors, and insulin pumps against various kinds of cybersecurity attacks. With medium to high threat levels, the table highlights the need for detecting malware injections and unauthorized access. Response times for critical issues such as DDoS attacks are significantly longer, indicating possible system vulnerabilities.

Table 6. Detection of Cybersecurity Threats in Pacemakers, Wearable Monitors, and Insulin Pumps

Device ID	Device Type	Threat Type	Detection Status	Risk Level	Response Time (ms)
D051	Pacemaker	Unauthorized Access	Detected	High	248.33
D052	Wearable Monitor	Firmware Tampering	Missed	Medium	319.76
D053	Blood Pressure Monitor	Signal Jamming	Detected	Low	153.29
D054	ECG Sensor	Malware Injection	Detected	Medium	230.11
D055	Insulin Pump	DDoS Attack	Missed	Critical	467.93
D056	Blood Glucose Meter	Data Breach	Detected	High	295.38
D057	ECG Sensor	Man-in-the-Middle	Missed	High	361.47
D058	Wearable Monitor	Unauthorized Access	Detected	Medium	188.24
D059	Pacemaker	Firmware Tampering	Detected	High	271.65
D060	Insulin Pump	Signal Jamming	Missed	Low	197.03

Table 7 still evaluates device security against different threats, such as DDoS attacks and firmware tampering. Devices such as pacemakers and ECG sensors have a combination of detected and undetected threats. The high-risk devices require more advanced detection systems since most of them have slow response times to critical attacks.

Table 7. Impact of DDoS Attacks and Firmware Tampering on Connected Medical Devices

Device ID	Device Type	Threat Type	Detection Status	Risk Level	Response Time (ms)
D061	ECG Sensor	Malware Injection	Missed	Critical	433.52
D062	Wearable Monitor	DDoS Attack	Detected	High	284.44
D063	Insulin Pump	Firmware Tampering	Detected	Medium	245.77
D064	Blood Pressure Monitor	Data Breach	Missed	High	311.08
D065	Blood Glucose Meter	Man-in-the-Middle	Detected	Medium	228.36
D066	Pacemaker	Signal Jamming	Detected	Low	138.92
D067	ECG Sensor	Unauthorized Access	Missed	High	356.31
D068	Insulin Pump	Malware Injection	Detected	Medium	202.65
D069	Wearable Monitor	Firmware Tampering	Missed	Medium	293.48
D070	Pacemaker	Data Breach	Detected	High	309.17

Table 8 explains the impact of signal jamming, illegal entry, and firmware tampering on connected medical devices. The response time also differs considerably with some being delayed in responding to harmful attacks. The table marks the variation of security measures with different devices pointing out an area of need to improve in certain categories.

Table 8. Cybersecurity Challenges: Signal Jamming and Unauthorized Access in Medical Devices

Device ID	Device Type	Threat Type	Detection Status	Risk Level	Response Time (ms)
D071	Blood Glucose Meter	DDoS Attack	Missed	Critical	498.23
D072	Blood Pressure Monitor	Man-in-the-Middle	Detected	Medium	265.14
D073	ECG Sensor	Signal Jamming	Detected	Low	142.05
D074	Wearable Monitor	Malware Injection	Detected	Medium	225.67
D075	Pacemaker	Firmware Tampering	Missed	High	337.29
D076	Insulin Pump	Data Breach	Detected	High	276.33
D077	ECG Sensor	Man-in-the-Middle	Missed	Medium	308.49

continued on following page

Table 8. Continued

Device ID	Device Type	Threat Type	Detection Status	Risk Level	Response Time (ms)
D078	Blood Glucose Meter	Unauthorized Access	Detected	Medium	197.54
D079	Wearable Monitor	DDoS Attack	Detected	High	265.67
D080	Pacemaker	Malware Injection	Missed	High	356.81

Table 9 is a similar analysis but for malware injection detection and signal jamming. Pacemakers and blood glucose meters are some of the devices that are plagued by a combination of risks of different levels of severity. It can be seen from the table that although there are certain devices which are more susceptible to unauthorized access, there are certain devices which can be more susceptible to firmware and malware.

Table 9. Malware Injections and Unauthorized Access in Connected Medical Devices

Device ID	Device Type	Threat Type	Detection Status	Risk Level	Response Time (ms)
D081	Blood Pressure Monitor	Data Breach	Detected	High	298.90
D082	Insulin Pump	Man-in-the-Middle	Missed	Medium	324.10
D083	ECG Sensor	Firmware Tampering	Detected	High	277.21
D084	Wearable Monitor	Unauthorized Access	Missed	High	345.18
D085	Pacemaker	Signal Jamming	Detected	Low	147.64
D086	Blood Glucose Meter	Malware Injection	Missed	Critical	414.28
D087	Insulin Pump	DDoS Attack	Detected	High	266.42
D088	Blood Pressure Monitor	Firmware Tampering	Missed	Medium	301.55
D089	ECG Sensor	Signal Jamming	Detected	Low	159.80
D090	Pacemaker	Data Breach	Detected	Medium	248.09

Table 10 presents the analysis based on the detection of DDoS attacks, illegal access, and signal blocking. Insulin pumps and glucose meters are some devices that have higher risk factors because their vulnerabilities are not being detected in certain situations. Response times indicate the challenge to address such serious issues in a timely manner

Table 10. Response Time and Risk Levels in Detection of DDoS and Malware Attacks in Medical Devices

Device ID	Device Type	Threat Type	Detection Status	Risk Level	Response Time (ms)
D091	Wearable Monitor	Firmware Tampering	Missed	Medium	327.48
D092	Blood Glucose Meter	Unauthorized Access	Detected	High	234.01
D093	Insulin Pump	Malware Injection	Missed	High	384.92
D094	ECG Sensor	Man-in-the-Middle	Detected	Medium	213.84
D095	Blood Pressure Monitor	Signal Jamming	Detected	Low	163.70
D096	Pacemaker	Firmware Tampering	Detected	High	297.02
D097	Wearable Monitor	Data Breach	Missed	Critical	409.56
D098	Insulin Pump	DDoS Attack	Detected	High	273.33
D099	ECG Sensor	Unauthorized Access	Detected	Medium	222.47
D100	Blood Glucose Meter	Man-in-the-Middle	Missed	Medium	316.71

CONCLUSION

The research suggests an adaptive and intelligent method to combat networked medical device-based cyber attacks on privacy and cybersecurity through a Bi-Stacked ANN model. Led by a carefully trained dataset, successful preprocessing operations, and PSO-based feature extraction, the model was able to learn successfully sophisticated patterns of cyber attacks and device vulnerabilities. Performance demonstrated that Bi-Stacked ANN had the greatest precision and dependability in foreseeing and categorizing future likely security intrusions. The method not only aggregates the threat identification but also enables the possible realization of the important risk factors interacting medical device networks. The system provides real-time monitoring, warning, and data-driven decision support for healthcare facilities and device manufacturers. In the future, edge computing, federated learning, or blockchain technologies can be incorporated to further strengthen security and safeguard privacy. In the future, this book is spreading out an increasingly connected world into a safer and more stable atmosphere in health care.

REFERENCES

Abdolkhani, R., Gray, K., Borda, A., & DeSouza, R. (2019). Patient-generated health data management and quality challenges in remote patient monitoring. *JAMIA Open*, *2*, 471–478. PMID: 32025644

Adel, E., El-Sappagh, S., Barakat, S., & Elmogy, M. (2019). Ontology-based electronic health record semantic interoperability: A survey. In Dey, N., Ashour, A. S., Fong, S. J., & Borra, S. (Eds.), *Advances in Ubiquitous Sensing Applications for Healthcare, U-Healthcare Monitoring Systems* (pp. 315–352). Academic Press.

Adler-Milstein, J., & Nong, P. (2019). Early experiences with patient-generated health data: Health system and patient perspectives. *Journal of the American Medical Informatics Association : JAMIA*, *26*, 952–959. PMID: 31329886

Alshaikh, F., Ramzan, F., Rawaf, S., & Majeed, A. (2014). Social network sites as a mode to collect health data: A systematic review. *Journal of Medical Internet Research*, *16*, e171. PMID: 25048247

Blondon, K., & Ehrler, F. (2022). Design Considerations for the Use of Patient-Generated Health Data in the Electronic Medical Records. In *Challenges of Trustable AI and Added-Value on Health* (p. 229). IOS Press.

Bourke, A., Dixon, W. G., Roddam, A., Lin, K. J., Hall, G. C., Curtis, J. R., van der Veer, S. N., Soriano-Gabarró, M., Mills, J. K., & Major, J. M. (2020). Incorporating patient-generated health data into pharmacoepidemiological research. *Pharmacoepidemiology and Drug Safety*, *29*, 1540–1549. PMID: 33146896

Brown, R., Coventry, L., Sillence, E., Blythe, J., Stumpf, S., Bird, J., & Durrant, A. C. (2022). Collecting and sharing self-generated health and lifestyle data: Understanding barriers for people living with long-term health conditions—A survey study. *Digital Health*, *8*. PMID: 35284085

Carroll, J., Hopper, L., Farrelly, A. M., Lombard-Vance, R., Bamidis, P. D., & Konstantinidis, E. I. (2021). A scoping review of augmented/virtual reality health and wellbeing interventions for older adults: Redefining immersive virtual reality. *Frontiers in Virtual Reality*, *2*, 655338.

Cohen, D. J., Keller, S. R., Hayes, G. R., Dorr, D. A., Ash, J. S., & Sittig, D. F. (2016). Integrating patient-generated health data into clinical care settings or clinical decision-making: Lessons learned from project healthdesign. *JMIR Human Factors*, *3*, e5919. PMID: 27760726

Dinh-Le, C., Chuang, R., Chokshi, S., & Mann, D. (2019). Wearable health technology and electronic health record integration: Scoping review and future directions. *JMIR mHealth and uHealth, 7*, e12861. PMID: 31512582

El Amrani, L., Engberink, A. O., Ninot, G., Hayot, M., & Carbonnel, F. (2017). Connected health devices for health care in French general medicine practice: Cross-sectional study. *JMIR mHealth and uHealth, 5*, e7427. PMID: 29269336

Foster, C., Schinasi, D., Kan, K., Macy, M., Wheeler, D., & Curfman, A. (2022). Remote monitoring of patient-and family-generated health data in pediatrics. *Pediatrics, 149*, e2021054137. PMID: 35102417

Goharinejad, S., Goharinejad, S., Hajesmaeel-Gohari, S., & Bahaadinbeigy, K. (2022). The usefulness of virtual, augmented, and mixed reality technologies in the diagnosis and treatment of attention deficit hyperactivity disorder in children: An overview of relevant studies. *BMC Psychiatry, 22*, 1–13. PMID: 34983446

Guanais, F., Doubova, S. V., Leslie, H. H., Perez-Cuevas, R., Garcia-Elorrio, E., & Kruk, M. E. (2018). Patient-centered primary care and self-rated health in 6 Latin American and Caribbean countries: Analysis of a public opinion cross-sectional survey. *PLoS Medicine, 15*, e1002673. PMID: 30300422

Hu, V., Chen, E., Bridgeman, M., & Jariwala, S. (2022). Utility of Patient-Generated Health Data and Artificial Intelligence in the Prediction of Asthma Exacerbations. *The Journal of Allergy and Clinical Immunology, 149*, AB185.

Huang, Y., Upadhyay, U., Dhar, E., Kuo, L. J., & Syed-Abdul, S. (2022). A Scoping Review to Assess Adherence to and Clinical Outcomes of Wearable Devices in the Cancer Population. *Cancers (Basel), 14*, 4437. PMID: 36139602

Hull, S. (2015). Patient-generated health data foundation for personalized collaborative care. *CIN Comput. Inform. Nurs., 33*, 177–180. PMID: 25974360

Hunt, L. M., Bell, H. S., Baker, A. M., & Howard, H. A. (2017). Electronic health records and the disappearing patient. *Medical Anthropology Quarterly, 31*, 403–421. PMID: 28370246

Kashani, M. H., Madanipour, M., Nikravan, M., Asghari, P., & Mahdipour, E. (2021). A systematic review of IoT in healthcare: Applications, techniques, and trends. *Journal of Network and Computer Applications, 192*, 103164.

Khatiwada, P., & Yang, B. (2022). *An Overview on Security and Privacy of Data in IoMT Devices: Performance Metrics, Merits, Demerits, and Challenges*. pHealth.

Kim, K. K., Jalil, S., & Ngo, V. (2019). Improving self-management and care coordination with person-generated health data and mobile health. In *Consumer Informatics and Digital Health: Solutions for Health and Health Care* (pp. 221–243). Springer.

Korjian, S., & Gibson, C. M. (2022). Digital technologies and the democratization of clinical research: Social media, wearables, and artificial intelligence. *Contemporary Clinical Trials*, *117*, 106767. PMID: 35462032

Krist, A. H., Tong, S. T., Aycock, R. A., & Longo, D. R. (2017). Engaging patients in decision-making and behavior change to promote prevention. *Information Services & Use*, *37*, 105–122. PMID: 28972524

Kumar, A., & Deepak, G. (2020). HeTOnto: A Novel Approach for Conceptualization, Modeling, Visualization, and Formalization of Domain Centric Ontologies for Heat Transfer. *Proceedings of the CONECCT 2020—6th IEEE International Conference on Electronics, Computing and Communication Technologies*, 1–6.

Lavallee, D. C., Lee, J. R., Austin, E., Bloch, R., Lawrence, S. O., McCall, D., Munson, S. A., Nery-Hurwit, M. B., & Amtmann, D. (2020). mHealth and patient-generated health data: Stakeholder perspectives on opportunities and barriers for transforming healthcare. *mHealth*, *6*, 8. PMID: 32190619

Liu, L., Stroulia, E., Nikolaidis, I., Miguel-Cruz, A., & Rincon, A. R. (2016). Smart homes and home health monitoring technologies for older adults: A systematic review. *International Journal of Medical Informatics*, *91*, 44–59. PMID: 27185508

Magnan, S. (2021). Social determinants of health 201 for health care: Plan, do, study, act. NAM Perspect.

Martin, R. L., & Irrgang, J. J. (2007). A survey of self-reported outcome instruments for the foot and ankle. *The Journal of Orthopaedic and Sports Physical Therapy*, *37*, 72–84. PMID: 17366962

McGinnis, J. M., Olsen, L. A., Goolsby, W. A., & Grossmann, C. (2011). *Clinical Data as the Basic Staple of Health Learning: Creating and Protecting a Public Good: Workshop Summary*. National Academies Press.

Medina, S. G., & Isomursu, M. (2023). The Use of Patient-Generated Health Data From Consumer-Grade Mobile Devices in Clinical Workflows: Protocol for a Systematic Review. *JMIR Research Protocols*, *12*, e39389. PMID: 36848208

Melstrom, L. G., Rodin, A. S., Rossi, L. A., Fu, P.Jr, Fong, Y., & Sun, V. (2021). Patient-generated health data and electronic health record integration in oncologic surgery: A call for artificial intelligence and machine learning. *Journal of Surgical Oncology*, *123*, 52–60. PMID: 32974930

Mozzaquatro, B. A., Agostinho, C., Goncalves, D., Martins, J., & Jardim-Goncalves, R. (2018). An Ontology-Based Cybersecurity Framework for the Internet of Things. *Sensors (Basel), 18*, 3053. PMID: 30213085

Muhammad Sayem, A. S., Hon Teay, S., Shahariar, H., Luise Fink, P., & Albarbar, A. (2020). Review on smart electro-clothing systems (SeCSs). *Sensors (Basel), 20*, 587. PMID: 31973123

Nagpal, M. S., Barbaric, A., Sherifali, D., Morita, P. P., & Cafazzo, J. A. (2021). Patient-Generated Data Analytics of Health Behaviors of People Living With Type 2 Diabetes: Scoping Review. *JMIR Diabetes, 6*, e29027. PMID: 34783668

Neches, R., Fikes, R. E., Finin, T., Gruber, T., Patil, R., Senator, T., & Swartout, W. R. (1991). Enabling Technology for Knowledge Sharing. *AI Magazine, 12*, 36–56.

Noy, N. F., & McGuinness, D. L. (2001). *Ontology Development 101: A Guide to Creating Your First Ontology*. Stanford University.

Omoloja, A., & Vundavalli, S. (2021). Patient-generated health data: Benefits and challenges. *Current Problems in Pediatric and Adolescent Health Care, 51*, 101103. PMID: 34799255

Park, Y. R., Lee, Y., Kim, J. Y., Kim, J., Kim, H. R., Kim, Y. H., Kim, W. S., & Lee, J. H. (2018). Managing patient-generated health data through mobile personal health records: Analysis of usage data. *JMIR mHealth and uHealth, 6*, e9620. PMID: 29631989

Petersen, C. (2021). Use of patient-generated health data for shared decision-making in the clinical environment: Ready for prime time. *mHealth, 7*, 39. PMID: 34345616

Petersen, C., & DeMuro, P. (2015). Legal and regulatory considerations associated with use of patient-generated health data from social media and mobile health (mHealth) devices. *Applied Clinical Informatics, 6*, 16–26. PMID: 25848410

Pinto, H. S., & Martins, J. P. (2004). Ontologies: How can They be Built? *Knowledge and Information Systems, 6*, 441–464.

Rahi, P., Sood, S. P., Bajaj, R., & Kumar, Y. (2021). Air quality monitoring for Smart eHealth system using firefly optimization and support vector machine. *International Journal of Information Technology : an Official Journal of Bharati Vidyapeeth's Institute of Computer Applications and Management, 13*, 1847–1859.

Rudolph, S. (2011). Foundations of Description Logics. In. Lecture Notes in Computer Science: Vol. 6848. *Reasoning Web. Semantic Technologies for the Web of Data. Reasoning Web 2011*. Springer.

Schütz, A. E., Fertig, T., & Weber, K. (2021). Defining a Core Ontology for Medical Devices in Germany to Ensure Semantic Interoperability. In Simian, D., & Stoica, L. F. (Eds.), *Modelling and Development of Intelligent Systems. MDIS 2020. Communications in Computer and Information Science* (Vol. 1341). Springer.

Shi, Q., Yang, Y., Sun, Z., & Lee, C. (2022). Progress of advanced devices and internet of things systems as enabling technologies for smart homes and health care. *ACS Materials Au*, *2*, 394–435. PMID: 36855708

Subramanian, H. (2023). A Decentralized Marketplace for Patient-Generated Health Data: Design Science Approach. *Journal of Medical Internet Research*, *25*, e42743. PMID: 36848185

Szeredi, P., Lukácsy, G., & Benkő, T. (2014). *Description Logic. The Semantic Web Explained The Technology and Mathematics behind Web 3.0*. Cambridge University Press.

Tang, Z., Pei, S., Peng, X., Zhuang, F., Zhang, X., & Hoehndorf, R. (2022). TAR: Neural Logical Reasoning across TBox and ABox. arXiv:2205.14591.

Tiase, V. L., Hull, W., McFarland, M. M., Sward, K. A., Del Fiol, G., Staes, C., Weir, C., & Cummins, M. R. (2020). Patient-generated health data and electronic health record integration: A scoping review. *JAMIA Open*, *3*, 619–627. PMID: 33758798

Tricoli, A., Nasiri, N., & De, S. (2017). Wearable and miniaturized sensor technologies for personalized and preventive medicine. *Advanced Functional Materials*, *27*, 1605271.

Trifan, A., Oliveira, M., & Oliveira, J. L. (2019). Passive sensing of health outcomes through smartphones: Systematic review of current solutions and possible limitations. *JMIR mHealth and uHealth*, *7*, e12649. PMID: 31444874

Wilson, J., Heinsch, M., Betts, D., Booth, D., & Kay-Lambkin, F. (2021). Barriers and facilitators to the use of e-health by older adults: A scoping review. *BMC Public Health*, *21*, 1–12. PMID: 34399716

Wu, D. T., Xin, C., Bindhu, S., Xu, C., Sachdeva, J., Brown, J. L., & Jung, H. (2020). Clinician perspectives and design implications in using patient-generated health data to improve mental health practices: Mixed methods study. *JMIR Formative Research*, *4*, e18123. PMID: 32763884

Zeng, N., & Gao, Z. (2017). Health wearable devices and physical activity promotion. In *Technology in Physical Activity and Health Promotion* (pp. 148–164). Taylor & Francis.

Zhu, X., Liu, B., Zhu, C., Ding, Z., & Yao, L. (2023). Approximate Reasoning for Large-Scale ABox in OWL DL Based on Neural-Symbolic Learning. *Mathematics*, *11*, 495.

Chapter 14

Understanding Perceived Risks and Drivers of Health Technology Adoption From User and Physician Perspectives

Suphan Nasir
https://orcid.org/0000-0002-2302-334X
Istanbul University, Turkey

Yiğit Yurder
https://orcid.org/0000-0002-3064-374X
Istanbul University, Turkey

ABSTRACT

Health technologies have become essential tools for both users and healthcare professionals in modern healthcare systems. These innovations enable real-time health monitoring, fostering proactive and personalized care. For doctors, such devices enhance diagnostic accuracy and streamline patient management. Meanwhile, users benefit from increased awareness of their health status, leading to improved well-being and preventive behaviors. This study examines user and physician perceptions of wearable health devices and applications integrated with them. By assessing the perceptions of both users and professionals, the research contributes to an understanding of the key drivers of technology adoption. The findings reveal that while users rate the benefits of technology highly, they are concerned about privacy and data security. Physicians, on the other hand, have significant concerns about the

DOI: 10.4018/979-8-3373-1514-0.ch014

protection and sharing of data with third parties. The study highlights the need to reduce perceived risks and address users' security concerns for effective adoption of wearable health devices.

1. INTRODUCTION

Computer and mobile technologies are rapidly advancing and becoming indispensable in our daily lives. The increasing popularity of mobile technologies has given rise to wearable technologies. Health technology significantly influences and benefits various industries, including healthcare, military, fitness, and entertainment. Health technologies, or wearable devices, are electronic computers that can be worn on the body as either an accessory or an integral part of clothing. A wearable device that is seamlessly integrated into an individual's attire or personal accessories has the ability to store and process data, facilitating real-time data exchange between the network and the device.

As the wearables market transforms, the worldwide wearables market continued its upward trajectory. According to the International Data Corporation (IDC) Worldwide Quarterly Wearable Device Tracker, The wearables market began 2024 with a growth spurt as global shipments of wearable devices grew 8.8% year over year in the first quarter (1Q24) to 113.1 million units (IDC Worldwide Quarterly Wearables Tracker, June 4, 2024) and worldwide wearable device shipments are forecast to grow 6.1% year over year in 2024 to 537.9 million units. Smartwatches are expected to face an annual decline of 3% in 2024, but are projected to recover in 2025 with a growth of 4.8%. This decline may raise some concerns, but it is important to note that this is mainly due to the situation in India. India has been an important market for low-cost smartwatches in recent years. The smartwatch market in the country is flooded with many white label products and is expected to consolidate in the short term. Excluding India, the global smartwatch market is expected to grow by 9.9%. Moreover, average selling prices (ASPs) of smartwatches are projected to increase by 5.7% in 2024. (IDC Worldwide Quarterly Wearables Tracker, September 27, 2024).

There has also been a remarkable surge in the development of mobile health applications for users. Wearable health devices and mobile health apps are still at a nascent stage, yet they are pivotal in the realm of healthcare innovation. Most wearable technologies are utilized for monitoring health and fitness activities. Nowadays, smartphones are equipped with advanced sensors and processors capable of tracking movements and conducting medical measurements such as heart rate, calories burned, blood sugar, cholesterol, and more. Health and fitness mobile applications on our smartphones, in conjunction with wearable technologies, empower users to gather, store, and share nearly all types of health information. Mobile health applications not only facilitate the tracking of real-time health data but also provide reminders for medication times for those who need to take drugs regularly. Furthermore, mobile health applications that integrate with wearable technologies enable physicians to monitor their patients' health data around the clock from anywhere. Keeping track of patients' health information allows physicians to intervene early when necessary. In summary, wearable technologies like smartwatches, fitness bands, and health and fitness mobile applications enable both users and their physicians to monitor real-time health and fitness data. Additionally, the information collected is utilized for follow-up and treatment purposes by physicians.

There is a significant surge of interest in utilizing mobile health applications and wearable sensors for the purpose of remote health monitoring, as well as enhancing patient adherence to treatment guidelines. Numerous companies are creating products that capture and archive data regarding biological parameters (like blood pressure, weight, and glucose levels) and behaviors (including mobility and medication intake). This can assist healthcare providers in monitoring patients who have or are susceptible to severe health incidents. It is anticipated that mobile health applications and patient monitoring devices for health services will lead to improved healthcare outcomes and reduced costs.

As computer and mobile technologies continue to advance at a rapid pace, it is essential to grasp the dynamics of computer-human interaction. Given that users' acceptance, adoption, and intention to utilize wearable health products are anticipated to increase in the near future, this paper seeks to explore the views of both users and physicians regarding the utilization of mobile applications powered by advanced wearable technology in the health sector. To forecast, elucidate, and enhance user acceptance of cutting-edge health products, we must gain a deeper understanding of the reasons behind individuals' acceptance or rejection of these technologies. In order to comprehend users' acceptance, adoption, and intention to use these advanced health products, a model has been formulated by incorporating the Technology Acceptance Model (TAM).

2. LITERATURE REVIEW

Since implementation of information systems as well as development of new products especially technological products are costly, companies need to understand the factors that facilitate use of new technologies in order to be successful in launching new technological products. Thus in the literature there are attempts to group factors into a model to explain adoption of new technologies. Technology Acceptance Model (TAM) is proposed by Davis (1989) and Davis, Bagozzi and Warshaw (1989) to explain acceptance of technology behavior of users. TAM is based on the social psychology theories that are Theory of Reasoned Action (TRA) developed by Ajzen and Fishbein (1975) and Theory of Planned Behaviour (TPB) developed by Ajzen (1985).

Technology acceptance model, a commonly used model while analyzing the information technologies adoption context, applies the TRA and TPB to explain the acceptance and usage behaviour of technology (Davis 1989). TAM aims to *"provide an explanation of the determinants of technology acceptance that is general, capable of explaining usage behaviour across a broad range of systems or end-user computing technologies and user populations, while at the same time being both parsimonious and theoretically justified"* (Davis et al., 1989). TAM establishes a theory that a person's behavioural intention to accept a new technology is determined by the person's attitude toward the use of the technology. Two beliefs determine attitude: perceived ease of use and perceived usefulness thus the model theorises that perceived usefulness and perceived ease of use are the most necessary components in explaining technology acceptance. According to the TAM, these two variables determine individual's behavioural intention to adopt a technology, attitude toward using it, and actual use of the technology (see Figure 1) (Davis, Bagozzi and Warshaw, 1989).

Although TAM is a useful model, critical reviews of TAM suggest that significant factors are not included in the model (Legris et al, 2003). There are many attempts to extent the model in order to contribute the understanding user adoption behavior in the literature. Venkatesh and Davis (2000) develop and test a theoretical extension of the TAM that explains perceived usefulness and usage intentions in terms of social influence and cognitive instrumental processes and they referred the extended model as TAM2 (Venkatesh and Davis, 2000). Pavlou (2003) proposes to integrate the trust and risk with the TAM to understand the consumer acceptance of electronic commerce (Pavlou, 2003). There are attempts to extend TAM with integrating subjective norm (Schepers and Wetzels, 2007; Venkatesh and Morris, 2000), risk (Featherman and Pavlou, 2003; Crespo et al., 2009; Wu and Wang, 2005; Luo et al., 2010), trust (v et al., 2003; Ha and Stoel, 2009; Kesharwani and Singh, 2012), prior experience (Oh et al., 2003; Taylor and Todd, 1995), social influence (Malhotra and Galletta, 1999), flow theory (Koufaris, 2002; Lu et al., 2009), task-technology fit (Dishaw and Strong, 1999; Klopping and McKinney, 2004; Pagani, 2006), expectation confirmation model (Thong et al., 2006; Lee, 2010), compatibility (Wu and Wang, 2005; Vijavasarathy, 2004; Schaper and Pervan, 2007), self-efficacy (Mun and Hwang, 2003; Venkatesh and Davis, 1996; Venkatesh, 2000), intrinsic motivation (Venkatesh, 2000, Mun and Hwang, 2003; Lee and Cheung, 2005), goal orientation (Mun and Hwang, 2003), and uncertainty avoidance (Cardon and Marshall, 2008; Hwang, 2005; Hwang and Lee, 2012).

According to prior studies, TAM is used to determine the users' acceptance and usage intentions of various technologies like smartphones (Park and Chen, 2007), online banking technologies (Lee, 2009), online shopping (Ha and Stoel, 2009), wearable technologies (Chae, 2009; Turhan, 2012), e-health care systems (Holden and Karsh, 2010) and so on.

In summary, TAM adapts the belief, attitude, intention, behaviour relationship for adaptation of technological advances. The two factors perceived ease of use and perceived usefulness are cognitions regarding the innovation. While perceived usefulness is the individual's cognitive evaluation of the utility offered by the new technology, perceived ease of use is an indicator of the cognitive energy needed to be expended to use the innovation. Further, perceived usefulness is influenced by perceived ease of use because if the technology is easier to use, it is perceived to be more useful.

Figure 1. Technology Acceptance Model

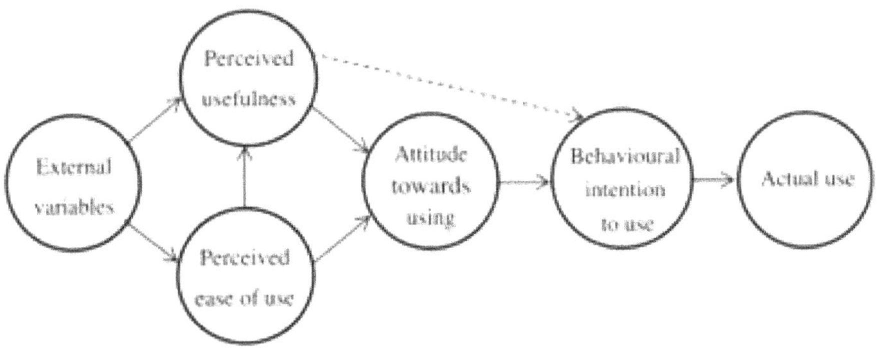

Finally, TAM has become one of the most influential behavioural models in information and communication technologies (ICT) studies. The most important strengths of TAM are associated with the consistency combined with its predictive power hence it makes easy to adjust to the various type of situations.

2.1. Perceived Usefulness

Researchers acknowledge that the beliefs of the individuals are the foundation for attitudes toward technology adoption (Brown and Venkatesh, 2005; Ajzen, 1991). Perceived usefulness is included by researchers as an individual belief that influences attitude and it is described as "*the prospective user's subjective probability that using a specific application system will increase his or her performance*" (Davis, 1989). Perceived usefulness is explained as the beliefs of individuals' that technology usage will improve the performance on the relative task (Taylor & Todd, 1995). Perceived usefulness has been accepted as the most influential and powerful factor for predicting technology usage intention and acceptance (Venkatesh et al., 2003; Featherman & Pavlou, 2003). The findings of major studies reveal the fact that perceived usefulness has positive influence on attitude towards using and intention to use technology (Davis, Bagozzi, & Warshaw, 1989; Mathieson, 1991; Taylor & Todd, 1995; Pikkarainen et al., 2004; Liao et al., 2007; Park & Chen, 2007). According to Davis (1989) perceived usefulness can be directly affected by an external variable such as relative advantage. If the adopted innovation will provide a relative advantage over the individuals who did not adopt the technology, the innovation will be perceived useful by the individual. Perceived usefulness generally measured by four factors: effectiveness, productivity, overall usefulness and performance of new technology (Legris et al., 2003).

2.2. Perceived Ease of Use

One of the most important factors in every individual's life is knowledge. Knowledge represents an individual's educational level, lifelong experiences and social information that the person imposed in daily life. Knowledge assumes critical role in the ease of use perception at various levels of technology acceptance. The challenging items of knowledge, such as learning and individual's perceived abilities, are the factors which determines the person's perception of ease of using a complex technology innovation (Martins & Kellermans, 2004; Gardner & Amoroso, 2004).

Perceived ease of use in TAM, is described as *"the degree to which a person believes that using a particular system would be free of effort"* (Davis, 1989). Davis (1989) identifies a person's educational level as an influential factor for technology acceptance. The educational level factor does not include the practical knowledge that is learned from social environment and life experiences. According to Davis, the level of new technology adoption influenced by not only educational level but also communication at the social life.

The social norm is affected by the perceived ease of use through the information that shared. The person may have the knowledge to perceive a technology to be easy to use but may not have the required abilities. Davis (1989) also posits that a new technology adopter observes and wants to try the use of innovations before decide to adopt or not to adopt. The person must have the new technology available in order to try using it and observe its operations. The technology availability is a major influential for the perception of ease of use.

Although intention to use is predicted by perceived usefulness, perceived ease of use is secondary and acts through perceived usefulness in TAM (Davis, Bagozzi, and Warshaw, 1989; Venkatesh and Davis, 2000). Keil, Beranek, and Konsynski

(1995) state that usefulness has more influence than ease of use in determining new technology adoption. More interestingly, some studies do not include perceived ease of use as a component of expected future adoption (Hu et al., 1999; Subramanian, 1994). Perceived ease of use is measured by six factors in the origin model, and these six factors are: easy to become skilful, easiness to learn, clarity, overall easiness to use, controllability, and flexibility of new technology (Davis, 1989).

Perceived usefulness and perceived ease of use were the main components in the original technology acceptance model. Previous studies which used TAM revealed that the individual's perceptions of usefulness and ease of use could be positive but some of them did not adopt technology innovations. Researchers described a third main perception factor which is affecting the decisions of adoption, named intent to use the technology (Davis, 1989; Lee, 2004).

2.3. Attitude Towards Using and Behavioral Intention to Use

Behavioural intention is a primary factor in TPB and continues as a component in TAM. Lin et al. (2006) states that subjective norms and behavioural attitudes effect the intention to use a technology as specified in TPB. Davis (1989) described intention to use as a part of adopters' personality. While innovators and early adopters have significantly strong intention to use, the laggards and the other late adopters tend to keep their intentions until more information about the innovation is accessible (Davis, 1989). Availability and accessibility of technology are main influents on a person's intention to accept the technology and also technology availability has effect on accessibility in terms of cost and time (Lee, 2004).

Attitude is conceptualised as the person's negative or positive feelings about adopting the new technology; on the other hand, behavioural intention refers the person's conscious thoughts to perform or not perform some specified future behaviour (Venkatesh and Davis, 2000). In other words, attitude explains the desire level to use a new technology of the individual (Lederer et al., 2000). In the literature the effect of behavioural beliefs such as perceived usefulness and perceived ease of use on technology adoption is determined the individuals' attitudes towards the technology, their intention to adopt the technology, and actual usage of the technology (Baron, Patterson, and Harris, 2006).

2.4. Perceived Risk

Perceived risk is generally feeling uncertainty regarding the probability of negative effects of using a service or product. In the early studies, It has been described as *"the expectation of losses associated with purchase and acts as an inhibitor to the purchase behaviour"* (Peter and Ryan, 1976) and *"a combination of uncertainty plus seriousness of outcome involved''* (Bauer, 1967). Perceived risk theory has been used to understand consumers' behaviour, and it is defined as a probability of loss when the desired result is pursued (Featherman and Pavlou, 2003). Early technology adoption literature about perceived risk enters the ICT adoption decision when the status of the decision create discomfort, anxiety and feelings of uncertainty (Dowling and Staelin, 1994), anxiety pain (Taylor, 1974) and cognitive dissonance (Germunden, 1985). The dissonance appears from the individual's evaluation of the service or product's risks, utility, benefits and costs. Potential increased technological performance efficiencies are the utility gains whereas problems related with performance are representing risks. On the other hand, other studies only focus on the potential advantages such as perceived ease of use and perceived usefulness that seem more important for the technology adoption. However, there are also potential losses that are attributable to technology adoption. Later, the technology adoption literature begins to include various risk facets within the technology acceptance model (Featherman and Pavlou, 2003; Pavlou, 2003; Wu and Wang, 2005; Lee, 2009; Luo et al., 2010). Featherman and Pavlou (2003) review the literature, and identify and describe various risk facets as following:

- Performance risk: *''The possibility of the product malfunctioning and not performing as it was designed and advertised and therefore failing to deliver the desired benefits.''* (Grewal et al., 1994)
- Time risk: Consumers may lose time when giving bad purchase decision by wasting time on research and making the purchase decision, learning how to use the new technology and finally replacing it if it does not meet the expectations of the user.
- Financial risk: *''The potential monetary outlay associated with the initial purchase price as well as the subsequent maintenance cost of the product''* (Grewal et al., 1994). After the study of Grewal et al. more current studies about financial services expand the context by including the potential financial losses related to fraud.
- Psychological risk: The risk that the product's performance and selection may have a negative effect on the individual's self-perception or peace of mind. The potential loss of ego because of the frustration of not accomplishing the buying goal.
- Social risk: Possibility of losing status in a social group due to purchasing a product or service which seem foolish or untrendy.
- Privacy risk: Possibility of losing control over personal private information, like when the information about the individual is used without his or her permission or knowledge. The worst case is where the consumer's identity is used to perform fraud transactions.

– Physical risk (safety): the probability of the adopted product's threat to human life
– Overall risk: Perceived risk when the individual evaluates all the criteria together.

In addition to the perceived ease of use, perceived usefulness and compatibility variables, perceived risk facets have to be included into TAM. Privacy, performance, psychological and physical risk dimensions are important components that have to be considered while analyzing wearable technology acceptance and intention to use wearable technologies.

2.5. Compatibility

The initial characterization of compatibility, as outlined by Rogers (1995), states that "compatibility is the extent to which an innovation is seen as aligning with the established values, previous experiences, and requirements of prospective adopters." Compatibility has been examined as a factor in the adoption of innovations and has been employed as an independent variable that influences other factors (Karahanna et al., 2006; Lee, 2004; Wu & Wu, 2005). An innovation or technology may either align or conflict with societal norms, previously acquired knowledge, or consumer demands (Rogers, 1995). Compatibility plays a crucial role in shaping the decisions made by users regarding technology acceptance (Rogers, 1995; Taylor & Todd, 1995; Chau & Hu, 2001). According to Chau and Hu (2001), compatibility appears to significantly affect perceived usefulness but does not impact perceived ease of use. As previously mentioned, the perceived relative advantage strongly influences how compatible the innovation is with an individual's lifestyle and environment, which in turn enhances the intention to adopt the innovation (Wu & Wu, 2005; Karahanna et al., 2006).Karahanna et al. categorized compatibility into two forms: cognitive compatibility and operational compatibility. Cognitive compatibility is described in line with Rogers' (1995) assertion that past experiences shape technology acceptance decisions. Conversely, operational compatibility emphasizes the perceived value of the new technology in achieving the individual's goals. Clearly, compatibility plays a vital role in shaping users' intentions and attitudes toward the adoption and utilization of technology.

2.6. Health Technologies and TAM

The researches about health care technologies usually focuses on technology design and implementing the technology on existing system (Holden and Karsh, 2010), however these researches fall short on explaining the end users' adaptation to use these health care technologies. After the development of the TAM, it was applied to health care researches to predict and explain the end users' reactions to the health care technologies. Nevertheless, the generic form of TAM is not a model specifically designed for healthcare technologies. Healthcare technologies focuses on supporting and improving physicians' patient care. Most of the previous health care technology researches have focused on physicians' technology acceptance (Allen et al., 1995; Gschwendter et al., 1997; Malringer et al., 1996; Malringer et al., 1998; Mitchell et al., 1996). These researches focused many different healthcare technologies; spoken dialog technology helping to get notes during endoscopic examinations (Barker et al., 2003), telemedicine technology (Hu et al., 1999; Chau and Hu, 2001; Chau and Hu, 2002), internet-based health applications (Chismar and Wiley-patton, 2002), radiology picture archiving and communication system (Duyck et al., 2008), mobile medicine information system (Nadal et al., 2020; Han et al., 2005), online evaluation system for patient assessment (Horan et al., 2004), internet-based e-medical records (Liu and Ma, 2006; Liu and Ma, 2012), electronic nursing care plans (Rawstorne et al., 2000), mobile healthcare systems (Wu et al., 2007), health information technology (Rahimi et al., 2018; Ahlan and Ahmad, 2014; Melas et al., 2011; Pai and Huang, 2011), e-health for ambulatory care (Dünnebeil et al., 2012), wearable health technologies(Talukder et al., 2020; Meier et al., 2020; Ahmad et al., 2020), digital transformation in healthcare (Stoumpos et al., 2023), privacy concerns (Dhagarra et al., 2020) information and communication technology (Schaper and Pervan, 2007; Yarbrough and Smith, 2007). However earlier investigations of user acceptance of healthcare technologies had small sample sizes on physician side. Therefore, technology acceptance and healthcare technologies integration need to be represented in reliable way.

Wearable health technology is a cutting edge in the technology industry, moreover, due to the general public's low acceptance to the original wearable technology models, there has been limited empirical researches that analyses the users' attitudes, purchase intentions and adoption of wearable technologies. Jung, Kim and Choi (2016) explored how much potential consumers value various smart watch attributes by examining brand, price, communication, shape and size perceptions. According to study shape and communication are more critical factors influencing the consumers. Ko, Sung, & Yun (2009) examined the effects of benefits and perceived risks on purchase intentions and attitudes for wearable technologies like smart shoes and jacket. The study also shows that attitude towards purchase intention is influenced positively by compatibility and is influenced negatively by technologies' perceived complexity. On the other hand, Turhan (2012), Nasir and Yurder(2015) used technology acceptance model and theory of planned behavior in the context of wearable technologies adoption. In Turhan's study, smart bra and t-shirt products are used for the research. The findings of the study show that perceived usefulness has a mediate influence on purchase intention through its effect on attitude. Park and Chen (2007) claims the fact that while the perceived usefulness increases, individual's attitude toward adopting the wearable technology increases, and this will positively influence their intention to use. In another research, Chae (2009) used extended technology acceptance model in the context of wearable technologies. Chae also confirmed that perceived usefulness is the most important variable that positively influences individuals' attitudes towards wearable technologies adoption. Lunney, Cunnigham and Eastin (2016), examines the wearable fitness technology adoption by using TAM. Chuah et al.'s(2016) study also reveals that perceived usefulness and visibility are important factors that drive adoption intention and suggest that smart watches represent a type of fashion. Thus, in wearable technology adoption, perceived usefulness is described as how much individuals believe the new technology can be the part of their daily life.

3. METHODOLOGY

As wearable health devices continue to gain prominence in the realm of health technology, it is anticipated that users' acceptance, adoption, and intention to utilize wearable health products will increase in the forthcoming future. Mobile health applications are projected to emerge as one of the most lucrative applications. The purpose of this paper is to uncover the motivations influencing the decision to adopt mobile health applications that are compatible with wearable technologies. This study aims to provide a more profound understanding of the motivations that guide individuals in their choice to embrace advanced wearable health technologies by utilizing the Technology Acceptance Model (TAM) as the foundational framework. Furthermore, this paper will examine whether there is a disparity between the perceptions of users and healthcare professionals regarding mobile health applications that integrate with wearable technologies. To gain insights into the acceptance, adoption, and intention to use these advanced health products among both users and physicians, a measurement scale has been developed by incorporating the Technology Acceptance Model (TAM). This study posits that an individual's intention to utilize wearable health devices is primarily influenced by perceived usefulness, perceived risk, and perceived compatibility.

Although numerous previous studies have concentrated on the factors that influence the adoption of wearable health technologies, there is a scarcity of empirical research that concurrently examines both the enabling factors (positive influences) and resistance factors (negative influences) that facilitate users and physicians in embracing advanced wearable health products. This paper investigates and synthesizes the various aspects of perceived usefulness of advanced wearable health products to delineate enabling factors. Additionally, drawing from perceived risk theory, three specific dimensions of risk—physical (safety), security/privacy, and performance—are incorporated with the technology acceptance model to identify the resistance factors affecting users' and physicians' intentions to utilize advanced wearable health products.

In this study, "Voice of Body" was presented, a hypothetical scenario of a health application and wearable technology integrated with wearable health technologies. This application, which works with wearable devices like smartwatches or another device that can be worn, continuously collects users' health data and transmits this information to healthcare professionals at regular intervals. The application monitors users' health data such as heart rate, physical activity level, sleep patterns, etc. and presents this information to physicians through an interface, thus facilitating health management. In our research, a survey was conducted to assess the perceptions of both physicians and users about this system.

The survey was designed to measure users' and healthcare professionals' views on wearable technologies, perceived usefulness, perceived risk, compatibility, and intention to use. The survey was conducted with 417 physicians and 373 users across Turkey and analyzed to reveal the differences in perceptions between different variables for both groups. Respondents' agreement to the statements was measured on a seven-point Likert scales, ranging from ''disagree strongly" (1) to ''agree strongly" (7). The data obtained were evaluated using statistical analysis methods and the differences in perceptions between the two groups were analyzed with t-tests. In this way, it was determined what differences the "Voice of Body" application created in the perceptions of users and physicians regarding health data.

The questionnaire is divided into two sections. The first section collects fundamental data regarding the characteristics of the respondents, including gender, age, education, occupation, and experience with high-tech wearable products. The second section of the questionnaire is designed around the constructs of perceived usefulness, perceived risk, and intention to use. The perceived usefulness scale is tailored to highlight the advantages of high-tech wearable technologies, drawing from the measurements established by Davis (1989), Taylor and Todd (1995), Venkatesh and Davis (2000), Venkatesh et al. (2003), and Cocosila et al. (2009). This scale for perceived usefulness includes ten items. Additionally, scales for performance risk, security/privacy risk, and physical risk are created to address the specific dangers associated with using high-tech wearable technologies. The perceived risk scale comprises six items, which are adapted from the work of Featherman and Pavlou (2003), Flavian and Guinaliu (2006), Lim (2003), and Laroche et al. (2004). Finally, the scales measuring attitude toward using and behavioral intention to use high-tech wearable technologies consist of six items, adapted from Davis (1989), Taylor and Todd (1995), Moore and Benbasat (1991), and Pae and Huyun (2002).

4. FINDINGS

Among users, the number of female participants was 199 (53,4%), while that of male participants was 174 (46,6%). The user participants' age range is mostly between 18-44 (80,3%). With respect to education, 355 (95,4%) participants were "4-year college graduate or above". 95% of the participants were smart phone owners and descriptive statistics indicated that 160 (43,8%) of the participants had healthcare applications on their phones while 74 (19,7%) of them had chronic health problems. On the other hand, the descriptive statistics of the physicians shows that 305 (73,5%) of the participants were specialist and 344 (82,7%) participants were between 25-54 age range.

4.1 Reliability

The reliability statistics obtained from the Table 1. show that the scales used for both users and physicians have a high level of reliability. Among users, variables such as perceived usefulness (Cronbach's Alpha = 0.961) and compatibility (Cronbach's Alpha = 0.926) show excellent reliability, while perceived risk (Cronbach's Alpha = 0.756) and intention to use (Cronbach's Alpha = 0.915) also show high reliability. For physicians, perceived usefulness (Cronbach's Alpha = 0.960) and compatibility (Cronbach's Alpha = 0.911) variables similarly show high reliability. The perceived risk (Cronbach's Alpha = 0.766) variable also achieves an acceptable level of reliability among physicians. Overall, these results support the validity and reliability of the scales measuring the perceptions of both groups, increasing the potential of the study to provide reliable findings. The cronbach's alpha values were found to be above the threshold of 0.70 (Table 1.), as remarked by Nunnaly and Bernstein (1994).

Table 1. Reliability Statistics

	Reliability Statistics	
Users	**Cronbach's Alpha**	**Item Number**
Perceived Usefulness	,961	10
Perceived Risk	,756	7
Intention to use	,915	6
Physicians		
Perceived Usefulness	,960	10

continued on following page

Table 1. Continued

	Reliability Statistics	
Users	**Cronbach's Alpha**	**Item Number**
Perceived Risk	,766	7
Intention to use	,911	6

4.2 Perceived Usefulness

The results obtained from the Table 2. reflect the views of the participants and physicians on the perceived usefulness of the "Voice of Body" (VOB) application. When the data obtained from a total of 373 participants for all variables are analyzed, it is seen that the participants expressed the idea that VOB helps them lead a healthy and active life with an average score of 5.04.

With an average score of 5.32, the participants evaluated that VOB makes exercising more conscious and healthier by monitoring health data. The perception that the application increases performance and efficiency is supported with an average score of 5.00. In particular, the opinion that VOB improves the quality of life of individuals with chronic diseases stands out with an average score of 5.07.

The score indicating that individuals think that they have become healthier by monitoring their biometric data is 5.13. Moreover, the importance of VOB for providing daily biometric data checks and timely reminders of medication use reached the highest level with a mean score of 5.54. The perception that VOB saves lives by providing early warnings of health anomalies is noteworthy with a mean score of 5.30. Participants evaluated the convenience provided by VOB with a score of 5.39.

Table 2. Usefulness perception of physicians and users

	Physicians			Users		
Perceived Usefulness	**N**	**Mean**	**Std. Deviation**	**N**	**Mean**	**Std. Deviation**
VOB helps to live in healthy and active way.	417	4.92	1.58	373	5.04	1.59
VOB helps to make exercise consciously and in a healthy way by tracking health data.	417	5.37	1.45	373	5.32	1.53
VOB improves performance and effectiveness.	417	4.91	1.57	373	5.00	1.56
VOB improves the life quality of people especially who has chronic illnesses.	417	4.84	1.55	373	5.07	1.64
VOB helps people become more healthy by monitoring biometric data.	417	4.93	1.56	373	5.13	1.61
VOB ensures daily biometric data control and medicine usage on time.	417	5.49	1.43	373	5.54	1.53

continued on following page

Table 2. Continued

Perceived Usefulness	Physicians			Users		
	N	Mean	Std. Deviation	N	Mean	Std. Deviation
VOB saves lives by providing early warning about abnormalities in health.	417	5.12	1.63	373	5.30	1.65
VOB is useful	417	5.25	1.52	373	5.46	1.55
VOB provides convenience	417	5.22	1.55	373	5.39	1.59
Using VOB is important	417	4.52	1.59	373	4.30	1.70

Finally, the statement "Using VoB is important" was answered by the participants with a mean score of 4.30, indicating a lower perception of the importance of VoB. Overall, these results suggest that respondents highly rated the positive health effects of VoB and emphasized the importance of its benefits.

On the other hand, the views of the physicians on the perceived usefulness of the VoB. When the data obtained from 417 physicians were analyzed, the perception that VoB helps them lead a healthy and active life was expressed with an average score of 4.92. This score indicates that the participants generally have a positive view on the effect of VoB in supporting a healthy life. The perception that VOB helps them monitor their health data and exercise in a conscious and healthy way was emphasized with a mean score of 5.37. Physicians support the perception that VOB improves performance and efficiency with a mean score of 4.91. In addition, the opinion that VOB improves the quality of life of individuals with chronic diseases is noteworthy with a mean score of 4.84.

Respondents indicated that VoB helps people become healthier by tracking biometric data with a mean score of 4.93. The importance of VoB in providing daily biometric data checks and timely reminders of medication use was the highest rated element with a mean score of 5.49. Furthermore, the perception of VoB's potential to save lives by providing early warnings of health anomalies was supported with a mean score of 5.12. Physicians also indicated that VoB is generally useful with a mean score of 5.25, while its convenience was rated with a mean score of 5.22. Finally, the statement "It is important to use VoB" was answered by the respondents with an average score of 4.52, indicating a lower perception of the importance of VoB. Overall, these results suggest that respondents highly rated the positive health effects of VoB and valued the benefits of the app.

Finally, according to normality tests its seen that the data does not distributed normally. Because of non-normal distribution, Mann Whitney U test was used to analyse the differences between physicians' and users' perceptions. Mann Whitney U test indicates that 3 items of perceived usefulness differ significantly between two groups. *Improving life quality of people who has chronic illness* (p= 0,023), *helping people become healthier by monitoring data* (p=0,041) and *VOB is useful* (p=0,024) statements differ significantly between physicians and users.

4.3 Perceived Risk

The data obtained from the Table 3. reflects the perceived risk levels of users and physicians regarding the "Voice of Body" (VoB) application. Analyzing the data obtained from 373 participants in total, the participants' perception of the reliability of the health data provided by VoB remains at a relatively low level with an average score of 3.84. This indicates that users have some uncertainties about the accuracy and reliability of the data provided by VoB. Concerns about VoB's performance were expressed with an average score of 4.02. Participants are concerned that the application may not work as expected. The perception that VoB may share personal information with third parties shows the highest perception of risk with a mean score of 4.96. This high score reveals that users' privacy concerns are an important factor.

Furthermore, the perception that VoB may not protect the confidentiality of private information was identified with a mean score of 4.74. Participants were also concerned that the app may use their personal health data without permission, with a mean score of 4.39. The perception that carrying VOB on the body is dangerous and risky in terms of health remains at a lower level with an average score of 3.72.

Finally, the perception that the use of VoB can cause anxiety and tension was rated by the participants with a mean score of 4.06. This reflects the emotional burden and uncertainty that users feel when using the app. Overall, these results suggest that users have various risk perceptions of the VoB app and are particularly concerned about data security and privacy. These findings reveal important factors that may influence the adoption of the app by users.

Table 3. Perceived risk of physicians and users

	Physicians			Users		
Perceived Risk	**N**	**Mean**	**Std. Deviation**	**N**	**Mean**	**Std. Deviation**
VOB provides reliable health data	417	4,06	1,46	373	3,84	1,45
VOB might not perform well and properly	417	4,33	1,64	373	4,02	1,61
VOB may share personal information to third parties (e.g. insurance and medicine companies)	417	5,36	1,70	373	4,96	1,88
VOB can not protect the confidentiality of private information	417	5,18	1,77	373	4,74	1,82
VOB can use personal health data without permission	417	4,34	2,28	373	4,39	2,10
Carrying VOB on body is dangerous and risky for health	417	3,42	1,59	373	3,72	1,69
Using VOB creates anxiety and tension	417	4,42	1,70	373	4,06	1,76

It also shows the perceived risk levels of physicians regarding the VoB. According to the data, reliability of the health data provided by VOB was determined with a mean score of 4.06. This result indicates that physicians have some uncertainty about the accuracy of the data provided by the application. Concerns about the performance of VOB were expressed with an average score of 4.33. Physicians are concerned that the app may not live up to expectations. Moreover, the perception that VOB may share personal information with third parties shows the highest risk perception among physicians with a mean score of 5.36. This high score emphasizes the sensitivity of healthcare professionals regarding privacy and data security.

The perception that VOB cannot protect the confidentiality of private information stands out with an average score of 5.18. Physicians are more concerned that the app may use their patients' data without permission. This risk perception is associated with the ethical responsibilities of healthcare professionals and their sensitivity to patients' privacy.

The perception that carrying VoB on the body is dangerous and risky for health remains at a lower level among physicians with a mean score of 3.42. This suggests that physicians are less concerned about the effects of the practice on physical health. Finally, the perception that the use of VoB can cause anxiety and tension was rated by physicians with a mean score of 4.42. This reflects the emotional burden and stressors that physicians feel when using the tech. Overall, these results suggest that physicians have various risk perceptions of the VoB app and are particularly concerned about data security and privacy. These findings highlight important factors that may influence the adoption and use of the tech by healthcare professionals.

For the perceived risk items, Mann Whitney U test indicates that 6 items of the variable differ significantly between physicians and users. VOB provides reliable health data (p=0,001), VOB might not perform well and properly (p=0,032), VOB may share personal information to third parties (p=0,006), VOB can't protect the confidentiality of private information (p=0,001), carrying VOB on body is dangerous and risky for health (p=0,008) and using VOB creates anxiety and tension (p=0,009) items differ significantly between physicians and users.

Physicians' perception of the risks associated with wearable health technologies is higher than users' perception of the risks associated with wearable health technologies. Physicians' "physical risk perception" related to wearable health technologies is that the collected health information can be shared with third parties (privacy risk), the confidentiality of private information cannot be protected (privacy risk), and that it can cause anxiety and tension (psychological risk), Although physicians' perception of "performance risk" related to wearable health technologies is not as intense as "privacy risk perception", it is higher compared to users' perception of "performance risk".

4.4 Intention to Use

As seen on Table 4., respondents gave an average score of 4.30 to the statement "Buying VoB is a smart idea". This sows that, in general, users evaluate the benefits of the VoB and find this technology sensible. However, the mean score for the statement "I intend to purchase and use VoB in the near future" was 3.28. This result suggests that users are hesitant to purchase VoB immediately and perhaps need more information. Users' response to the statement "I would like to use VoB for trial purposes" is indicative of a very high evaluation with a mean score of 4.87. This shows that users are willing to try VoB to see its functionality and benefits. The mean score for the statement "I will use VoB in the future" is 4.68, which reflects users' willingness to use this technology in the future.

Table 4. Usage intention of users and physicians

	Physicians			Users		
Usage Intention	**N**	**Mean**	**Std. Deviation**	**N**	**Mean**	**Std. Deviation**
Buying VOB is a wise idea.	373	4,30	1,46	417	3,99	1,44
Have intention to buy and use VOB in the near future	373	3,28	1,77	417	2,97	1,71
Want to use VOB on a trial basis to see how it works	373	4,87	1,83	417	4,82	1,82
Will use VOB in the future	373	4,68	1,64	417	4,55	1,55
Many people will use VOB in the future	373	5,06	1,51	417	4,93	1,49
It is worth to buy VOB technologies	373	4,41	1,63	417	4,28	1,55

Moreover, the statement "Many people will use VoB in the future" has one of the highest values with a mean score of 5.06. This indicates that users have a positive belief that VoB will reach a large user base in the future. Finally, the response to the statement "It is worthwhile to buy VoB technologies" is evaluated with a mean score of 4.41, suggesting that users consider the cost of VoB benefits and think that it makes sense to invest in these technologies.

Table 4. also pictures the usage intentions of physicians. For the statement "Buying VoB is a smart idea", physicians gave an average score of 3.99. This indicates that while physicians generally recognize the benefits of VoB, they have some uncertainty about the value of the application.

However, the mean score for the statement "I intend to purchase and use VoB in the near future" was 2.97. This low score suggests that physicians are undecided about purchasing VOB immediately and need more information or experience in this regard. The response to the statement "I would like to use VOB for trial purposes" is indicative of a very high evaluation with a mean score of 4.82. This shows that physicians are willing to try VOB to see its functionality and benefits. The mean for the statement "I will use VOB in the future" is 4.55, which reflects the willingness of physicians to use this technology in the future.

Also, the statement "Many people will use VoB in the future" stands out with a mean score of 4.93. This indicates that physicians have a positive belief that VoB will reach a large user base in the future. Finally, the response to the statement "It is valuable to buy VoB technologies" is evaluated with an average score of 4.28. This result reveals that physicians consider the cost of the benefits offered by VoB and think that it makes sense to invest in these technologies.

For the usage intention items, Mann Whitney U test indicates that 2 items of the variable differ significantly between physicians and users. *Buying VOB is a wise idea* (p=0,004) and *have intention to buy and use VOB in the near future* (p=0,013) items differ significantly between physicians and users.

4.5 Cluster Analysis

In this study, cluster analysis was conducted to better understand the perceptions and attitudes of both physicians and users towards VOB technology. This analysis, based on key variables such as perceived usefulness, perceived risk, intention to use and compatibility of the technology, divided both groups into subgroups with different characteristics and tendencies. Through this method, the similarities and differences in physicians' and patients' perspectives on technology were analyzed in detail and appropriate strategic recommendations were developed for these groups. The results of the analysis show how health technologies receive different reactions according to user profiles and provide important clues to facilitate the adoption process.

Table 5. Cluster Analysis (Physicians)

	Cluster		
	1	**2**	**3**
Perceived Usefulness	6,07	3,18	4,89
Perceived Risk	4,33	3,56	5,06
Intention to Use	5,33	2,75	3,55
Distances between Final Cluster Centers			
Cluster	1	2	3
1		3,951	2,255
2	3,951		2,409
3	2,255	2,409	

Table 6. Analysis of usefulness vs. risk

Anova						
	Cluster		Error			
	Mean Square	df	Mean Square	df	F	Sig.
Perceived Usefulness	239,190	2	0,572	401	418,425	0,000
Peceived Risk	56,739	2	0,858	401	66,148	0,000
Intention to Use	234,376	2	0,638	401	367,292	0,000

Physicians' Cluster 1: High Engagement Group

Physicians in this group strongly see the positive impacts of VOB technology on healthcare. Perceived benefit (6.07) and intention to use (5.33) are quite high. The potential benefits of the technology outweigh concerns about the risks, although there is a moderate perceived risk (4.33).

This group consists of professionals who are open to innovation and believe that technology can improve patient care processes. They are attracted by the increased efficiency and performance that VOB can provide, while minor concerns about risks do not prevent them from adopting the technology. These physicians can support solutions to improve quality of life, especially for chronically ill patients. For this group, additional features can be offered to increase the benefits of the technology and incentives can be provided to improve the user experience. The loyalty of this group can be increased with trainings or special content for advanced use of VOB technology.

Physicians' Cluster 2: Low Engagement Group

Physicians in this group find it difficult to believe in the benefits of VOB technology. Perceived benefit (3.18) and intention to use (2.75) are the lowest. Although the perceived risk (3.56) is lower than the other groups, this does not help them to adopt the technology.

This group consists of physicians who do not find technology meaningful for healthcare or see its applications as limited. The low perceived benefits are a clear indication of their apathy. Therefore, it is important to clearly emphasize the benefits of technology in communication strategies targeting this group. The tangible health benefits of technology should be more clearly demonstrated and user-friendly experiences offered. Free trial opportunities or low-cost entry options can attract this group.

Physicians' Cluster 3: Balanced Skeptics

Physicians in this group perceive the benefits (4.89) and intention to use (3.55) of the VOB technology at a moderate level. However, their perceived risk level (5.06) is quite high. They have serious concerns about data security, privacy and reliability of the technology.

This group consists of Physicians who carefully consider both the potential benefits and risks of technology. Although they have a balanced approach, their high perception of risk limits their adoption of the technology. Providing clear information and solutions regarding security and privacy to address the concerns of this group in particular could increase adoption. Data privacy and reliability guarantees should be emphasized to reduce the security concerns of this group. Their trust in technology can be increased by offering customized information and support services.

Table 7. Cluster Analysis (Users)

	Cluster		
	1	**2**	**3**
Perceived Usefulness	6,31	5,23	3,22
Perceived Risk	4,30	4,59	3,78
Intention to Use	5,67	4,23	2,35
Compatibility	5,44	3,32	1,70
Distances between Final Cluster Centers			
Cluster	1	2	3
1		2,800	5,897
2	2,800		3,290
3	5,897	3,290	

Table 8. Perceived usefulness vs. risk

Anova						
	Cluster		**Error**			
	Mean Square	**df**	**Mean Square**	**df**	**F**	**Sig.**
Perceived Usefulness	227,444	2	0,672	362	338,227	0,000
Perceived Risk	16,358	2	1,144	362	14,302	0,000
Intention to Use	266,301	2	0,505	362	527,620	0,000
Compatibility	363,396	2	0,780	362	466,030	0,000

User (Patient) Cluster 1: Strong Intention to Use

Perceived Usefulness (6.31): In this cluster, the benefits of VOB such as health monitoring, improving quality of life and providing convenience are perceived quite high. Users think that VOB meets their needs.

Compatibility (5.44): The level of compliance is quite high. This cluster is likely to consist of individuals who have chronic health problems or who need to track their health data regularly. VoB seems to be suitable for the lifestyle and needs of these individuals.

Perceived Risk (4.30): There is a medium level of risk perception. Although issues such as security concerns and sharing personal health data are important, these individuals think that the perception of benefit and compatibility overrides these concerns.

Intention to Use (5.67): Intention to use is quite high. It is clear that VOB technology offers a meaningful solution for these users.

This group consists of individuals who care about health monitoring and improving quality of life, perceive the technology positively and have a strong desire to use it. This group has the highest potential as a target audience. This group of innovative and health-monitoring-sensitive individuals should be the primary target of the marketing strategy. Messages that further emphasize product benefits can be used.

User (Patient) Cluster 2: Medium Usefulness - Undecided Users

Perceived Usefulness (5.23): Perception of usefulness is moderate. This group recognizes some of the benefits of VOB, but is not fully convinced about the impact of the technology.

Compatibility (3.32): Perception of compatibility is low to moderate. It can be assumed that these individuals do not have a chronic health problem or do not need to track their health data regularly. It is felt that VOB is not fully compatible with their lifestyle.

Perceived Risk (4.59): Risk perceptions are high. Security concerns and protection of personal data are a determining factor in this group's reservations towards VOB.

Intention to Use (4.23): Intention to use is low to medium. This group can be convinced if risks are reduced and benefits are better explained.

This group can be defined as undecided users. This group consists of individuals who are open to health technologies but need to be convinced. More information on risk management and compliance issues will be critical to win this group over. Campaigns can be designed for this group with reassuring content that increases risk management and compliance.

User (Patient) Cluster 3: Low Usefulness and Compatibility - Rejecting Users

Perceived Usefulness (3.22): Perception of usefulness is low. This group does not find the benefits offered by VOB meaningful and has a negative view of the technology.

Compatibility (1.70): Perception of compatibility is very low. These individuals do not have chronic health problems or do not feel a need to monitor their health data. VOB is not seen as compatible with their needs.

Perceived Risk (3.78): Perceptions of risk are the highest. This group considers security and privacy concerns very important and these concerns greatly influence their usage decisions.

Intention to Use (2.35): Intention to use is quite low. These individuals are almost completely reluctant to purchase or try VOB.

This group consists of individuals who have a negative view of health technologies and believe that the risks outweigh the benefits. Rather than focusing on this group, it would be more effective to invest in the other two groups. A group that is distant from technology and does not feel the need. Instead of spending resources to target this group, it would be more effective to target other groups better.

5. CONCLUSION

This study aims to examine user and physician perceptions of wearable health technologies and their integrated mobile applications. The findings reflect both users' and physicians' perceptions of the health applications and wearable health tech, contributing to an understanding of the key drivers of adoption of these technologies. Participants' perceptions highlight the benefits of tech in terms of monitoring and managing health data, but also reveal concerns about privacy and data security.

Users highly rated the benefits of VOB for health management. However, low scores on intention to use indicate that users are hesitant to make an immediate purchase. This reveals that there is a lack of knowledge and a need to increase awareness in the adoption of wearable health technologies. In particular, education and information activities are important to positively influence users' perceptions of the technology.

Assessments from the physicians' perspective show that there are more significant concerns about privacy and security issues. In particular, concerns about sharing personal health data with third parties and maintaining confidentiality may negatively affect physicians' intention to use VOB. These findings emphasize the importance of security and privacy in the adoption of technology by healthcare professionals, and also highlight the ethical dimension of technology use in healthcare.

The results of the cluster analysis revealed that there are different user profiles among both doctors and patients in terms of perceptions, risk assessments and usage intentions towards the VOB technology. The analysis showed that users' propensity to adopt the technology varies significantly according to perceived usefulness and risk levels. In particular, high perceived usefulness and low perceived risk resulted in a strong intention to use, while a distant approach towards the technology was observed in groups with high perceived risk. These results highlight the importance of user-centered strategies to ensure wider adoption of health technologies and provide guidance for technology developers to develop customized communication and trust-building policies for different target audiences.

In conclusion, wearable health technologies offer important opportunities for both users and healthcare professionals. However, for effective adoption of these technologies, perceived risks need to be reduced and users' safety concerns need to be addressed. In addition to the benefits offered by mobile health applications, it is important to consider the psychological effects of these applications on users.

Future research should examine the impact of wearable health technologies on users in more depth. In particular, investigating differences in perceptions between different demographic groups, social norms and cultural factors influencing technology adoption are important topics to be emphasized. Furthermore, studies on long-term user experiences and their impact on health outcomes can provide valuable insights into technology development processes. Finally, the development of comprehensive strategies that address users' safety concerns will increase the adoption of health technologies.

REFERENCES

Ahlan, A. R., & Ahmad, B. I. E. (2014). User acceptance of health information technology (HIT) in developing countries: A conceptual model. *Procedia Technology, 16*, 1287–1296.

Ahmad, A., Rasul, T., Yousaf, A., & Zaman, U. (2020). Understanding factors influencing elderly diabetic patients' continuance intention to use digital health wearables: Extending the technology acceptance model (TAM). *Journal of Open Innovation, 6*(3), 81.

Ajzen, I. (1991). The theory of planned behavior. *Organizational Behavior and Human Decision Processes, 50*, 179–211.

Ajzen, M. & Fishbein, M. (1975). Belief, attitude, intention and behavior: An introduction to theory and research. Academic Press.

Allen, A., Hayes, J., Sadasivan, R., & Williamson, S.K., & Wittman, C. (1995). A pilot study of the physician acceptance of teleoncology. *Journal of Telemedicine and Telecare, 1*(1), 34–37. PMID: 9375117

Barker, D. J., van Schaik, P., Simpson, D. S., & Corbett, W. A. (2003). Evaluating a spoken dialogue system for recording clinical observations during an endoscopic examination. *Medical Informatics and the Internet in Medicine, 28*, 85–97. PMID: 14692586

Baron, S., Patterson, A., & Harris, K. (2006). Beyond technology acceptance: Understanding consumer practice. *International Journal of Service Industry Management, 17*(2), 111–135.

Bauer, R. (1967). Consumer behavior as risk taking. In Cox, D. (Ed.), *Risk Taking and Information Handling in Consumer Behavior*. Harvard University Press.

Chae, J. M. (2009). Clothing & Textiles: Consumer acceptance model of smart clothing according to innovation. *International Journal of Human Ecology, 10*(1), 23–33.

Chau, P. Y. K., & Hu, P. J. (2001). Information technology acceptance by individual professionals: A model comparison approach. *Decision Sciences, 32*(4), 699–719.

Chau, P. Y. K., & Hu, P. J. H. (2002). Examining a model of information technology acceptance by individual professionals: An exploratory study. *Journal of Management Information Systems, 18*, 191–229.

Chismar, W. G., & Wiley-Patton, S. (2002) Test of the technology acceptance model for the internet in pediatrics. *Proceedings of the annual symposium of the American medical informatics association*, 155–9.

Chuah, S. H. W., Rauschnabel, P. A., Krey, N., Nguyen, B., Ramayah, T., & Lade, S. (2016). Wearable technologies: The role of usefulness and visibility in smartwatch adoption. *Computers in Human Behavior, 65*, 276–284.

Davis, F. D. (1989). Perceived usefulness, perceived ease of use, and user acceptance of information technology. *Management Information Systems Quarterly*, 319–340.

Davis, F. D., Bagozzi, R. P., & Warshaw, P. R. (1989). User acceptance of computer technology: A comparison of two theoretical models. *Management Science, 35*(8), 982–1003.

Dhagarra, D., Goswami, M., & Kumar, G. (2020). Impact of trust and privacy concerns on technology acceptance in healthcare: An Indian perspective. *International Journal of Medical Informatics, 141*, 104164. PMID: 32593847

Dowling, G., & Staelin, R. (1994). A model of perceived risk and intended risk-handling activity. *The Journal of Consumer Research, 21*, 119–134.

Dünnebeil, S., Sunyaev, A., Blohm, I., Leimeister, J. M., & Krcmar, H. (2012). Determinants of physicians' technology acceptance for e-health in ambulatory care. *International Journal of Medical Informatics, 81*(11), 746–760. PMID: 22397989

Duyck, P., Pynoo, B., Devolder, P., Voet, T., Adang, L., & Vercruysse, J. (2008). User acceptance of a picture archiving and communication system. Applying the unified theory of acceptance and use of technology in a radiological setting. *Methods of Information in Medicine, 47*, 149–156. PMID: 18338086

Featherman, M. S., & Pavlou, P. A. (2003). Predicting e-services adoption: A perceived risk facets perspective. *International Journal of Human-Computer Studies, 59*(4), 451–474.

Gefen, D. (2003). TAM or just plain habit: A look at experienced online shoppers. *Journal of Organizational and End User Computing, 15*(3), 1–13.

Germunden, H. G. (1985). Perceived risk and information search: A systematic meta-analysis of empirical evidence. *International Journal of Research in Marketing, 2*, 79–100.

Grewal, D., Gotlieb, J., & Marmorstein, H. (1994). The moderating effects of message framing and source credibility on the price-perceived risk relationship. *The Journal of Consumer Research, 21*, 145–153.

Han, S., Mustonen, P., Seppänen, M., & Kallio, M. (2005). *Does fragmenting of working time and working space influence the acceptance of mobile technology? A case of Finnish physicians*. Turku Centre for Computer Science.

Horan, T. A., Tulu, B., Hilton, B., & Burton, J. (2004) Use of online systems in clinical medical assessments: an analysis of physician acceptance of online disability evaluation systems. In: *Proceedings of the 37th Hawaii international conference on system sciences*; p. 1–10.

Hu, P. J. H., Chau, P. Y. K., Sheng, O. R. L., & Tam, K. Y. (1999). Examining the technology acceptance model using physician acceptance of telemedicine technology. *Journal of Management Information Systems*, *16*, 91–112.

Jung, Y., Kim, S., & Choi, B. (2016). Consumer valuation of the wearables: The case of smartwatches. *Computers in Human Behavior*, *63*, 899–905.

Karahanna, E., Agarwal, R., & Angst, C. (2006). Reconceptualizing compatibility beliefs in technology acceptance research. *Management Information Systems Quarterly*, *30*(4), 781–804.

Keil, M., Beranek, P., & Konsynski, B. (1995). Usefulness and ease of use: Field study evidence regarding tasks considerations. *Decision Support Systems*, *13*(1), 75–91.

Ko, E., Sung, H., & Yun, H. (2009). Comparative Analysis of Purchase Intentions Toward Smart Clothing Between Korean and US Consumers. *Clothing & Textiles Research Journal*, *27*(4), 259–273.

Lederer, A., Maupin, D., Sena, M., & Zhuang, Y. (2000). The technology acceptance model and the World Wide Web. *Decision Support Systems*, *29*, 269–282.

Lee, M. C. (2009). Factors influencing the adoption of internet banking: An integration of TAM and TPB with perceived risk and perceived benefit. *Electronic Commerce Research and Applications*, *8*(3), 130–141.

Legris, P., Ingham, J., & Collerette, P. (2003). Why do people use information technology? A critical review of the technology acceptance model. *Information & Management*, *40*(3), 191–204.

Liu, L., & Ma, Q. (2006). Perceived system performance: A test of an extended technology acceptance model. *The Data Base for Advances in Information Systems*, *37*, 51–59.

Luo, X., Li, H., Zhang, J., & Shim, J. P. (2010). Examining multi-dimensional trust and multi-faceted risk in initial acceptance of emerging technologies: An empirical study of mobile banking services. *Decision Support Systems*, *49*, 222–234.

Mathieson, K. (1991). Predicting user intentions: Comparing the technology acceptance model with the theory of planned behavior. *Information Systems Research, 2*(3), 173–191.

Melas, C. D., Zampetakis, L. A., Dimopoulou, A., & Moustakis, V. (2011). Modeling the acceptance of clinical information systems among hospital medical staff: An extended TAM model. *Journal of Biomedical Informatics, 44*(4), 553–564. PMID: 21292029

Mitchell, B.R., Mitchell, J.G., & Disney, A.P. (1996). User adoption issues in renal telemedicine. *Journal of Telemedicine and Telecare, 2*(2), 81-86.

Nadal, C., Sas, C., & Doherty, G. (2020). Technology acceptance in mobile health: Scoping review of definitions, models, and measurement. *Journal of Medical Internet Research, 22*(7), e17256. PMID: 32628122

Nasir, S., & Yurder, Y. (2015). Consumers' and physicians' perceptions about high tech wearable health products. *Procedia: Social and Behavioral Sciences, 195*, 1261–1267.

Pai, F. Y., & Huang, K. I. (2011). Applying the technology acceptance model to the introduction of healthcare information systems. *Technological Forecasting and Social Change, 78*(4), 650–660.

Park, Y., & Chen, J. V. (2007). Acceptance and adoption of the innovative use of smartphone. *Industrial Management & Data Systems, 107*(9), 1349–1365.

Pavlou, P. A. (2003). Consumer acceptance of electronic commerce: Integrating trust and risk with the technology acceptance model. *International Journal of Electronic Commerce, 7*(3), 101–134.

Peter, J., & Ryan, M. (1976). An investigation of perceived risk at the brand level. *JMR, Journal of Marketing Research, 13*, 184–188.

Pikkarainen, T., Pikkarainen, K., Karjaluoto, H., & Pahnila, S. (2004). Consumer acceptance of online banking: An extension of the technology acceptance model. *Internet Research, 14*(3), 224–235.

Rahimi, B., Nadri, H., Afshar, H. L., & Timpka, T. (2018). A systematic review of the technology acceptance model in health informatics. *Applied Clinical Informatics, 9*(03), 604–634. PMID: 30112741

Rawstorne, P., Jayasuriya, R., & Caputi, P. (2000) Issues in predicting and explaining usage behaviors with the technology acceptance model and the theory of planned behavior when usage is mandatory. *Proceedings of the 21st international conference on information systems*, 35–44.

Rogers, E. M. (1995). *Diffusion o f Innovations*. The Free Press.

Schaper, L. K., & Pervan, G. P. (2007). ICT and OTs: A model of information and communication technology acceptance and utilisation by occupational therapists. *International Journal of Medical Informatics*, *76*, S212–S221. PMID: 16828335

Stoumpos, A. I., Kitsios, F., & Talias, M. A. (2023). Digital transformation in healthcare: Technology acceptance and its applications. *International Journal of Environmental Research and Public Health*, *20*(4), 3407. PMID: 36834105

Talukder, M. S., Sorwar, G., Bao, Y., Ahmed, J. U., & Palash, M. A. S. (2020). Predicting antecedents of wearable healthcare technology acceptance by elderly: A combined SEM-Neural Network approach. *Technological Forecasting and Social Change*, *150*, 119793.

Taylor, J. (1974). The role of risk in consumer behavior. *Journal of Marketing*, *38*, 54–60.

Turhan, G. (2012). An assessment towards the acceptance of wearable technology to consumers in Turkey: The application to smart bra and t-shirt products. *Journal of the Textile Institute*, *104*(4), 375–395.

Venkatesh, V., & Davis, F. D. (2000). A theoretical extension of the technology acceptance model: Four longitudinal field studies. *Management Science*, *46*(2), 186–204.

Venkatesh, V., Morris, M. G., Davis, G. B., & Davis, F. D. (2003). User acceptance of information technology: Toward a unified view. *Management Information Systems Quarterly*, 425–478.

Wu, I., & Wu, K. (2005). A hybrid technology acceptance approach for exploring e-CRM adoption in organizations. *Behaviour & Information Technology*, *24*(4), 303–316.

Wu, J. H., & Wang, S. C. (2005). What drives mobile commerce?: An empirical evaluation of the revised technology acceptance model. *Information & Management*, *42*(5), 719–729.

Wu, J.-H., Wang, S.-C., & Lin, L.-M. (2007). Mobile computing acceptance factors in the healthcare industry: A structural equation model. *International Journal of Medical Informatics*, *76*, 66–77. PMID: 16901749

Yarbrough, A. K., & Smith, T. B. (2007). Technology acceptance among physicians: A new take on TAM. *Medical Care Research and Review : MCRR*, *64*(6), 650–672. PMID: 17717378

Compilation of References

Abaszadeh, F., Ashoub, M. H., Khajouie, G., & Amiri, M. (2023). Nanotechnology development in surgical applications: Recent trends and developments. *European Journal of Medical Research*, *28*(1). Advance online publication. DOI: 10.1186/s40001-023-01429-4 PMID: 38001554

Abdolkhani, R., Gray, K., Borda, A., & DeSouza, R. (2019). Patient-generated health data management and quality challenges in remote patient monitoring. *JAMIA Open*, *2*, 471–478. PMID: 32025644

Abid, M. H., Ashraf, R., Mahmood, T., & Faisal, C. M. N. (2023). Multi-modal medical image classification using deep residual network and genetic algorithm. *PLoS One*, *18*(6), e0287786. Advance online publication. DOI: 10.1371/journal.pone.0287786

Acharya, R., Patil, T. V., Dutta, S. D., Lee, J., Ganguly, K., Kim, H., Randhawa, A., & Lim, K. (2024). Single-Walled Carbon Nanotube-Based Optical Nano/Biosensors for biomedical applications: Role in bioimaging, disease diagnosis, and biomarkers detection. *Advanced Materials Technologies*, *9*(20). Advance online publication. DOI: 10.1002/admt.202400279

Adel, E., El-Sappagh, S., Barakat, S., & Elmogy, M. (2019). Ontology-based electronic health record semantic interoperability: A survey. In Dey, N., Ashour, A. S., Fong, S. J., & Borra, S. (Eds.), *Advances in Ubiquitous Sensing Applications for Healthcare, U-Healthcare Monitoring Systems* (pp. 315–352). Academic Press.

Adiuku, N., Avdelidis, N. P., Tang, G., & Plastropoulos, A. (2024). Advancements in Learning-Based Navigation Systems for Robotic Applications in MRO Hangar [Review]. *Sensors (Basel)*, *24*(5), 1377. https://www.mdpi.com/1424-8220/24/5/1377 PMID: 38474913

Adler, D. A., Tseng, E., Moon, K. C., Young, J. Q., Kane, J. M., Moss, E., & Choudhury, T. (2022). Burnout and the Quantified Workplace: Tensions around Personal Sensing Interventions for Stress in Resident Physicians. *Proceedings of the ACM on Human-computer Interaction, 6*(CSCW2), 1-48.

Adler-Milstein, J., & Nong, P. (2019). Early experiences with patient-generated health data: Health system and patient perspectives. *Journal of the American Medical Informatics Association : JAMIA, 26*, 952–959. PMID: 31329886

Adnan, M., Kalra, S., Cresswell, J. C., Taylor, G. W., & Tizhoosh, H. R. (2022). Federated Learning And Differential Privacy For Medical Image Analysis. *Scientific Reports, 12*, 1953. PMID: 35121774

Afeef, S., Tolfrey, K., Zakrzewski-Fruer, J. K., & Barrett, L. A. (2023). Performance of the FreeStyle Libre Flash Glucose Monitoring System during an Oral Glucose Tolerance Test and Exercise in Healthy Adolescents. *Sensors (Basel), 23*(9), 4249. DOI: 10.3390/s23094249 PMID: 37177452

Aggarwal, A., Tam, C. C., Wu, D., Li, X., & Qiao, S. (2023). Artificial Intelligence–Based Chatbots for Promoting Health Behavioral Changes: Systematic Review. *Journal of Medical Internet Research, 25*, e40789.

Ahammed, S., Hassan, N., Cheragee, S. H., & Islam, A. Z. M. T. (2021). An iot-based real-time remote health monitoring system. *International Journal of Research Engineering Science, 8*(3), 23–29.

Ahlan, A. R., & Ahmad, B. I. E. (2014). User acceptance of health information technology (HIT) in developing countries: A conceptual model. *Procedia Technology, 16*, 1287–1296.

Ahmad, A., Rasul, T., Yousaf, A., & Zaman, U. (2020). Understanding factors influencing elderly diabetic patients' continuance intention to use digital health wearables: Extending the technology acceptance model (TAM). *Journal of Open Innovation, 6*(3), 81.

Ahsan, M. M., & Siddique, Z. (2022). Industry 4.0 in Healthcare: A systematic review. *International Journal of Information Management Data Insights, 2*(1), 100079. DOI: 10.1016/j.jjimei.2022.100079

Ajzen, M. & Fishbein, M. (1975). Belief, attitude, intention and behavior: An introduction to theory and research. Academic Press.

Ajzen, I. (1991). The theory of planned behavior. *Organizational Behavior and Human Decision Processes, 50*, 179–211.

Al Kuwaiti, A., Nazer, K., Al-Reedy, A., Al-Shehri, S., Al-Muhanna, A., Subbarayalu, A. V., Al Muhanna, D., & Al-Muhanna, F. A. (2023). A Review of the Role of Artificial Intelligence in Healthcare. *Journal of Personalized Medicine, 13*(6), 951.

Alanazi, A. (2022). Using machine learning for healthcare challenges and opportunities. *Informatics in Medicine Unlocked, 30*, 100924.

Albee, D. T., & Hunter, M. R. (2022). AARP. In *Encyclopedia of Gerontology and Population Aging* (pp. 1–4). Springer International Publishing.

Albelwi, S. (2021). Survey on self-supervised learning: Auxiliary pretext tasks and contrastive learning methods in imaging. *Entropy (Basel, Switzerland), 24*(4). Advance online publication. DOI: 10.3390/e24040551

Albustanji, R. N., Elmanaseer, S., & Alkhatib, A. A. A. (2023). Robotics: Five Senses plus One—An Overview. *Robotics (Basel, Switzerland), 12*(3), 68. https://www.mdpi.com/2218-6581/12/3/68

Al-Dhaen, F., Hou, J., Rana, N. P., & Weerakkody, V. (2023). Advancing the Understanding of the Role of Responsible AI in the Continued Use of IoMT in Healthcare. *Information Systems Frontiers, 25*(6), 2159–2178.

Aldoseri, A., Al-Khalifa, K. N., & Hamouda, A. M. (2023). Re-Thinking Data Strategy and Integration for Artificial intelligence: Concepts, opportunities, and challenges. *Applied Sciences (Basel, Switzerland), 13*(12), 7082. DOI: 10.3390/app13127082

Alhashmi, S., Salloum, S. A., & Mhamdi, C. (2019). Implementing artificial intelligence in the United Arab Emirates healthcare sector: An extended technology acceptance model. *International Journal of Information Technology and Language Studies, 3*(3), 27–42.

Ali, Y. H., Chooralil, V. S., Balasubramanian, K., Manyam, R. R., Raju, S. K., Sadiq, A. T., & Farhan, A. K. (2023). Optimization system based on convolutional neural network and internet of medical things for early diagnosis of lung cancer. *Bioengineering (Basel, Switzerland), 10*(3), 320. DOI: 10.3390/bioengineering10030320 PMID: 36978711

Allen, A., Hayes, J., Sadasivan, R., & Williamson, S.K., & Wittman, C. (1995). A pilot study of the physician acceptance of teleoncology. *Journal of Telemedicine and Telecare, 1*(1), 34–37. PMID: 9375117

Almurashi, A. M., Rodriguez, E., & Garg, S. K. (2023). Emerging Diabetes Technologies: Continuous Glucose Monitors/Artificial Pancreases. *Journal of the Indian Institute of Science, 103*(1), 205–230. DOI: 10.1007/s41745-022-00348-3 PMID: 37362851

Al-Sammarraie, S. Z., Bratchenko, L. A., Tupikova, E. N., Skuratova, M. A., Wang, S., Lebedev, P. A., & Bratchenko, I. A. (2024). Human blood plasma SERS analysis using silver nanoparticles for cardiovascular diseases detection. *Journal of Biomedical Photonics & Engineering, 10*(1), 010301. DOI: 10.18287/jbpe24.10.010301

Alsanie, S., Ibrahim, K., Lim, S., & Wootton, S. (2024). Understanding the nature and scale of low-intake dehydration on 'Medicine for Older People' wards at University Hospital Southampton: A mixed-methods study. *Proceedings of the Nutrition Society, 83*(OCE2), E214.

Alshaikh, F., Ramzan, F., Rawaf, S., & Majeed, A. (2014). Social network sites as a mode to collect health data: A systematic review. *Journal of Medical Internet Research, 16*, e171. PMID: 25048247

Altman, J., Jones, G., Ahmed, S., Sharma, S., & Sharma, A. (2023). Tear Film MicroRNAs as potential biomarkers: A review. *International Journal of Molecular Sciences, 24*(4), 3694. DOI: 10.3390/ijms24043694 PMID: 36835108

Alyami, A. A. (2018). *Smart e-health system for real-time tracking and monitoring of patients, staff and assets for healthcare decision support in Saudi Arabia* (Doctoral dissertation, Staffordshire University).

Amal, H., Leja, M., Funka, K., Skapars, R., Sivins, A., Ancans, G., Liepniece-Karele, I., Kikuste, I., Lasina, I., & Haick, H. (2015). Detection of precancerous gastric lesions and gastric cancer through exhaled breath. *Gut, 65*(3), 400–407. DOI: 10.1136/gutjnl-2014-308536 PMID: 25869737

Amparore, D., De Cillis, S., Colombo, M., Garzena, V., Sica, M., Checcucci, E., & Porpiglia, F. (2025). TYTOCARE™ home telemonitoring device after radical cystectomy to optimise postoperative outcomes. *BJU International, 135*(6), 960–968. PMID: 39725555

Anand, M., & Garg, A. (2021). Recent advancements in self-supervised paradigms for visual feature representation. arXiv. https://arXiv.org/abs/2111.02042

Ansari, M. A., Mohd-Naim, N. F., & Ahmed, M. U. (2024). Electrochemical nanoaptasensor based on graphitic carbon Nitride/Zirconium Dioxide/Multiwalled carbon nanotubes for matrix metalloproteinase-9 in human serum and saliva. *ACS Applied Bio Materials, 7*(3), 1579–1587. DOI: 10.1021/acsabm.3c01075 PMID: 38386014

Apoorva, S., Nguyen, N., & Sreejith, K. R. (2024). Recent developments and future perspectives of microfluidics and smart technologies in wearable devices. *Lab on a Chip, 24*(7), 1833–1866. DOI: 10.1039/d4lc00089g PMID: 38476112

Arduini, F. (2024). Wireless real-time monitoring of oestradiol in sweat. *Nature Nanotechnology, 19*(3), 271–272. DOI: 10.1038/s41565-024-01611-7 PMID: 38366226

Argaw, S. T., Troncoso-Pastoriza, J. R., Lacey, D., Florin, M., Calcavecchia, F., Anderson, D., Burleson, W. P., Vogel, J., O'Leary, C., & Eshaya-Chauvin, B. (2020). Cybersecurity of Hospitals: Discussing the challenges and working towards mitigating the risks. *BMC Medical Informatics and Decision Making, 20*, 146. PMID: 32620167

Arkhypova, V., Soldatkin, O., Soldatkin, A., & Dzyadevych, S. (2023). Electrochemical biosensors based on enzyme inhibition effect. *Chemical Record (New York, N.Y.), 24*(2). Advance online publication. DOI: 10.1002/tcr.202300214 PMID: 37639188

Ashraf, F. B., Alam, S. M. M., & Sakib, S. M. (2024). Enhancing breast cancer classification via histopathological image analysis: Leveraging self-supervised contrastive learning and transfer learning. *Heliyon, 10*(2), e24123. Advance online publication. DOI: 10.1016/j.heliyon.2024.e24123

Astillo, P. V., Choudhary, G., Duguma, D. G., Kim, J., & You, I. (2021). TrMAps: Trust Management in Specification-Based Misbehavior Detection System for IMD-Enabled Artificial Pancreas System. *IEEE Journal of Biomedical and Health Informatics, 25*, 3763–3775. PMID: 33651704

Ateeq, A., Al-Refaei, A. A. A., Alzoraiki, M., Milhem, M., Al-Tahitah, A. N., & Ibrahim, A. (2024). Sustaining Organizational Outcomes in Manufacturing Firms: The Role of HRM and Occupational Health and Safety. *Sustainability, 16*(3), 1035.

Auwal, A. M. (2023). *IoT integration in telemedicine: Investigating the role of Internet of things devices in facilitating remote patient monitoring and data transmission.*

Azizipour, N.. (2020). Evolution of biochip technology: A review from lab-on-a-chip to organ-on-a-chip. *Micromachines, 11*(6), 599. DOI: 10.3390/mi11060599 PMID: 32570945

Bacha, A., & Shah, H. H. (2025). AI-Powered Virtual Health Assistants: Transforming Patient Care and Engagement. *Global Insights in Artificial Intelligence and Computing, 1*(1), 15–30.

Bae, G., Kim, M., Lee, A., Ji, S., Jang, M., Yim, S., Song, W., Lee, S. S., Yoon, D. H., & An, K. (2021). Nanometric lamination of zinc oxide nanofilms with gold nanoparticles for self-perceived periodontal disease sensors. *Composites. Part B, Engineering, 230*, 109490. DOI: 10.1016/j.compositesb.2021.109490

Bahari, H., Hasanzadeh, M., Kohansal, F., Peirovi, B., & Shadjou, N. (2024a). Smartphone-assisted immunosensing of cancer biomarkers in human biofluids using poly (methyl methacrylate) decorated by triangular silver nanoparticles. *Journal of Photochemistry and Photobiology A Chemistry*, *457*, 115882. DOI: 10.1016/j.jphotochem.2024.115882

Bai, H., Cao, M., Huang, P., & Shan, J. (2021). Self-supervised semi-supervised learning for data labeling and quality evaluation. arXiv. https://arXiv.org/abs/2111.10932

Bai, N., Xue, Y., Chen, S., Shi, L., Shi, J., Zhang, Y., & Guo, C. F. (2023). A robotic sensory system with high spatiotemporal resolution for texture recognition. *Nature Communications*, *14*(1), 7121. DOI: 10.1038/s41467-023-42722-4 PMID: 37963866

Ballard, Z. S., Joung, H., Goncharov, A., Liang, J., Nugroho, K., Di Carlo, D., Garner, O. B., & Ozcan, A. (2020). Deep learning-enabled point-of-care sensing using multiplexed paper-based sensors. *NPJ Digital Medicine*, *3*(1). Advance online publication. DOI: 10.1038/s41746-020-0274-y PMID: 32411827

Ballouhey, Q., Esposito, C., Taghavi, K., Lardy, H., Berte, N., Abbo, O., & Blanc, T. (2025). Robot-assisted Surgery in Pediatric Patients: Results of a French Multicenter Study on 1401 Patients. *Journal of Pediatric Surgery*, *60*(8), 162397. DOI: 10.1016/j.jpedsurg.2025.162397 PMID: 40472888

Bao, W., Jin, Y., Huang, C., & Peng, W. (2021). CT image classification of invasive depth of gastric cancer based on 3D-DPN structure. *The 11th International Workshop on Computer Science and Engineering (WCSE 2021)*, 115–121. DOI: 10.18178/wcse.2021.06.018

Barker, D. J., van Schaik, P., Simpson, D. S., & Corbett, W. A. (2003). Evaluating a spoken dialogue system for recording clinical observations during an endoscopic examination. *Medical Informatics and the Internet in Medicine*, *28*, 85–97. PMID: 14692586

Baron, S., Patterson, A., & Harris, K. (2006). Beyond technology acceptance: Understanding consumer practice. *International Journal of Service Industry Management*, *17*(2), 111–135.

Bartoletti, I. (2019). AI in healthcare: Ethical and privacy challenges. In *Artificial Intelligence in Medicine: 17th Conference on Artificial Intelligence in Medicine, AIME 2019, Poznan, Poland, June 26–29, 2019* [Springer International Publishing.]. *Proceedings*, *17*, 7–10.

Basulo-Ribeiro, J., & Teixeira, L. (2024). The Future of Healthcare with Industry 5.0: Preliminary Interview-Based Qualitative Analysis. *Future Internet, 16*(3), 68. https://www.mdpi.com/1999-5903/16/3/68

Bathirappan, K., Pandurengan, D. B., Nawaz, J. Y., & Arulrajan, J. R. (2022, October). Patient monitoring and medicine dispenser robot. In *AIP Conference Proceedings* (Vol. 2494, No. 1). AIP Publishing.

Bauer, R. (1967). Consumer behavior as risk taking. In Cox, D. (Ed.), *Risk Taking and Information Handling in Consumer Behavior*. Harvard University Press.

Bayoumy, R. E., El-Ragehy, N. A., Hassan, N. Y., & Mahmoud, A. M. (2024). Disposable Point-of-Care Electrochemical Sensor for Uric Acid Determination in Human Urine Utilizing a Pencil Graphite Electrode Modified with Polydopamine/ Gold Nanoparticles. *Journal of the Electrochemical Society, 171*(2), 027506. DOI: 10.1149/1945-7111/ad2281

Beatto, T. G., Gomes, W. E., Etchegaray, A., Gupta, R., & Mendes, R. K. (2023). Dopamine levels determined in synthetic urine using an electrochemical tyrosinase biosensor based on ZnO@Au core–shell. *RSC Advances, 13*(47), 33424–33429. DOI: 10.1039/d3ra06277e PMID: 38025875

Benedetti, T. M., Somerville, S. V., Wordsworth, J., Yamamoto, Y., Schuhmann, W., Tilley, R. D., & Gooding, J. J. (2024). An artificial enzyme: How nanoconfinement allows the selective electrochemical detection of glucose directly in whole blood. *Advanced Functional Materials, 34*(30). Advance online publication. DOI: 10.1002/ adfm.202400322

Besnik, Q. (2020). *The Framework of a Real-time Patient Monitoring System* (Doctoral dissertation, Budapesti Corvinus Egyetem).

Bhende, P. M. (2020). *Quality of Work Life of Employees in Banking Sector-A Study of Bank Managers and Staff in Goa* (Doctoral dissertation, Goa University).

Bilsen, M. P., Treep, M. M., Aantjes, M. J., Van Andel, E., Stalenhoef, J. E., Van Nieuwkoop, C., Leyten, E. M., Delfos, N. M., Van Uhm, J. I., Sijbom, M., Akintola, A. A., Numans, M. E., Achterberg, W. P., Mooijaart, S. P., Van Der Beek, M. T., Cobbaert, C. M., Conroy, S. P., Visser, L. G., & Lambregts, M. M. (2023). Diagnostic accuracy of urine biomarkers for urinary tract infection in older women: A case-control study. *Clinical Microbiology and Infection, 30*(2), 216–222. DOI: 10.1016/j.cmi.2023.09.023 PMID: 37805035

Biswas, P., Sikander, S., & Kulkarni, P. (2023). Recent advances in robot-assisted surgical systems. *Biomedical Engineering Advances, 6*, 100109. DOI: 10.1016/j.bea.2023.100109

Bi, Y., Sun, M., Wang, J., Zhu, Z., Bai, J., Emran, M. Y., Kotb, A., Bo, X., & Zhou, M. (2023). Universal fully integrated wearable sensor arrays for the multiple electrolyte and metabolite monitoring in raw sweat, saliva, or urine. *Analytical Chemistry, 95*(16), 6690–6699. DOI: 10.1021/acs.analchem.3c00361 PMID: 36961950

Blondon, K., & Ehrler, F. (2022). Design Considerations for the Use of Patient-Generated Health Data in the Electronic Medical Records. In *Challenges of Trustable AI and Added-Value on Health* (p. 229). IOS Press.

Boffa, M., Vassio, L., Mellia, M., Drago, I., Milan, G., Ben Houidi, Z., & Rossi, D. (2022). On using pretext tasks to learn representations from network logs. *Proceedings of the 1st International Workshop on Native Network Intelligence*, 21–26. DOI: 10.1145/3565009.3568682

Bora, G. S., Narain, T. A., Sharma, A. P., Mavuduru, R. S., Devana, S. K., Singh, S. K., & Mandal, A. K. (2020). Robot-assisted surgery in India: A SWOT analysis. *Indian Journal of Urology : IJU : Journal of the Urological Society of India, 36*(1). https://journals.lww.com/indianjurol/fulltext/2020/36010/robot_assisted_surgery_in_india__a_swot_analysis.1.aspx PMID: 31983817

Boscarelli, A., Giglione, E., Caputo, M. R., Guida, E., Iaquinto, M., Scarpa, M. G., & Schleef, J. (2023). Robotic-assisted surgery in pediatrics: What is evidence-based?-a literature review. *Translational Pediatrics, 12*(2), 271–279. DOI: 10.21037/tp-22-338 PMID: 36891357

Bose, P. (2025, March). *The future of hospital care with smart bed technology. News-Medical.* Retrieved June 20, 2025, from https://www.news-medical.net/health/The-Future-of-Hospital-Care-Embracing-Smart-Bed-Technology.aspx

Bourke, A., Dixon, W. G., Roddam, A., Lin, K. J., Hall, G. C., Curtis, J. R., van der Veer, S. N., Soriano-Gabarró, M., Mills, J. K., & Major, J. M. (2020). Incorporating patient-generated health data into pharmacoepidemiological research. *Pharmacoepidemiology and Drug Safety, 29*, 1540–1549. PMID: 33146896

Bowers, H., & Cheer, J. M. (2017). Yoga tourism: Commodification and western embracement of eastern spiritual practice. *Tourism Management Perspectives, 24*, 208–216. DOI: 10.1016/j.tmp.2017.07.013

Bozorgtabar, B., Mahapatra, D., Vray, G., & Thiran, J.-P. (2020). SALAD: Self-supervised aggregation learning for anomaly detection on X-rays. In *MICCAI 2020* (pp. 468–478). Medical image computing and computer assisted intervention. Springer. DOI: 10.1007/978-3-030-59725-2_45

Brasier, N., Frobert, O., De Ieso, F., Meyer, D., Kowatsch, T., & Ghaffari, R. (2024). The potential of wearable sweat sensors in heart failure management. *Nature Electronics*, *7*(3), 182–184. DOI: 10.1038/s41928-024-01136-w

Brinza, M., Schröder, S., Ababii, N., Gronenberg, M., Strunskus, T., Pauporte, T., Adelung, R., Faupel, F., & Lupan, O. (2023). Two-in-One sensor based on PV4D4-Coated TIO2 films for food spoilage detection and as a breath marker for several diseases. *Biosensors (Basel)*, *13*(5), 538. DOI: 10.3390/bios13050538 PMID: 37232899

Brown, R., Coventry, L., Sillence, E., Blythe, J., Stumpf, S., Bird, J., & Durrant, A. C. (2022). Collecting and sharing self-generated health and lifestyle data: Understanding barriers for people living with long-term health conditions—A survey study. *Digital Health*, *8*. PMID: 35284085

Buczak, A. L., & Guven, E. (2016). A Survey of Data Mining and Machine Learning Methods for Cyber Security Intrusion Detection. *IEEE Communications Surveys and Tutorials*, *18*, 1153–1176.

Budhiraja, S., & Kant, S. (2020). Challenges associated with work-life balance: A meta-analysis. *J. Strat. Human Res. Manag*, *9*, 11–16.

Bustillo, A., Reis, R., & Machado, A. R., & Others. (2022). Improving the accuracy of machine-learning models with data from machine test repetitions. *Journal of Intelligent Manufacturing*, *33*(1), 203–221. DOI: 10.1007/s10845-020-01661-3

Cáceres, C., Heusser, B., Garnham, A., & Moczko, E. (2023). The major hypotheses of Alzheimer's disease: Related Nanotechnology-Based Approaches for its diagnosis and treatment. *Cells*, *12*(23), 2669. DOI: 10.3390/cells12232669 PMID: 38067098

Canadian Healthcare Technology. (2025, April). *AI-powered robots take the stage at HIMSS.* Canadian Healthcare Technology, 30(3). Retrieved June 23, 2025, from https://www.canhealth.com/wp-content/uploads/2025/03/Canadian-Healthcare-Technology-2025-03-1.pdf

Caron, M., Misra, I., Mairal, J., Goyal, P., Bojanowski, P., & Joulin, A. (2020). Unsupervised learning of visual features by contrasting cluster assignments. *Advances in Neural Information Processing Systems*, *33*, 9912–9924.

Carroll, J., Hopper, L., Farrelly, A. M., Lombard-Vance, R., Bamidis, P. D., & Konstantinidis, E. I. (2021). A scoping review of augmented/virtual reality health and wellbeing interventions for older adults: Redefining immersive virtual reality. *Frontiers in Virtual Reality*, *2*, 655338.

Castro, E. M. J., & Faria Araújo, N. M. (2020). Impact of the Fourth Industrial Revolution on the Health Sector: A Qualitative Study. *Healthcare Informatics Research*, *26*(4), 328–334. DOI: 10.4258/hir.2020.26.4.328 PMID: 33190467

Catherine, S., Suresh, N. V., Mangaiyarkarasi, T., & Jenefa, L. (2025). Unveiling the Enigma of Shadow: Ethical Difficulties in the Field of AI. In *Navigating Data Science: Unleashing the Creative Potential of Artificial Intelligence* (pp. 57-67). Emerald Publishing Limited.

Center for Internet Security (CIS). (2017). *Cyber Attacks: In the Healthcare Sector; Center for Internet Security*. CIS.

CGCompliance. (2025, February). *A complete guide to HIPAA compliance services: Protecting patient data effectively*. CGCompliance. Retrieved June 20, 2025, from https://info.cgcompliance.com/blog/a-complete-guide-to-hipaa-compliance-services-protecting-patient-data-effectively

Chae, J. M. (2009). Clothing & Textiles: Consumer acceptance model of smart clothing according to innovation. *International Journal of Human Ecology*, *10*(1), 23–33.

Chaitanya, K., Erdil, E., Karani, N., & Konukoglu, E. (2020). Contrastive learning of global and local features for medical image segmentation with limited annotations. *34th Conference on Neural Information Processing Systems (NeurIPS 2020)*. DOI: 10.48550/arXiv.2006.10511

Charnysh, E., Pal, S., Reader, J. M., Uhlmann, W. R., McCain, S., Sanghavi, K., Blasco, D., Brandt, R., Feero, W. G., Ferber, R., Giri, V. N., Hendy, K., Prince, A. E. R., Lee, C., & Roberts, J. S. (2024). Health care utilization and behavior changes after workplace genetic testing at a large US health care system. *Genetics in Medicine*, *26*(8), 101160. DOI: 10.1016/j.gim.2024.101160 PMID: 38733246

Chaudhary, V., Taha, B. A., Lucky, N., Rustagi, S., Khosla, A., Papakonstantinou, P., & Bhalla, N. (2024). Nose-on-Chip Nanobiosensors for early detection of lung cancer breath biomarkers. *ACS Sensors*, *9*(9), 4469–4494. DOI: 10.1021/acssensors.4c01524 PMID: 39248694

Chaudhry, U. H., Arshad, R., Abbas, N. N., & Zeerak, A. A. (2023). Data Leakage In Business And Fintech. In *Handbook Of Research On Cybersecurity Issues And Challenges For Business And Fintech Applications*. IGI Global.

Chau, P. Y. K., & Hu, P. J. (2001). Information technology acceptance by individual professionals: A model comparison approach. *Decision Sciences*, *32*(4), 699–719.

Chau, P. Y. K., & Hu, P. J. H. (2002). Examining a model of information technology acceptance by individual professionals: An exploratory study. *Journal of Management Information Systems*, *18*, 191–229.

Cheese, P. (2021). *The New World of Work: Shaping a Future that Helps People, Organizations and Our Societies to Thrive*. Kogan Page Publishers.

Chen, T., & Guestrin, C. (2016). XGBoost: A Scalable Tree Boosting System. In *Proceedings of the KDD '16: 22nd ACM SIGKDD International Conference on Knowledge Discovery and Data Mining*. Association for Computing Machinery.

Chen, Y., Ding, J., Li, D., & Chen, Z. (2021). Joint BERT Model Based Cybersecurity Named Entity Recognition. *Proceedings of the ICSIM 2021: 2021 The 4th International Conference on Software Engineering and Information Management*, 236–242.

Chen, J., Li, K., & Philip, S. Y. (2021). Privacy-Preserving Deep Learning Model For Decentralized Vanets Using Fully Homomorphic Encryption And Blockchain. *IEEE Transactions on Intelligent Transportation Systems*, *23*, 11633–11642.

Chen, L., Bentley, P., Mori, K., Misawa, K., Fujiwara, M., & Rueckert, D. (2019). Self-supervised learning for medical image analysis using image context restoration. *Medical Image Analysis*, *58*, 101539. Advance online publication. DOI: 10.1016/j.media.2019.101539

Chen, T., Kornblith, S., Norouzi, M., & Hinton, G. (2020). A simple framework for contrastive learning of visual representations. arXiv. https://arXiv.org/abs/2002.05709

Chen, X., Ding, M., Wang, X., Xin, Y., Mo, S., Wang, Y., Han, S., Luo, P., Zeng, G., & Wang, J. (2022). Context autoencoder for self-supervised representation learning. arXiv. https://arXiv.org/abs/2202.03026

Chen, X., Fan, H., Girshick, R., & He, K. (2020). Improved baselines with momentum contrastive learning. arXiv. https://arXiv.org/abs/2003.04297

Chhillar, M., Kukkar, D., Deep, A., Yadav, A. K., & Kim, K. (2023). Zn2+/GNPs nanocomposite for highly selective colorimetric detection of creatinine in urine samples of CKD patients. *Inorganic Chemistry Communications*, *158*, 111618. DOI: 10.1016/j.inoche.2023.111618

Chhillar, M., Kukkar, D., Yadav, A. K., & Kim, K. (2024). Nitrogen doped carbon dots and gold nanoparticles mediated FRET for the detection of creatinine in human urine samples. *Spectrochimica Acta Part a Molecular and Biomolecular Spectroscopy, 321*, 124752. DOI: 10.1016/j.saa.2024.124752 PMID: 38945007

Chismar, W. G., & Wiley-Patton, S. (2002) Test of the technology acceptance model for the internet in pediatrics. *Proceedings of the annual symposium of the American medical informatics association*, 155–9.

Choi, P. J., Oskouian, R. J., & Tubbs, R. S. (2018). Telesurgery: Past, Present, and Future. *Cureus, 10*(5), e2716. DOI: 10.7759/cureus.2716 PMID: 30079282

Chuah, S. H. W., Rauschnabel, P. A., Krey, N., Nguyen, B., Ramayah, T., & Lade, S. (2016). Wearable technologies: The role of usefulness and visibility in smartwatch adoption. *Computers in Human Behavior, 65*, 276–284.

Chung, H., Jaga, A., & Lambert, S. (2022). Possibilities for change and new frontiers: Introduction to the work and family researchers network special issue on advancing equality at work and home. *Community Work & Family, 25*(1), 1–12.

Ciampi, M., De Pietro, G., Masciari, E., & Silvestri, S. (2020). Some Lessons Learned Using Health Data Literature for Smart Information Retrieval. *Proceedings of the 35th Annual ACM Symposium on Applied Computing*, 931–934.

Citron, D. K., & Solove, D. J. (2022). Privacy Harms. *Bul Rev., 102*, 793.

Cohen, R. A., & Mykyta, L. (2024). Prescription Medication Use, Coverage, and Nonadherence Among Adults Age 65 and Older: United States, 2021–2022. Academic Press.

Cohen, D. J., Keller, S. R., Hayes, G. R., Dorr, D. A., Ash, J. S., & Sittig, D. F. (2016). Integrating patient-generated health data into clinical care settings or clinical decision-making: Lessons learned from project healthdesign. *JMIR Human Factors, 3*, e5919. PMID: 27760726

Cordas, C. M., Nunes, M. J., Valério, G. N., Samhan-Arias, A., Krippahl, L., Moura, J. J. G., Santos, G., Sousa, J. P., & Rouco, C. (2023). Sweat as a testing analytical fluid for emotions and stress biomarkers detection. In *Smart innovation, systems and technologies* (pp. 77–85). DOI: 10.1007/978-981-19-7689-6_7

Cornelissen, S., & van der Putten, J. A. (2021). Evaluating self-supervised learning methods for downstream classification of neoplasia in Barrett's esophagus. *2021 IEEE International Conference on Image Processing (ICIP)*, 66–70. DOI: 10.1109/ICIP42928.2021.9506042

Coventry, L., & Branley, D. (2018). Cybersecurity in healthcare: A narrative review of trends, threats and ways forward. *Maturitas*, *113*, 48–52. PMID: 29903648

Cruz, J. N., Da Silva Souza Filho, A. P., Oliveira, M. E. C., Pereira, D. S., & De Oliveira, M. S. (2021). Nanosensor for the detection of malaria parasite. In *Elsevier eBooks* (pp. 107–116). DOI: 10.1016/b978-0-12-821100-7.00024-8

Cuevas, C. A. G., Alvarado, G. A. D., González, C. J., Peña, C. F. P., & Castro, L. E. C. (2025). Scientific evolution of robotic surgery in urogenital diseases: Bibliometric analysis. *Journal of Robotic Surgery*, *19*(1), 219. DOI: 10.1007/s11701-025-02359-5 PMID: 40377820

Czarniak, N., Kamińska, J., Matowicka-Karna, J., & Koper-Lenkiewicz, O. (2023). Cerebrospinal Fluid–Basic Concepts Review. *Biomedicines*, *11*(5), 1461. DOI: 10.3390/biomedicines11051461 PMID: 37239132

Da Silva, S. M. S. D., Ferreira, C. L., Rizzato, J. M. B., Toledo, G. D. S., Furukawa, M., Rovai, E. S., Nogueira, M. S., & De Carvalho, L. F. D. C. E. S. (2024). Infrared spectroscopy for fast screening of diabetes and periodontitis. *Photodiagnosis and Photodynamic Therapy*, *46*, 104106. DOI: 10.1016/j.pdpdt.2024.104106 PMID: 38677501

Dagnino, G.. (2024). Robot-assistive minimally invasive surgery: Trends and future directions. *International Journal of Intelligent Robotics and Applications*, *8*, 812–826. DOI: 10.1007/s41315-024-00341-2

Dangi, S., Ghanshala, K., & Sharma, S. (2025b). LIFT: Lightweight incremental and federated techniques for live memory forensics and proactive malware detection. *International Journal of Advanced Computer Science and Applications*, *16*(4). Advance online publication. DOI: 10.14569/ijacsa.2025.0160445

Das, C., Das, S., Chugh, V., & Bhattacharjee, M. (2023). 3D Printed Design-Assisted Multilayered Graphene Oxide-Modified Polymer Glucose Sensor. *Advanced Engineering Materials*, *26*(1). Advance online publication. DOI: 10.1002/adem.202301067

Dave, S.. (2024). Advancements in healthcare through 3D-printed micro and nanosensors: Innovation, application, and prospects. *Hybrid Advances*, *7*, 100311. DOI: 10.1016/j.hybadv.2024.100311

Davis, F. D. (1989). Perceived usefulness, perceived ease of use, and user acceptance of information technology. *Management Information Systems Quarterly*, 319–340.

Davis, F. D., Bagozzi, R. P., & Warshaw, P. R. (1989). User acceptance of computer technology: A comparison of two theoretical models. *Management Science*, *35*(8), 982–1003.

De Castro, J. M. N. L. (2019). *Transforming Lives and the Healthcare Business: Remote Patient 5G-IoT Technology Monitoring Solution for the Home Hospitalization Service* (Master's thesis, Universidade Catolica Portuguesa (Portugal)).

De Jong, F. C., Iflé, I. G., Van Der Made, A. C., Kooper, D., De Jong, J. J., Franckena, M., Zuiverloon, T. C., Van Criekinge, W., Incrocci, L., Zwarthoff, E. C., & Boormans, J. L. (2024). A Genomic Urine Assay for Surveillance of Patients with Bladder Cancer Treated with Radiotherapy. *European Urology Open Science*, *62*, 131–139. DOI: 10.1016/j.euros.2024.02.009 PMID: 38496820

De Lima, L. T. F., Crawford, D. H., Broszczak, D. A., & Zhang, X., R, K. B., & Punyadeera, C. (2023). A salivary biomarker panel to detect liver cirrhosis. *iScience*, *26*(7), 107015. DOI: 10.1016/j.isci.2023.107015 PMID: 37360686

De Oliveira Filho, J. I., Faleiros, M. C., Ferreira, D. C., Mani, V., & Salama, K. N. (2023). Empowering Electrochemical Biosensors with AI: Overcoming Interference for Precise Dopamine Detection in Complex Samples. *Advanced Intelligent Systems*, *5*(10). Advance online publication. DOI: 10.1002/aisy.202300227

Dehaene, O., Camara, A., Moindrot, O., de Lavergne, A., & Courtiol, P. (2020). Self-supervision closes the gap between weak and strong supervision in histology. *ML4H 2020 NeurIPS Workshop*. /arXiv.2012.03583DOI: 10.48550

Dermody, G., Wadsworth, D., Dunham, M., Glass, C., & Fritz, R. (2024). Factors Affecting Clinician Readiness to Adopt Smart Home Technology for Remote Health Monitoring: Systematic Review. *JMIR Aging*, *7*(1), e64367. PMID: 39012852

Devgan, K., Sharma, S., Jangra, D., & Sharma, S. (2025b). Artificial Intelligence-Enabled Apple Disease Monitoring System for environmental protection and resource conservation. In Advances in computational intelligence and robotics book series (pp. 271–300). https://doi.org/DOI: 10.4018/979-8-3373-3246-8.ch011

Devi, S., Merchant, Z. A. M., Siddiqui, M. S., & Lobo, M. (2019). Artificial intelligence based personal assistant. *Asian J. Converg. Technol.*, *5*(1), 1–4.

Devliyal, S., Goyal, H. R., & Sharma, S. (2025b). ICDRET: A dynamic cyber risk estimation technique for intelligent Cyber-Physical Systems in PCS. *The Open Bioinformatics Journal*, *18*(1). Advance online publication. DOI: 10.2174/0118750362380269250502062754

Dey, M. (2025, January 28). *Surgical Robotics Statistics and Facts*. Electro IQ. https://electroiq.com/stats/surgical-robotics-statistics-and-facts/

Dhagarra, D., Goswami, M., & Kumar, G. (2020). Impact of trust and privacy concerns on technology acceptance in healthcare: An Indian perspective. *International Journal of Medical Informatics*, *141*, 104164. PMID: 32593847

Dhar, M., Mittal, K., Pathania, M., & Kalra, S. (2023). Dehydration in Elderly: Revisiting the Assessment and Management Strategies. *The Journal of the Association of Physicians of India*, *71*(12), 47–50.

Di Sarno, C., Formicola, V., Sicuranza, M., & Paragliola, G. (2013). Addressing Security Issues of Electronic Health Record Systems through Enhanced SIEM Technology. *Proceedings of the 2013 International Conference on Availability, Reliability and Security*, 646–653.

Dinh-Le, C., Chuang, R., Chokshi, S., & Mann, D. (2019). Wearable health technology and electronic health record integration: Scoping review and future directions. *JMIR mHealth and uHealth*, *7*, e12861. PMID: 31512582

Dixit, P., & Silakari, S. (2021). Deep Learning Algorithms for Cybersecurity Applications: A Technological and Status Review. *Computer Science Review*, *39*, 100317.

Dixon, D.. (2024). Unveiling the influence of AI predictive analytics on patient outcomes: A comprehensive narrative review. *Cureus*, *16*(5), e59954. DOI: 10.7759/cureus.59954 PMID: 38854327

Dobbs, T. D., Cundy, O., Samarendra, H., Khan, K., & Whitaker, I. S. (2017). A Systematic Review of the Role of Robotics in Plastic and Reconstructive Surgery-From Inception to the Future. *Frontiers in Surgery*, *4*, 66. DOI: 10.3389/fsurg.2017.00066 PMID: 29188219

DocTime. (n.d.). *Online doctor consultation & telehealth in BD*. https://doctime.com.bd/

Doersch, C., Gupta, A., & Efros, A. A. (2015). Unsupervised visual representation learning by context prediction. *Proceedings of the IEEE International Conference on Computer Vision (ICCV)*, 1422–1430. DOI: 10.1109/ICCV.2015.167

Donahue, J., Krähenbühl, P., & Darrell, T. (2016). Adversarial feature learning. arXiv. https://arXiv.org/abs/1605.09782

Dong, J., Roth, A., & Su, W. J. (2022). Gaussian Differential Privacy. *J. R. Stat. Soc. Ser. B. Statistical Methodology*, *84*, 3–37.

Dong, T., Pires, N. M. M., Yang, Z., & Jiang, Z. (2022). Advances in electrochemical biosensors based on nanomaterials for protein biomarker detection in saliva. *Advancement of Science, 10*(6). Advance online publication. DOI: 10.1002/advs.202205429 PMID: 36585368

Dosovitskiy, A., Fischer, P., Springenberg, J. T., Riedmiller, M., & Brox, T. (2015). Discriminative unsupervised feature learning with exemplar convolutional neural networks. *IEEE Transactions on Pattern Analysis and Machine Intelligence, 38*(9), 1734–1747. DOI: 10.1109/TPAMI.2015.2496141

Dosovitskiy, A., Springenberg, J. T., Riedmiller, M., & Brox, T. (2014). Discriminative unsupervised feature learning with convolutional neural networks. *Advances in Neural Information Processing Systems, 27*, 766–774.

Doulgeris, J. J., Gonzalez-Blohm, S. A., Filis, A. K., Shea, T. M., Aghayev, K., & Vrionis, F. D. (2015). Robotics in Neurosurgery: Evolution, Current Challenges, and Compromises. *Cancer Control : Journal of the Moffitt Cancer Center, 22*(3), 352–359. DOI: 10.1177/107327481502200314 PMID: 26351892

Dowling, G., & Staelin, R. (1994). A model of perceived risk and intended risk-handling activity. *The Journal of Consumer Research, 21*, 119–134.

Dünnebeil, S., Sunyaev, A., Blohm, I., Leimeister, J. M., & Krcmar, H. (2012). Determinants of physicians' technology acceptance for e-health in ambulatory care. *International Journal of Medical Informatics, 81*(11), 746–760. PMID: 22397989

Duyck, P., Pynoo, B., Devolder, P., Voet, T., Adang, L., & Vercruysse, J. (2008). User acceptance of a picture archiving and communication system. Applying the unified theory of acceptance and use of technology in a radiological setting. *Methods of Information in Medicine, 47*, 149–156. PMID: 18338086

Dwivedi, Y. K.. (2022). Metaverse beyond the hype: Multidisciplinary perspectives on emerging challenges, opportunities, and agenda for research, practice and policy. *International Journal of Information Management, 66*, 102542. DOI: 10.1016/j.ijinfomgt.2022.102542

Dwork, C. (2006). Differential Privacy. In *International Colloquium On Automata, Languages, And Programming*. Springer.

Dwork, C., Mcsherry, F., Nissim, K., & Smith, A. (2006). Calibrating Noise To Sensitivity In Private Data Analysis. In *Proceedings Of The Theory Of Cryptography: Third Theory Of Cryptography Conference, Tcc 2006*. Springer.

Ebersole, J. L., Hasturk, H., Huber, M., Gellibolian, R., Markaryan, A., Zhang, X. D., & Miller, C. S. (2024). Realizing the clinical utility of saliva for monitoring oral diseases. *Periodontology 2000, 95*(1), 203–219. DOI: 10.1111/prd.12581 PMID: 39010260

Eckhardt, C. M., Madjarova, S. J., & Williams, R. J., & Others. (2022). Unsupervised machine learning methods and emerging applications in healthcare. *Knee Surgery, Sports Traumatology, Arthroscopy : Official Journal of the ESSKA, 31*(2), 376–387. DOI: 10.1007/s00167-022-07233-7

El Amrani, L., Engberink, A. O., Ninot, G., Hayot, M., & Carbonnel, F. (2017). Connected health devices for health care in French general medicine practice: Cross-sectional study. *JMIR mHealth and uHealth, 5*, e7427. PMID: 29269336

Eldakak, A., Alremeithi, A., & Dahiyat, E. (2024). Civil liability for the actions of autonomous AI in healthcare: An invitation to further contemplation. *Humanities & Social Sciences Communications, 11*, 305. DOI: 10.1057/s41599-024-02806-y

Emerging Nano-Theranostic Strategies against Non-Alcoholic Fatty Liver Disease: a review. (2023). *Iranian Journal Materials Science and Engineering* (Vols. 1–1, pp. 1–28). DOI: 10.22068/ijmse.2861

Ericsson, L., Gouk, H., & Hospedales, T. M. (2021). How well do self-supervised models transfer? *Proceedings of the IEEE/CVF Conference on Computer Vision and Pattern Recognition (CVPR)*, 5414–5423. DOI: 10.1109/CVPR46437.2021.00537

Esposito, C., Masieri, L., Di Mento, C., Cerulo, M., Del Conte, F., Coppola, V., & Escolino, M. (2025). Seven years of pediatric robotic-assisted surgery: Insights from 105 procedures. *Journal of Robotic Surgery, 19*(1), 157. DOI: 10.1007/s11701-025-02257-w PMID: 40232570

Fairag, M.. (2024). Robotic revolution in surgery: Diverse applications across specialties and future prospects review article. *Cureus, 16*(1), e52148. DOI: 10.7759/cureus.52148 PMID: 38344598

Fallica, A. (2022). Smart working: measurement of sustainability impact. Academic Press.

Fan, X., Wang, Y., Zhang, S., Xing, Y., Li, J., Ma, X., & Ma, J. (2025). Orthopedic surgical robotic systems in knee arthroplasty: A comprehensive review. *Frontiers in Bioengineering and Biotechnology, 13*, 1523631. DOI: 10.3389/fbioe.2025.1523631 PMID: 40051834

Farley, A., Wang, J., & Marshall, J. A. (2022). How to pick a mobile robot simulator: A quantitative comparison of CoppeliaSim, Gazebo, MORSE and Webots with a focus on accuracy of motion. *Simulation Modelling Practice and Theory, 120*, 102629.

Feather Staff. (2025, May 28). *HIPAA compliance guide for evaluating medical IoT devices*. AskFeather. Retrieved June 20, 2025, from https://www.askfeather.com/resources/hipaa-evaluation-of-medical-iot-devices

Featherman, M. S., & Pavlou, P. A. (2003). Predicting e-services adoption: A perceived risk facets perspective. *International Journal of Human-Computer Studies, 59*(4), 451–474.

Fedorov, A. (2021). Tasting the cake: Evaluating self-supervised generalization on out-of-distribution multimodal MRI data. *RobustML Workshop ICLR 2021*. DOI: 10.48550/arXiv.2103.12808

Felfeliyan, B., Forkert, N. D., Hareendranathan, A., Cornel, D., Zhou, Y., Kuntze, G., Jaremko, J. L., & Ronsky, J. L. (2023). Self-supervised-RCNN for medical image segmentation with limited data annotation. *Computerized Medical Imaging and Graphics, 109*, 102297. Advance online publication. DOI: 10.1016/j.compmedimag.2023.102297

Ferreira, D. C.. (2023). Patient satisfaction with healthcare services and the techniques used for its assessment: A systematic literature review and a bibliometric analysis. *Healthcare (Basel), 11*(5), 639. DOI: 10.3390/healthcare11050639 PMID: 36900644

Flatebø, S., Tran, V. N., Wang, C. E. A., & Bongo, L. A. (2024). Social robots in research on social and cognitive development in infants and toddlers: A scoping review. *PLoS One, 19*(5), e0303704. DOI: 10.1371/journal.pone.0303704 PMID: 38748722

Foster, C., Schinasi, D., Kan, K., Macy, M., Wheeler, D., & Curfman, A. (2022). Remote monitoring of patient-and family-generated health data in pediatrics. *Pediatrics, 149*, e2021054137. PMID: 35102417

Gaboriau, T., Dubois, R., Foucque, B., Malet, F., & Schweitzer, C. (2023). 24-Hour monitoring of intraocular pressure fluctuations using a contact lens sensor: Diagnostic performance for glaucoma progression. *Investigative Ophthalmology & Visual Science, 64*(3), 3. DOI: 10.1167/iovs.64.3.3 PMID: 36862120

Ganesh, S., Dhinakaran, A. K., Premnath, P., Venkatakrishnan, K., & Tan, B. (2023). Label-Free Saliva Test for Rapid Detection of Coronavirus Using Nanosensor-Enabled SERS. *Bioengineering (Basel, Switzerland), 10*(3), 391. DOI: 10.3390/bioengineering10030391 PMID: 36978782

Gao, C., Liu, X., Peven, M., Unberath, M., & Reiter, A. (2018). Learning to See Forces: Surgical Force Prediction with RGB-Point Cloud Temporal Convolutional Networks. In *Lecture notes in computer science* (pp. 118–127). DOI: 10.1007/978-3-030-01201-4_14

Gao, C., Zhang, X., & Liu, H. (2021). Data and knowledge-driven named entity recognition for cyber security. *Cybersecurity*, *4*, 9.

Gao, Z., Wanyama, T., Singh, I., Gadhrri, A., & Schmidt, R. (2020). From Industry 4.0 to Robotics 4.0 - A Conceptual Framework for Collaborative and Intelligent Robotic Systems. *Procedia Manufacturing*, *46*, 591–599. DOI: 10.1016/j.promfg.2020.03.085

Garcia-Rey, S., Gil-Hernandez, E., Gunatilake, U. B., Basabe-Desmonts, L., & Benito-Lopez, F. (2023). Development of an alginate/TiO2-based microfluidic biosystem for chrono-sampling and sensing of glucose in artificial sweat. *Sensors and Actuators. B, Chemical*, *382*, 133514. DOI: 10.1016/j.snb.2023.133514

Garg, M., Guo, H., Maclam, E., Zhanov, E., Samudrala, S., Pavlov, A., Rahman, M. S., Namkoong, M., Moreno, J. P., & Tian, L. (2024). Molecularly Imprinted Wearable Sensor with Paper Microfluidics for Real-Time Sweat Biomarker Analysis. *ACS Applied Materials & Interfaces*, *16*(35), 46113–46122. DOI: 10.1021/acsami.4c10033 PMID: 39178237

Gefen, D. (2003). TAM or just plain habit: A look at experienced online shoppers. *Journal of Organizational and End User Computing*, *15*(3), 1–13.

Gentry, C. (2009). Fully Homomorphic Encryption Using Ideal Lattices. *Proceedings Of The Forty-First Annual Acm Symposium On Theory Of Computing*, 169–178.

Gerber, M. J., Pettenkofer, M., & Hubschman, J.-P. (2020). Advanced robotic surgical systems in ophthalmology. *Eye*, *34*(9), 1554–1562. DOI: 10.1038/s41433-020-0837-9 PMID: 32152518

Germunden, H. G. (1985). Perceived risk and information search: A systematic meta-analysis of empirical evidence. *International Journal of Research in Marketing*, *2*, 79–100.

Ghaffarian, S. M., & Shahriari, H. R. (2017). Software Vulnerability Analysis and Discovery Using Machine-Learning and Data-Mining Techniques: A Survey. *ACM Computing Surveys*, *50*, 56.

Ghafouri, T., & Manavizadeh, N. (2023). A 3D-printed millifluidic device for triboelectricity-driven pH sensing based on ZnO nanosheets with super-Nernstian response. *Analytica Chimica Acta, 1267*, 341342. DOI: 10.1016/j.aca.2023.341342 PMID: 37257971

Ghorbian, M., Ghobaei-Arani, M., Babaei, M. R., & Ghorbian, S. (2025). Nanotechnology and nanosensors in personalized healthcare: A comprehensive review. *Sensing and Bio-Sensing Research, 100740*. Advance online publication. DOI: 10.1016/j.sbsr.2025.100740

Ghosh, T. N., Rotake, D., Kumar, S., Kaur, I., & Singh, S. G. (2023). Tear-based MMP-9 detection: A rapid antigen test for ocular inflammatory disorders using vanadium disulfide nanowires assisted chemi-resistive biosensor. *Analytica Chimica Acta, 1263*, 341281. DOI: 10.1016/j.aca.2023.341281 PMID: 37225335

Gidaris, S., Singh, P., & Komodakis, N. (2018). Unsupervised representation learning by predicting image rotations. arXiv. https://arXiv.org/abs/1803.07728

Goetz, L. H.. (2018). Personalized medicine: Motivation, challenges, and progress. *Fertility and Sterility*, *109*(6), 952–963. DOI: 10.1016/j.fertnstert.2018.05.006 PMID: 29935653

Goharinejad, S., Goharinejad, S., Hajesmaeel-Gohari, S., & Bahaadinbeigy, K. (2022). The usefulness of virtual, augmented, and mixed reality technologies in the diagnosis and treatment of attention deficit hyperactivity disorder in children: An overview of relevant studies. *BMC Psychiatry*, *22*, 1–13. PMID: 34983446

Goldberg, S. G., Johnson, G. A., & Shriver, S. K. (2024). Regulating Privacy Online: An Economic Evaluation Of The Gdpr. *American Economic Journal. Economic Policy*, *16*, 325–358.

Goodfellow, I., Pouget-Abadie, J., Mirza, M., Xu, B., Warde-Farley, D., Ozair, S., Courville, A., & Bengio, Y. (2014). Generative adversarial nets. *Advances in Neural Information Processing Systems*, *27*, 2672–2680.

Goud, N. (2017). *Malware and Ransomware Attack on Medical Devices*. Cybersecurity Insiders.

Grewal, D., Gotlieb, J., & Marmorstein, H. (1994). The moderating effects of message framing and source credibility on the price-perceived risk relationship. *The Journal of Consumer Research*, *21*, 145–153.

Grill, J.-B., Strub, F., Altché, F., Tallec, C., Richemond, P., Buchatskaya, E., & Doersch, C., & Others. (2020). Bootstrap your own latent: A new approach to self-supervised learning. *Advances in Neural Information Processing Systems*, *33*, 21271–21284.

Guanais, F., Doubova, S. V., Leslie, H. H., Perez-Cuevas, R., Garcia-Elorrio, E., & Kruk, M. E. (2018). Patient-centered primary care and self-rated health in 6 Latin American and Caribbean countries: Analysis of a public opinion cross-sectional survey. *PLoS Medicine*, *15*, e1002673. PMID: 30300422

Guang, P., Huang, W., Guo, L., Yang, X., Huang, F., Yang, M., Wen, W., & Li, L. (2020). Blood-based FTIR-ATR spectroscopy coupled with extreme gradient boosting for the diagnosis of type 2 diabetes. *Medicine*, *99*(15), e19657. DOI: 10.1097/md.0000000000019657 PMID: 32282717

Guarducci, S., Jayousi, S., Caputo, S., & Mucchi, L. (2025). Key Fundamentals and Examples of Sensors for Human Health: Wearable, Non-Continuous, and Non-Contact Monitoring Devices. *Sensors (Basel)*, *25*(2), 556.

Gudiño-Ochoa, A., García-Rodríguez, J. A., Ochoa-Ornelas, R., Cuevas-Chávez, J. I., & Sánchez-Arias, D. A. (2024). Noninvasive Diabetes Detection through Human Breath Using TinyML-Powered E-Nose. *Sensors (Basel)*, *24*(4), 1294. DOI: 10.3390/s24041294 PMID: 38400451

Gu, J., Wang, Z., Kuen, J., Ma, L., Shahroudy, A., Shuai, B., Liu, T., Wang, X., Wang, G., Cai, J., & Chen, T. (2018). Recent advances in convolutional neural networks. *Pattern Recognition*, *77*, 354–377. DOI: 10.1016/j.patcog.2017.10.013

Gul, F., Rahiman, W., & Nazli Alhady, S. S. (2019). A comprehensive study for robot navigation techniques. *Cogent Engineering*, *6*(1), 1632046. DOI: 10.1080/23311916.2019.1632046

Gupta, K., Sharma, D. K., Datta Gupta, K., & Kumar, A. (2022). A Tree Classifier Based Network Intrusion Detection Model for Internet of Medical Things. *Computers & Electrical Engineering*, *102*, 108158.

Gyles, C. (2019). Robots in medicine. *The Canadian Veterinary Journal = La Revue Vétérinaire Canadienne*, *60*(8), 819–820. PMID: 31391598

Hady, A.A., Ghubaish, A., Salman, T., Unal, D., & Jain, R. (2020). Intrusion Detection System for Healthcare Systems Using Medical and Network Data: A Comparison Study. IEEE Access, 8, 106576–106584.

Haghighi, F., Taher, M. R. H., Zhou, Z., Gotway, M. B., & Liang, J. (2021). Transferable visual words: Exploiting the semantics of anatomical patterns for self-supervised learning. *IEEE Transactions on Medical Imaging*, *40*(10), 2857–2868. DOI: 10.1109/TMI.2021.3067770

Halperin, D., Heydt-Benjamin, T. S., Ransford, B., Clark, S. S., Defend, B., Morgan, W., Fu, K., Kohno, T., & Maisel, W. H. (2008). Pacemakers and implantable cardiac defibrillators: Software radio attacks and zero-power defenses. *Proceedings of the 2008 IEEE Symposium on Security and Privacy*, 129–142.

Hamza, R., & Pradana, H. (2022). A Survey Of Intellectual Property Rights Protection In Big Data Applications. *Algorithms*, *15*, 418.

Han, S., Mustonen, P., Seppänen, M., & Kallio, M. (2005). *Does fragmenting of working time and working space influence the acceptance of mobile technology? A case of Finnish physicians*. Turku Centre for Computer Science.

Han, T., Xie, W., & Zisserman, A. (2020). Memory-augmented dense predictive coding for video representation learning. In *Computer vision – ECCV 2020* (pp. 312–329). Springer. DOI: 10.1007/978-3-030-58517-4_19

Hao, H., Didari, S., Woo, J. O., Moon, H., & Bangert, P. (2021). Highly efficient representation and active learning framework for imbalanced data and its application to COVID-19 X-ray classification. *Conference on Neural Information Processing Systems (NeurIPS 2021)*. DOI: 10.48550/arXiv.2012.04376

Haque, N. I., Rahman, M. A., Shahriar, M. H., Khalil, A. A., & Uluagac, A. S. (2021). A Novel Framework for Threat Analysis of Machine Learning-based Smart Healthcare Systems. arXiv:2103.03472.

Harky, A., & Hussain, S. M. A. (2019). Robotic Cardiac Surgery: The Future Gold Standard or An Unnecessary Extravagance? *Braz J Cardiovasc Surg, 34*(4), xii-xiii. DOI: 10.21470/1678-9741-2019-0194

Hart, L. A., Vo, S., Hanlon, J. T., Schmader, K. E., & Gray, S. L. (2025). Medication Use Quality and Safety in Older Adults: 2023 Update. *Journal of the American Geriatrics Society*.

Hasan, M. K., Ghazal, T. M., Saeed, R. A., Pandey, B., Gohel, H., Eshmawi, A., Abdel-Khalek, S., & Alkhassawneh, H. M. (2022). A Review On Security Threats, Vulnerabilities, And Counter Measures Of 5g Enabled Internet-Of-Medical-Things. *IET Communications*, *16*, 421–432.

Hassan, A., Sirshar, M., Akram, M. U., & Farooq, M. U. (2022). Analysis of multimodal representation learning across medical images and reports using multiple vision and language pre-trained models. *19th International Bhurban Conference on Applied Sciences and Technology (IBCAST)*, 337–342. DOI: 10.1109/IBCAST54850.2022.9990154

Hill, M. G., Sim, M., & Mills, B. (2020). The quality of diagnosis and triage advice provided by free online symptom checkers and apps in Australia. *The Medical Journal of Australia, 212*(11), 514–519.

Hirani, R., Noruzi, K., Khuram, H., Hussaini, A. S., Aifuwa, E. I., Ely, K. E., Lewis, J. M., Gabr, A. E., Smiley, A., Tiwari, R. K., & Etienne, M. (2024). Artificial Intelligence and Healthcare: A Journey through History, Present Innovations, and Future Possibilities. *Life (Chicago, Ill.), 14*(5), 557. DOI: 10.3390/life14050557 PMID: 38792579

Hoagland, A.. (2024). Challenges in promoting health equity and reducing disparities in access across new and established technologies. *The Canadian Journal of Cardiology, 40*(6), 1154–1167. DOI: 10.1016/j.cjca.2024.02.014 PMID: 38417572

Hofman, P. (2024). Liquid and tissue biopsies for lung cancer: Algorithms and perspectives. *Cancers (Basel), 16*(19), 3340. DOI: 10.3390/cancers16193340 PMID: 39409960

Holm, E. A. (2019). In defense of the black box. *Science, 364*, 26–27.

Hooshiar, M. H., Moghaddam, M. A., Kiarashi, M., Al-Hijazi, A. Y., & Hussein, A. F., Aalrikabi, H., Salari, S., Esmaelian, S., Mesgari, H., & Yasamineh, S. (2024). Recent advances in nanomaterial-based biosensor for periodontitis detection. *Journal of Biological Engineering, 18*(1). Advance online publication. DOI: 10.1186/s13036-024-00423-6 PMID: 38637787

Horan, T. A., Tulu, B., Hilton, B., & Burton, J. (2004) Use of online systems in clinical medical assessments: an analysis of physician acceptance of online disability evaluation systems. In: *Proceedings of the 37th Hawaii international conference on system sciences*; p. 1–10.

Hospital Management Asia. (2024, March 28). *Samsung Medical Centre's path to smart healthcare.* Retrieved June 23, 2025, from https://www.hospitalmanagementasia.com/tech-innovation/samsung-medical-centres-path-to-smart-healthcare/

Hossain, G. M. M., Jalal, A. H., Pala, N., & Alam, F. (2024a). Advancements in Glucose Monitoring: A Thin Film ZnO-Nanoflakes Based Highly Sensitive Wearable Biosensor for Noninvasive Sweat-Based Point-of-Care Monitoring for Diabetes. *ECS Transactions, 113*(13), 35–42. DOI: 10.1149/11313.0035ecst

Hossain, N. I., Sharma, A., & Sonkusale, S. (2023a). A wearable and multiplexed electrochemical sensor suite for Real-Time sweat ionic content and pH monitoring with IoT integration. *IEEE Sensors Letters*, *7*(9), 1–4. DOI: 10.1109/lsens.2023.3300827

Hsieh, W.-T., Lefort-Besnard, J., Yang, H.-C., Kuo, L.-W., & Lee, C.-C. (2020). Behavior score-embedded brain encoder network for improved classification of Alzheimer disease using resting state fMRI. *2020 42nd Annual International Conference of the IEEE Engineering in Medicine & Biology Society (EMBC)*, 5486–5489. DOI: 10.1109/EMBC44109.2020.9175690

Huang, Y., Upadhyay, U., Dhar, E., Kuo, L. J., & Syed-Abdul, S. (2022). A Scoping Review to Assess Adherence to and Clinical Outcomes of Wearable Devices in the Cancer Population. *Cancers (Basel)*, *14*, 4437. PMID: 36139602

Hu, B. (2023). Mass spectrometric analysis of exhaled breath: Recent advances and future perspectives. *Trends in Analytical Chemistry*, *168*, 117320. DOI: 10.1016/j.trac.2023.117320

Hu, H., Cui, J., & Wang, L. (2021). Region-aware contrastive learning for semantic segmentation. *Proceedings of the IEEE/CVF International Conference on Computer Vision (ICCV)*, 16291–16301. DOI: 10.1109/ICCV48922.2021.01599

Hull, S. (2015). Patient-generated health data foundation for personalized collaborative care. *CIN Comput. Inform. Nurs.*, *33*, 177–180. PMID: 25974360

Hunt, L. M., Bell, H. S., Baker, A. M., & Howard, H. A. (2017). Electronic health records and the disappearing patient. *Medical Anthropology Quarterly*, *31*, 403–421. PMID: 28370246

Hu, P. J. H., Chau, P. Y. K., Sheng, O. R. L., & Tam, K. Y. (1999). Examining the technology acceptance model using physician acceptance of telemedicine technology. *Journal of Management Information Systems*, *16*, 91–112.

Hu, R., Longo, U. G., Pittman, J., & Nazarian, A. (2025). Robotic Innovations in Orthopedics: A Growing Landscape, Challenges, and Implications for Care. *Osteology*, *5*(2), 13. https://www.mdpi.com/2673-4036/5/2/13

Hu, T., Khishe, M., Mohammadi, M., Parvizi, G.-R., Taher Karim, S. H., & Rashid, T. A. (2021). Real-time COVID-19 diagnosis from X-ray images using deep CNN and extreme learning machines stabilized by chimp optimization algorithm. *Biomedical Signal Processing and Control*, *68*, 102764. Advance online publication. DOI: 10.1016/j.bspc.2021.102764

Hu, V., Chen, E., Bridgeman, M., & Jariwala, S. (2022). Utility of Patient-Generated Health Data and Artificial Intelligence in the Prediction of Asthma Exacerbations. *The Journal of Allergy and Clinical Immunology*, *149*, AB185.

Hu, X., Mao, N., Yan, X., Huang, L., Liu, X., Yang, H., Sun, Q., Liu, X., & Jia, H. (2024). Non-invasive healthcare analytical platform based on organic electrochemical transistors. *Chemical Research in Chinese Universities*. Advance online publication. DOI: 10.1007/s40242-024-4176-4

Iftikhar, M.. (2024). Artificial intelligence: Revolutionizing robotic surgery [Review]. *Annals of Medicine and Surgery (London), 86*(9), 5401–5409. DOI: 10.1097/MS9.0000000000002426 PMID: 39238994

Iliashenko, O., Bikkulova, Z., & Dubgorn, A. (2019). Opportunities and challenges of artificial intelligence in healthcare. In *E3S Web of Conferences* (Vol. 110, p. 02028). EDP Sciences.

Ireland, S. G. (2022). A Study on the Need for Investment in Employee Wellbeing in Small and Medium Enterprises (SMEs) In Bangalore, India.

Islam, P. (2024). Nanotechnology in development of next generation of stent and related medical devices: Current and future aspects. *Wiley Interdisciplinary Reviews: Nanomedicine and Nanobiotechnology, 16*(2), Article e1941. DOI: 10.1002/wnan.1941

Islam, S., Papastergiou, S., & Mouratidis, H. (2021). A Dynamic Cyber Security Situational Awareness Framework for Healthcare ICT Infrastructures. In *Proceedings of the PCI 2021: 25th Pan-Hellenic Conference on Informatics*. ACM.

Islam, S., Abba, A., Ismail, U., Mouratidis, H., & Papastergiou, S. (2022). Vulnerability prediction for secure healthcare supply chain service delivery. *Integrated Computer-Aided Engineering, 29*, 389–409.

Islam, S., Papastergiou, S., Kalogeraki, E. M., & Kioskli, K. (2022). Cyberattack Path Generation and Prioritisation for Securing Healthcare Systems. *Applied Sciences (Basel, Switzerland), 12*, 4443.

Jahangiri-Manesh, A., Mousazadeh, M., & Nikkhah, M. (2022a). Fabrication of chemiresistive nanosensor using molecularly imprinted polymers for acetone detection in gaseous state. *Iranian Polymer Journal, 31*(7), 883–891. DOI: 10.1007/s13726-022-01044-w

Jaiswal, A., Babu, A. R., Zadeh, M. Z., Banerjee, D., & Makedon, F. (2020). A survey on contrastive self-supervised learning. *Technologies, 9*(1), 2. Advance online publication. DOI: 10.3390/technologies9010002

Jana, A. (2021). Liver fibrosis and NAS scoring from CT images using self-supervised learning and texture encoding. *2021 IEEE 18th International Symposium on Biomedical Imaging (ISBI)*, 1553–1557. DOI: 10.1109/ISBI48211.2021.9433783

Jang, H., Sharma, A. B., Dan, U., Wong, J. H., Knight, Z. A., & Garrison, J. L. (2024). Dysregulation of the fluid homeostasis system by aging. *bioRxiv*.

Javaid, M.. (2022). Significance of machine learning in healthcare: Features, pillars and applications. *International Journal of Intelligent Networks, 3*, 58–73. DOI: 10.1016/j.ijin.2022.05.002

Javaid, M., Haleem, A., Pratap Singh, R., Rab, S., Suman, R., & Kumar, L. (2025). Utilization of Robotics for Healthcare: A Scoping Review. *Journal of Industrial Integration and Management, 10*(01), 43–65. DOI: 10.1142/s2424862222500154

Jayakumar, M., Jenefa, L., Dulloo, R., Jose, J. S., & Kumar, A. (2025, March). Smart and Sustainable Tourism Development: Contention convenience and accessibility using Artificial Intelligence, Internet of Things, Augmented Reality and Virtual Reality Technologies. In *2025 International Conference on Data Science, Agents & Artificial Intelligence (ICDSAAI)* (pp. 1-6). IEEE.

Jayakumar, M., Jenefa, L., Mishra, N., Kumar, A., & Sumitha, S. (2024, December). Artificial Intelligence In Digital Marketing Platform: Impact In Consumer Buying Behaviour. In *2024 International Conference on Emerging Research in Computational Science (ICERCS)* (pp. 1-6). IEEE.

Jenefa, L., Jayakumar, M., Catherine, S., Kumar, S. A., Tripathi, R., & Jeevitha, M. The Application of Artificial Intelligence and Robotics in Healthcare Services. In *Revolutionizing Healthcare Services* (pp. 27–45). CRC Press.

Jenefa, L., Kanchana, K., Jayakumar, M., & Kumar, A. (2024, December). The Impact of Artificial Intelligence for Developing Supply Chain Collaboration Performance: An Empirical Investigation. In *2024 International Conference on Emerging Research in Computational Science (ICERCS)* (pp. 1-4). IEEE.

Jenefa, L., & Ravikumar, S. (2024, September). Improving Diagnosis and Classification of Severity in Diabetic Retinopathy Using Transfer Learning. In *2024 International Conference on Integration of Emerging Technologies for the Digital World (ICIETDW)* (pp. 1-5). IEEE.

Jeon, H., Lee, W., Park, H., Lee, H., Kim, S., Kim, H., Jeon, B., & Park, K. (2017). Correction: Automatic classification of tremor severity in Parkinson's disease using a wearable device. Sensors 2017, 17, 2067. *Sensors (Basel), 18*(1), 33. DOI: 10.3390/s18010033 PMID: 29295543

Jeshuram, S. B., Ebenzer, K., & Jenefa, L. (2019). An Empirical Study on satisfaction towards selected herbal medicines. *History Research Journal, 5*, 30–36.

Jha, P., & Chaurasia, B. (2024). The art of neurosurgery: Precision beyond machines. *Annals of Medicine and Surgery (London), 86*(8), 4325–4326. DOI: 10.1097/ms9.0000000000002280 PMID: 39118761

Jian, G.-Z., Lin, G.-S., Wang, C.-M., & Yan, S.-L. (2021). Helicobacter pylori infection classification based on convolutional neural network and self-supervised learning. *2021 5th International Conference on Graphics and Signal Processing*, 60–64. DOI: 10.1145/3474906.3474915

Jin, C., Yang, S., Zheng, J., Chai, F., & Tian, M. (2024). Paper-based triple-readout nanosensor for point-of-care detection of glucose in urine. *Biosensors & Bioelectronics, 269*, 116931. DOI: 10.1016/j.bios.2024.116931 PMID: 39549311

Jing, L., & Tian, Y. (2020). Self-supervised visual feature learning with deep neural networks: A survey. *IEEE Transactions on Pattern Analysis and Machine Intelligence, 43*(11), 4037–4058. DOI: 10.1109/TPAMI.2020.2992393

Johnson, K. B.. (2020). Precision medicine, AI, and the future of personalized health care. *Clinical and Translational Science, 14*(1), 86–93. DOI: 10.1111/cts.12884 PMID: 32961010

Jordaens, S., Zwaenepoel, K., Tjalma, W., Deben, C., Beyers, K., Vankerckhoven, V., Pauwels, P., & Vorsters, A. (2023a). Urine biomarkers in cancer detection: A systematic review of preanalytical parameters and applied methods. *International Journal of Cancer, 152*(10), 2186–2205. DOI: 10.1002/ijc.34434 PMID: 36647333

Junaid, B. S.. (2022). Recent advancements in emerging technologies for healthcare management systems: A survey. *Healthcare (Basel), 10*(10), 1940. DOI: 10.3390/healthcare10101940 PMID: 36292387

Jung, Y., Kim, S., & Choi, B. (2016). Consumer valuation of the wearables: The case of smartwatches. *Computers in Human Behavior, 63*, 899–905.

Kadian, S., Kumari, P., Shukla, S., & Narayan, R. (2023). Recent advancements in machine learning enabled portable and wearable biosensors. *Talanta Open, 8*, 100267. DOI: 10.1016/j.talo.2023.100267

Kaissis, G. A., Makowski, M. R., Rückert, D., & Braren, R. F. (2020). Secure, Privacy-Preserving And Federated Machine Learning In Medical Imaging. *Nature Machine Intelligence, 2*, 305–311.

Kalra, N., Verma, P., & Verma, S. (2024). Advancements in AI based healthcare techniques with focus on diagnostic techniques. *Computers in Biology and Medicine, 179*, 108917. Advance online publication. DOI: 10.1016/j.compbiomed.2024.108917

Kapoor, A., Deguet, A., & Kazanzides, P. (2006). Software components and frameworks for medical robot control. *Proceedings 2006 IEEE International Conference on Robotics and Automation, 2006. ICRA 2006.*

Kapruwan, A., Sharma, S., & Goyal, H. R. (2025). ESCBR: Expert System Enabled Case-based Reasoning Approach in IDDCS for CIND. *Recent Patents on Engineering, 19.* Advance online publication. DOI: 10.2174/0118722121336689250116074945

Karahanna, E., Agarwal, R., & Angst, C. (2006). Reconceptualizing compatibility beliefs in technology acceptance research. *Management Information Systems Quarterly, 30*(4), 781–804.

Karnam, S. (2020). Self-supervised learning for segmentation using image reconstruction [Unpublished master's thesis]. Rochester Institute of Technology.

Kashani, M. H., Madanipour, M., Nikravan, M., Asghari, P., & Mahdipour, E. (2021). A systematic review of IoT in healthcare: Applications, techniques, and trends. *Journal of Network and Computer Applications, 192*, 103164.

Kaushik, K., Dahiya, S., & Sharma, R. (2021). Internet of things advancements in healthcare. In *Internet of things* (pp. 19–32). CRC Press.

Keil, M., Beranek, P., & Konsynski, B. (1995). Usefulness and ease of use: Field study evidence regarding tasks considerations. *Decision Support Systems, 13*(1), 75–91.

Ke, J., Shen, Y., Liang, X., & Shen, D. (2021). Contrastive learning based stain normalization across multiple tumor in histopathology. In *MICCAI 2021* (pp. 571–580). Medical image computing and computer assisted intervention. Springer. DOI: 10.1007/978-3-030-87199-4_54

Keras Team. (n.d.). Building autoencoders in Keras. Retrieved October 13, 2025, from https://blog.keras.io/building-autoencoders-in-keras.html

Kharitonov, E., Rivière, M., Synnaeve, G., Wolf, L., Mazaré, P.-E., Douze, M., & Dupoux, E. (2021). Data augmenting contrastive learning of speech representations in the time domain. *2021 IEEE Spoken Language Technology Workshop (SLT)*, 215–222. DOI: 10.1109/SLT48900.2021.9383605

Khatiwada, P., & Yang, B. (2022). *An Overview on Security and Privacy of Data in IoMT Devices: Performance Metrics, Merits, Demerits, and Challenges*. pHealth.

Kiio, L. K., Onyatta, J. O., Ndangili, P. M., Oloo, F., Santamaria, C., Montuenga, L. M., & Mbui, D. N. (2023). Ultrasensitive immunosensor for multiplex detection of cancer biomarkers carcinoembryonic antigen (CEA) and yamaguchi sarcoma viral oncogene homolog 1 (YES1) based on eco-friendly synthesized gold nanoparticles. *Talanta*, *266*, 124934. DOI: 10.1016/j.talanta.2023.124934 PMID: 37454512

Kim, H., Awofeso, O., Choi, S., Jung, Y., & Bae, E. (2016). Colorimetric analysis of saliva–alcohol test strips by smartphone-based instruments using machine-learning algorithms. *Applied Optics*, *56*(1), 84. DOI: 10.1364/ao.56.000084

Kim, K. K., Jalil, S., & Ngo, V. (2019). Improving self-management and care coordination with person-generated health data and mobile health. In *Consumer Informatics and Digital Health: Solutions for Health and Health Care* (pp. 221–243). Springer.

Kingma, D. P., & Welling, M. (2013). Auto-encoding variational bayes. arXiv. https://arXiv.org/abs/1312.6114

Knott, B., Venkataraman, S., Hannun, A., Sengupta, S., Ibrahim, M., & Van Der Maaten, L. (2021). Crypten: Secure Multi-Party Computation Meets Machine Learning. *Advances in Neural Information Processing Systems*, *34*, 4961–4973.

Ko, E., Sung, H., & Yun, H. (2009). Comparative Analysis of Purchase Intentions Toward Smart Clothing Between Korean and US Consumers. *Clothing & Textiles Research Journal*, *27*(4), 259–273.

Koh, A., Kang, D., Xue, Y., Lee, S., Pielak, R. M., Kim, J., Hwang, T., Min, S., Banks, A., Bastien, P., Manco, M. C., Wang, L., Ammann, K. R., Jang, K., Won, P., Han, S., Ghaffari, R., Paik, U., Slepian, M. J., & Rogers, J. A. (2016). A soft, wearable microfluidic device for the capture, storage, and colorimetric sensing of sweat. *Science Translational Medicine*, *8*(366). Advance online publication. DOI: 10.1126/scitranslmed.aaf2593 PMID: 27881826

Kohli, P., & Sharma, S. (2025b). EDGE Artificial Intelligence-Enabled 6G communication security system for connected vehicles in revolutionizing urban development and governance. In IGI Global eBooks (pp. 431–462). https://doi.org/DOI: 10.4018/979-8-3373-1375-7.ch015

Kondo, M., & Sonenshein, S. (2020). *Joy at work: Organizing your professional life*. Pan Macmillan.

Kong, X.. (2023). Advances of medical nanorobots for future cancer treatments. *Journal of Hematology & Oncology*, *16*(1), 74. DOI: 10.1186/s13045-023-01463-z PMID: 37452423

Kopalli, S. R.. (2025). Artificial intelligence in stroke rehabilitation: From acute care to long-term recovery. *Neuroscience*, *572*, 214–231. DOI: 10.1016/j.neuroscience.2025.03.017 PMID: 40068721

Korjian, S., & Gibson, C. M. (2022). Digital technologies and the democratization of clinical research: Social media, wearables, and artificial intelligence. *Contemporary Clinical Trials*, *117*, 106767. PMID: 35462032

Koukourikis, P., & Rha, K. H. (2021). Robotic surgical systems in urology: What is currently available? *Investigative and Clinical Urology*, *62*(1), 14–22. DOI: 10.4111/icu.20200387 PMID: 33381927

Krishnamoorthy, G., & Sistla, S. M. K. (2023). Exploring Machine Learning Intrusion Detection: Addressing security and Privacy Challenges in IoT - A Comprehensive review. *Journal of Knowledge Learning and Science Technology, 2*(2), 114–125. DOI: 10.60087/jklst.vol2.n2.p125

Krist, A. H., Tong, S. T., Aycock, R. A., & Longo, D. R. (2017). Engaging patients in decision-making and behavior change to promote prevention. *Information Services & Use*, *37*, 105–122. PMID: 28972524

Kubota, T., Ogawa, K., Yoshikawa, Y., & Ishiguro, H. (2022). Alignment of the attitude of teleoperators with that of a semi-autonomous android. *Scientific Reports*, *12*(1), 10473. DOI: 10.1038/s41598-022-13829-3 PMID: 35760935

Kumar, A., & Deepak, G. (2020). HeTOnto: A Novel Approach for Conceptualization, Modeling, Visualization, and Formalization of Domain Centric Ontologies for Heat Transfer. *Proceedings of the CONECCT 2020—6th IEEE International Conference on Electronics, Computing and Communication Technologies*, 1–6.

Kumar, D., Ram, R., & Sarkar, A. (2023). A smartphone enabled low-cost portable centrifuge integrated with a simple paper-based device for the estimation of plasma-albumin concentration. *Microchemical Journal*, *197*, 109822. DOI: 10.1016/j.microc.2023.109822

Kumari, M., Kumar, D., Bhattacharyya, R., & Banerjee, D. (2024). Whether Dye-Based methods are ready for microalbuminuria detection: A review of research in the field. *Indian Journal of Clinical Biochemistry : IJCB*. Advance online publication. DOI: 10.1007/s12291-024-01213-z

Kumari, S., Islam, M., & Gupta, A. (2023). Paper-based multiplex biosensors for inexpensive healthcare diagnostics: A comprehensive review. *Biomedical Microdevices*, *25*(2). Advance online publication. DOI: 10.1007/s10544-023-00656-0 PMID: 37133791

Kumari, S., Samara, M., Ramachandran, R. A., Gosh, S., George, H., Wang, R., Pesavento, R. P., & Mathew, M. T. (2023a). A review on Saliva-Based Health Diagnostics: Biomarker selection and future directions. *Deleted Journal*, *2*(1), 121–138. DOI: 10.1007/s44174-023-00090-z PMID: 37363139

Kumar, K. P.. (2024). Secure approach to sharing digitized medical data in a cloud environment. *Data Science and Management*, *7*(2), 108–118. DOI: 10.1016/j.dsm.2023.12.001

Kumar, P., Gupta, G. P., & Tripathi, R. (2021). An Ensemble Learning and Fog-Cloud Architecture-Driven Cyber-Attack Detection Framework for IoMT Networks. *Computer Communications*, *166*, 110–124.

Kumar, S., Singh, H., Feder-Kubis, J., & Nguyen, D. D. (2023). Recent advances in nanobiosensors for sustainable healthcare applications: A systematic literature review. *Environmental Research*, *238*, 117177. DOI: 10.1016/j.envres.2023.117177 PMID: 37751831

Kumar, Y., Koul, A., Singla, R., & Ijaz, M. F. (2023). Artificial intelligence in disease diagnosis: A systematic literature review, synthesizing framework and future research agenda. *Journal of Ambient Intelligence and Humanized Computing*, *14*(7), 8459–8486.

Kuwait Computer Services. (2024, March). *Smart IoT solution for hospital & health care*. Retrieved from https://www.kcs.com.kw/wp-content/uploads/2024/03/kcs_kuwait_iot_smart_hospital_monitoring.pdf

Kuwait Direct Investment Promotion Authority. (2022, June). *Sector opportunities*. Retrieved June 23, 2025, from https://kdipa.gov.kw/wp-content/uploads/2022/06/Sector-Opportunities-June2022.pdf

Kyrarini, M.. (2021). A survey of robots in healthcare. *Technologies*, *9*, 8. DOI: 10.3390/technologies9010008

Lavallee, D. C., Lee, J. R., Austin, E., Bloch, R., Lawrence, S. O., McCall, D., Munson, S. A., Nery-Hurwit, M. B., & Amtmann, D. (2020). mHealth and patient-generated health data: Stakeholder perspectives on opportunities and barriers for transforming healthcare. *mHealth*, *6*, 8. PMID: 32190619

Lederer, A., Maupin, D., Sena, M., & Zhuang, Y. (2000). The technology acceptance model and the World Wide Web. *Decision Support Systems*, *29*, 269–282.

Lee, J.W., Kang, H., Lee, Y., Choi, W., Eom, J., Deryabin, M., Lee, E., Lee, J., Yoo, D., & Kim, Y.S. (2022). Privacy-Preserving Machine Learning With Fully Homomorphic Encryption For Deep Neural Network. *IEEE Access, 10*, 30039–30054.

Lee, B., Lee, J., Lee, J., Hwang, Y., Bahn, H., Park, I., Jheon, S., & Lee, D. (2024). Breath analysis system with convolutional neural network (CNN) for early detection of lung cancer. *Sensors and Actuators. B, Chemical, 409*, 135578. DOI: 10.1016/j.snb.2024.135578

Lee, M. C. (2009). Factors influencing the adoption of internet banking: An integration of TAM and TPB with perceived risk and perceived benefit. *Electronic Commerce Research and Applications, 8*(3), 130–141.

Legris, P., Ingham, J., & Collerette, P. (2003). Why do people use information technology? A critical review of the technology acceptance model. *Information & Management, 40*(3), 191–204.

Lehne, M., & Sass, J. (2019). Essen wanger A, Schepers J, Thun S. Why digital medicine depends on interoperability. *Digital Medicine, 2*, 1–5.

Lengyel, B. C., Chinnadurai, P., Corr, S. J., Lumsden, A. B., & Bavare, C. S. (2024). Robot-assisted vascular surgery: Literature review, clinical applications, and future perspectives. *Journal of Robotic Surgery, 18*(1), 328. DOI: 10.1007/s11701-024-02087-2 PMID: 39174843

Leung, T., & Vyas, D. (2014). Robotic Surgery: Applications. *American Journal of Robotic Surgery, 1*(1), 1–64. PMID: 26501128

Li, Q., Ren, J., Zhang, Y., Song, C., Liao, Y., & Zhang, Y. (2023). Privacy-Preserving Dnn Training With Prefetched Meta-Keys On Heterogeneous Neural Network Accelerators. *Proceedings Of The Ieee 2023 60th Acm/Ieee Design Automation Conference (Dac),* 1–6.

Liao, C., Chen, X., & Fu, Y. (2023). Salivary analysis: An emerging paradigm for non-invasive healthcare diagnosis and monitoring. *Deleted Journal, 1*(3). Advance online publication. DOI: 10.1002/inmd.20230009

Li, C.. (2024). A review of IoT applications in healthcare. *Neurocomputing, 565*, 127017. DOI: 10.1016/j.neucom.2023.127017

Licci, M., Thieringer, F. M., Guzman, R., & Soleman, J. (2020). Development and validation of a synthetic 3D-printed simulator for training in neuroendoscopic ventricular lesion removal. *Neurosurgical Focus, 48*(3), E18.

Li, H., Ota, K., & Dong, M. (2018). Learning IoT in Edge: Deep Learning for the Internet of Things with Edge Computing. *IEEE Network, 32*, 96–101.

Li, M., & Others. (2025). Enhancing medical vision-language contrastive learning via inter-matching relation modelling. *IEEE Transactions on Medical Imaging*. Advance online publication. DOI: 10.1109/TMI.2024.3426738

Li, Q., & Zhang, Y. (2024). Confidential Federated Learning For Heterogeneous Platforms Against Client-Side Privacy Leakages. *Proceedings Of The Acm Turing Award Celebration Conference*, 239–241.

Liu, C., & Others. (2021). TN-USMA Net: Triple normalization-based gastrointestinal stromal tumors classification on multicenter EUS images with ultrasound-specific pretraining and meta attention. *Medical Physics*, *48*(11), 7199–7214. DOI: 10.1002/mp.15228

Liu, L., & Ma, Q. (2006). Perceived system performance: A test of an extended technology acceptance model. *The Data Base for Advances in Information Systems*, *37*, 51–59.

Liu, L., Stroulia, E., Nikolaidis, I., Miguel-Cruz, A., & Rincon, A. R. (2016). Smart homes and home health monitoring technologies for older adults: A systematic review. *International Journal of Medical Informatics*, *91*, 44–59. PMID: 27185508

Liu, T., Dong, Y., Chen, S., Zhou, J., Ma, Z., & Li, J. (2022). Battery-free, tuning circuit–inspired wireless sensor systems for detection of multiple biomarkers in bodily fluids. *Science Advances*, *8*(27). Advance online publication. DOI: 10.1126/sciadv.abo7049 PMID: 35857473

Liu, X., Liu, F., Jin, L., & Wu, J. (2024). Evolution of Neurosurgical Robots: Historical Progress and Future Direction. *World Neurosurgery*, *191*, 49–57. DOI: 10.1016/j.wneu.2024.08.008 PMID: 39116942

Liu, X., Zhang, F., Hou, Z., Mian, L., Wang, Z., Zhang, J., & Tang, J. (2021). Self-supervised learning: Generative or contrastive. *IEEE Transactions on Knowledge and Data Engineering*, *35*(1), 857–876. DOI: 10.1109/TKDE.2021.3095305

Liu, Y., Wang, F., Hu, H., Zhang, Z., Yang, H., Yao, X., Liu, H., & Zheng, J. (2025). A paper-based label-free plasmonic nanosensor for portable pre-diagnosis of multiple metabolic diseases. *Biosensors & Bioelectronics*, *275*, 117231. DOI: 10.1016/j.bios.2025.117231 PMID: 39946755

Longlong, J., & Tian, Y. (2019). Self-supervised visual feature learning with deep neural networks: A survey. arXiv. https://arXiv.org/abs/1902.06162

Lorre, G., Rabarisoa, J., Orcesi, A., Ainouz, S., & Canu, S. (2020). Temporal contrastive pretraining for video action recognition. *Proceedings of the IEEE Winter Conference on Applications of Computer Vision (WACV)*, 662–670. DOI: 10.1109/WACV45572.2020.9093418

Lu, G., Du, R. Y., & Peng, X. (2022). The impact of schedule consistency on shift worker productivity: An empirical investigation. *Manufacturing & Service Operations Management, 24*(5), 2780–2796.

Lugonja, N., Marinković, V., Pucarević, M., Miletić, S., Stojić, N., Crnković, D., & Vrvić, M. (2024). Human Milk—The Biofluid That Nourishes Infants from the First Day of Life. *Foods, 13*(9), 1298. DOI: 10.3390/foods13091298 PMID: 38731669

Luo, X., Li, H., Zhang, J., & Shim, J. P. (2010). Examining multi-dimensional trust and multi-faceted risk in initial acceptance of emerging technologies: An empirical study of mobile banking services. *Decision Support Systems, 49*, 222–234.

Maafa, I. M. (2025). Potential of zinc oxide nanostructures in biosensor application. *Biosensors (Basel), 15*(1), 61. DOI: 10.3390/bios15010061 PMID: 39852112

Madadi, Y., Delsoz, M., Khouri, A. S., Boland, M., Grzybowski, A., & Yousefi, S. (2024). Applications of artificial intelligence-enabled robots and chatbots in ophthalmology: Recent advances and future trends. *Current Opinion in Ophthalmology, 35*(3), 238–243. DOI: 10.1097/icu.0000000000001035 PMID: 38277274

Magnan, S. (2021). Social determinants of health 201 for health care: Plan, do, study, act. NAM Perspect.

Mahapatra, D., & Ge, Z. (2020). Training data independent image registration using generative adversarial networks and domain adaptation. *Pattern Recognition, 100*, 107109. Advance online publication. DOI: 10.1016/j.patcog.2019.107109

Mani, A., & Anirudhan, T. (2024). Electrochemical sensing of cortisol by gold nanoparticle incorporated carboxylated graphene oxide based molecularly imprinted polymer. *Chemical Engineering Journal, 493*, 152654. DOI: 10.1016/j.cej.2024.152654

Mansuri, R., Hirpara, F., & Dudhat, K. (2024). Diabetes Mellitus: Prevalence, knowledge and future consideration for the development of technological innovation. DOI: 10.22034/abec.2024.713505

Marbán, A., Casals, A., Fernández, J., & Amat, J. (2014). Haptic Feedback in Surgical Robotics: Still a Challenge. In Armada, M. A., Sanfeliu, A., & Ferre, M. (Eds.), *ROBOT2013: First Iberian Robotics Conference: Advances in Robotics,* Vol. 1 (pp. 245-253). Cham: Springer International Publishing.

Marchianò, V., Tricase, A., Macchia, E., Bollella, P., & Torsi, L. (2024). Self-powered wearable biosensor based on stencil-printed carbon nanotube electrodes for ethanol detection in sweat. *Analytical and Bioanalytical Chemistry*, *416*(24), 5303–5316. DOI: 10.1007/s00216-024-05467-7 PMID: 39134727

Marcolla, C., Sucasas, V., Manzano, M., Bassoli, R., Fitzek, F. H., & Aaraj, N. (2022). Survey On Fully Homomorphic Encryption, Theory, And Applications. *Proceedings of the IEEE*, *110*, 1572–1609.

Maric, T., Mikhaylov, G., Khodakivskyi, P., Bazhin, A., Sinisi, R., Bonhoure, N., & Goun, E. (2019). Bioluminescent-based imaging and quantification of glucose uptake in vivo. *Nature Methods*, *16*(6), 526–532. DOI: 10.1038/s41592-019-0421-z PMID: 31086341

Marques, L.. (2024). Advancing precision medicine: A review of innovative in silico approaches for drug development, clinical pharmacology and personalized healthcare. *Pharmaceutics*, *16*(3), 332. DOI: 10.3390/pharmaceutics16030332 PMID: 38543226

Martin, R. L., & Irrgang, J. J. (2007). A survey of self-reported outcome instruments for the foot and ankle. *The Journal of Orthopaedic and Sports Physical Therapy*, *37*, 72–84. PMID: 17366962

Martins, P., Matos, L., Moreira, A., Simões, M., & Silva, B. (2025). A transdisciplinary approach of the role of consciousness and spirituality in physics and healing. *Transdisciplinary Journal of Engineering & Science*, *16*. Advance online publication. DOI: 10.22545/2025/00273

Mascolini, A., Cardamone, D., Ponzio, F., Di Cataldo, S., & Ficarra, E. (2022). Exploiting generative self-supervised learning for the assessment of biological images with lack of annotations. *BMC Bioinformatics*, *23*(1), 374. Advance online publication. DOI: 10.1186/s12859-022-04845-1

Mathieson, K. (1991). Predicting user intentions: Comparing the technology acceptance model with the theory of planned behavior. *Information Systems Research*, *2*(3), 173–191.

Matsumoto, H., Tomoto, K., Kawase, G., Iitani, K., Toma, K., Arakawa, T., Mitsubayashi, K., & Moriyama, K. (2023). Real-Time Continuous Monitoring of Oral Soft Tissue Pressure with a Wireless Mouthguard Device for Assessing Tongue Thrusting Habits. *Sensors (Basel)*, *23*(11), 5027. DOI: 10.3390/s23115027 PMID: 37299753

Mavroeidis, V., & Bromander, S. (2017). Cyber Threat Intelligence Model: An Evaluation of Taxonomies, Sharing Standards, and Ontologies within Cyber Threat Intelligence. *Proceedings of the 2017 European Intelligence and Security Informatics Conference (EISIC)*, 91–98.

McCurdie, T., Taneva, S., Casselman, M., Yeung, M., McDaniel, C., Ho, W., & Cafazzo, J. (2012). mHealth consumer apps: The case for user-centered design. *Biomedical Instrumentation & Technology*, *46*(s2), 49–56.

McGinnis, J. M., Olsen, L. A., Goolsby, W. A., & Grossmann, C. (2011). *Clinical Data as the Basic Staple of Health Learning: Creating and Protecting a Public Good: Workshop Summary*. National Academies Press.

McKee, D., & Laulheret, P. (2021). *McAfee Enterprise ATR Uncovers Vulnerabilities in Globally Used B. Braun Infusion Pump*. Trellix.

McLean, G. (2021). Alexa, do voice assistants influence consumer brand engagement? Examining the role of AI-Powered voice assistants in influencing consumer brand engagement,

Medina, S. G., & Isomursu, M. (2023). The Use of Patient-Generated Health Data From Consumer-Grade Mobile Devices in Clinical Workflows: Protocol for a Systematic Review. *JMIR Research Protocols*, *12*, e39389. PMID: 36848208

Megarit, M. (2021, October 23). *3 ways smart hospitals will revolutionize the healthcare experience.* Michael Megarit. https://michaelmegarit.com/blog/smart-hospitals-will-revolutionize-the-healthcare-experience/

Mehra, P. S., Goyal, L. M., Dagur, A., & Dwivedi, A. K. (Eds.). (2022). *Healthcare Systems and Health Informatics: Using Internet of Things*. CRC Press.

Mehta, A., Cheng Ng, J., Andrew Awuah, W., Huang, H., Kalmanovich, J., Agrawal, A., & Isik, A. (2022). Embracing robotic surgery in low- and middle-income countries: Potential benefits, challenges, and scope in the future. *Annals of Medicine and Surgery (London)*, *84*, 104803. DOI: 10.1016/j.amsu.2022.104803 PMID: 36582867

Mei, H., & Tang, S. (2023). Robotic-assisted surgery in the pediatric surgeons' world: Current situation and future prospectives. *Frontiers in Pediatrics*, *11*, 1120831. DOI: 10.3389/fped.2023.1120831 PMID: 36865692

Melas, C. D., Zampetakis, L. A., Dimopoulou, A., & Moustakis, V. (2011). Modeling the acceptance of clinical information systems among hospital medical staff: An extended TAM model. *Journal of Biomedical Informatics*, *44*(4), 553–564. PMID: 21292029

Melstrom, L. G., Rodin, A. S., Rossi, L. A., Fu, P.Jr, Fong, Y., & Sun, V. (2021). Patient-generated health data and electronic health record integration in oncologic surgery: A call for artificial intelligence and machine learning. *Journal of Surgical Oncology, 123*, 52–60. PMID: 32974930

Memon, F. H., Inseok, K., Ahmed, F., Ali, W., Soomro, A. M., Memon, S. R., Memon, K. H., & Choi, K. H. (2023). A Comprehensive review of biosensor integration in microphysiological systems for online monitoring: Current challenges and future advancements. *ChemBioEng Reviews, 10*(5), 817–828. DOI: 10.1002/cben.202200066

Mendsaikhan, O., Hasegawa, H., Yamaguchi, Y., & Shimada, H. (2019). Identification of Cybersecurity Specific Content Using the Doc2Vec Language Model. *Proceedings of the 2019 IEEE 43rd Annual Computer Software and Applications Conference (COMPSAC)*, 1, 396–401.

Mennella, C.. (2024). Ethical and regulatory challenges of AI technologies in healthcare: A narrative review. *Heliyon, 10*(4), e26297. DOI: 10.1016/j.heliyon.2024.e26297 PMID: 38384518

Michel, O. (2025, January 31). *Webots R2025a* [Computer software]. Cyberbotics Ltd. https://www.cyberbotics.com/

Minaee, S., Boykov, Y. Y., Porikli, F., Plaza, A. J., Kehtarnavaz, N., & Terzopoulos, D. (2021). Image segmentation using deep learning: A survey. *IEEE Transactions on Pattern Analysis and Machine Intelligence, 44*(7), 3523–3542. DOI: 10.1109/TPAMI.2021.3059968

Minew. (n.d.). *Advanced Bluetooth IoT solutions for smart hospitals.* Retrieved June 23, 2025, from https://www.minew.com/solutions/smart-healthcare/

Mitchell, B.R., Mitchell, J.G., & Disney, A.P. (1996). User adoption issues in renal telemedicine. *Journal of Telemedicine and Telecare,* 2(2), 81-86.

Mitsubayashi, K. (2024). *Wearable biosensing in medicine and healthcare*. Springer Nature.

Mittal, M., Arora, M., Pandey, T., & Goyal, L. M. (2020). Image segmentation using deep learning techniques in medical images. In *Advancement of machine intelligence in interactive medical image analysis* (pp. 41–63). Springer. DOI: 10.1007/978-981-15-1100-4_3

Mohan, O., Banur, B. K. P., & Pawar, S. (2024, February). Integration of robotics and automation in supply chain: A comprehensive review. *Robotic Systems and Applications*, *4*(1), 1–19. DOI: 10.21595/rsa.2023.23349

Mojab, N. (2020). Real-world multi-domain data applications for generalizations to clinical settings. *2020 19th IEEE International Conference on Machine Learning and Applications (ICMLA)*, 677–684. DOI: 10.1109/ICMLA51294.2020.00112

Molla, G.. (2024). Revolutionizing personalized medicine: Synergy with multi-omics data generation, main hurdles, and future perspectives. *Biomedicines*, *12*(12), 2750. DOI: 10.3390/biomedicines12122750 PMID: 39767657

Mondal, I., Mansour, E., Zheng, Y., Gupta, R., & Haick, H. (2024). Self-Sustaining triboelectric nanosensors for Real-Time urine analysis in smart toilets. *Small*, *20*(42). Advance online publication. DOI: 10.1002/smll.202403385 PMID: 39031720

Moosavi-Dezfooli, S. M., Fawzi, A., & Frossard, P. (2016). DeepFool: a simple and accurate method to fool deep neural networks. In: *Proceedings of the IEEE Conference on Computer Vision and Pattern Recognition*; 2016 Jun 27–30; Las Vegas, NV. p. 2574–82.

Mori, M., & Geirsson, A. (2024). The way forward in research on robotic cardiac surgery: The need for transatlantic robotic cardiac surgery registry. *Annals of Cardiothoracic Surgery*, *13*(4), 376–378. https://www.annalscts.com/article/view/17105 PMID: 39157188

Mottaghi, A., Nikkhah, M., & Masroor, M. J. (2023). Lable-Free LSPR-Based colorimetric detection of A-Synuclein, a biomarker of Parkinson's disease, in saliva. *IEEE Sensors Journal*, *23*(6), 5713–5719. DOI: 10.1109/jsen.2023.3239887

Moulahoum, H., Ghorbanizamani, F., Beduk, T., Beduk, D., Ozufuklar, O., Celik, E. G., & Timur, S. (2023). Emerging trends in nanomaterial design for the development of point-of-care platforms and practical applications. *Journal of Pharmaceutical and Biomedical Analysis*, *235*, 115623. DOI: 10.1016/j.jpba.2023.115623 PMID: 37542827

Mozzaquatro, B. A., Agostinho, C., Goncalves, D., Martins, J., & Jardim-Goncalves, R. (2018). An Ontology-Based Cybersecurity Framework for the Internet of Things. *Sensors (Basel)*, *18*, 3053. PMID: 30213085

Mudireddy, D. R., Thakur, J., Vianney, N. J. M., Srivastava, S., Mathur, A., & Joseph, S. (2024). Prediction of blood glucose levels in diabetic and non-diabetic patients using Bi-RNN Transformers. *2021 IEEE International Conference on Electronics, Computing and Communication Technologies (CONECCT)*, 1–6. DOI: 10.1109/conecct62155.2024.10677194

Muhammad Sayem, A. S., Hon Teay, S., Shahariar, H., Luise Fink, P., & Albarbar, A. (2020). Review on smart electro-clothing systems (SeCSs). *Sensors (Basel), 20*, 587. PMID: 31973123

Mullins, L. B., Scutelnicu, G., & Charbonneau, É. (2022). A Qualitative Study of Pandemic-Induced Telework: Federal Workers Thrive, Working Parents Struggle. *Public Administration Quarterly*, *46*(3).

Murdoch, B. (2021). Privacy and artificial intelligence: Challenges for protecting health information in a new era. *BMC Medical Ethics*, *22*, 1–5.

Nadal, C., Sas, C., & Doherty, G. (2020). Technology acceptance in mobile health: Scoping review of definitions, models, and measurement. *Journal of Medical Internet Research*, *22*(7), e17256. PMID: 32628122

Nagpal, M. S., Barbaric, A., Sherifali, D., Morita, P. P., & Cafazzo, J. A. (2021). Patient-Generated Data Analytics of Health Behaviors of People Living With Type 2 Diabetes: Scoping Review. *JMIR Diabetes*, *6*, e29027. PMID: 34783668

Nandy, S., Adhikari, M., Khan, M. A., Menon, V. G., & Verma, S. (2022). An Intrusion Detection Mechanism for Secured IoMT Framework Based on Swarm-Neural Network. *IEEE Journal of Biomedical and Health Informatics*, *26*, 1969–1976. PMID: 34357873

Nasir, S., & Yurder, Y. (2015). Consumers' and physicians' perceptions about high tech wearable health products. *Procedia: Social and Behavioral Sciences*, *195*, 1261–1267.

Nayak, S. K., & Ojha, A. C. (2020). Data Leakage Detection And Prevention: Review And Research Directions. In *Machine Learning And Information Processing: Proceedings Of Icmlip 2019* (pp. 203–212). Springer.

Neches, R., Fikes, R. E., Finin, T., Gruber, T., Patil, R., Senator, T., & Swartout, W. R. (1991). Enabling Technology for Knowledge Sharing. *AI Magazine*, *12*, 36–56.

Nehme, J., Neville, J. J., & Bahsoun, A. N. (2017). The use of robotics in plastic and reconstructive surgery: A systematic review. *JPRAS Open*, *13*, 1–10. DOI: 10.1016/j.jpra.2017.03.005

Newaz, A. I., Sikder, A. K., Babun, L., & Uluagac, A. S. (2020). HEKA: A Novel Intrusion Detection System for Attacks to Personal Medical Devices. *Proceedings of the 2020 IEEE Conference on Communications and Network Security (CNS)*, 1–9.

Nguyen, N.-Q., & Le, T.-S. (2021). A semi-supervised learning method to remedy the lack of labeled data. *2021 15th International Conference on Advanced Computing and Applications (ACOMP)*, 78–84. DOI: 10.1109/ACOMP53746.2021.00019

Nifakos, S., Chandramouli, K., Nikolaou, C. K., Papachristou, P., Koch, S., Panaousis, E., & Bonacina, S. (2021). Influence of Human Factors on Cyber Security within Healthcare Organisations: A Systematic Review. *Sensors (Basel)*, *21*, 5119. PMID: 34372354

Nikolova, B. (2024). The 2030 Agenda for Sustainable Development: Goals and Implementation. *International Journal of Sustainability Policy & Practice*, *20*(2).

Ninaus, K., Diehl, S., & Terlutter, R. (2021). Employee perceptions of information and communication technologies in work life, perceived burnout, job satisfaction and the role of work-family balance. *Journal of Business Research*, *136*, 652–666.

Njor, E., Hasanpour, M. A., Madsen, J., & Fafoutis, X. (2024). A holistic review of the TinyML stack for predictive maintenance. *IEEE Access : Practical Innovations, Open Solutions*, *1*. Advance online publication. DOI: 10.1109/access.2024.3512860

Noroozi, M., & Favaro, P. (2016). Unsupervised learning of visual representations by solving jigsaw puzzles. In *Computer vision – ECCV 2016* (pp. 69–84). Springer. DOI: 10.1007/978-3-319-46466-4_5

Noroozi, M., Vinjimoor, A., Favaro, P., & Pirsiavash, H. (2018). Boosting self-supervised learning via knowledge transfer. *Proceedings of the IEEE/CVF Conference on Computer Vision and Pattern Recognition (CVPR)*, 9359–9367. DOI: 10.1109/CVPR.2018.00975

Noy, N. F., & McGuinness, D. L. (2001). *Ontology Development 101: A Guide to Creating Your First Ontology*. Stanford University.

Ochoa, J. J. (2023). *Occupational Burnout and Work-Life Balance Strategies Among Chaplains* (Doctoral dissertation, University of Arizona Global Campus).

Omoloja, A., & Vundavalli, S. (2021). Patient-generated health data: Benefits and challenges. *Current Problems in Pediatric and Adolescent Health Care*, *51*, 101103. PMID: 34799255

Onyeka, N. F. (2022). *Exploring Female Perspectives of Work-Life Balance and the Role of Organizational Culture* (Doctoral dissertation, Capella University).

Orringer, D. A., Golby, A., & Jolesz, F. (2012). Neuronavigation in the surgical management of brain tumors: Current and future trends. *Expert Review of Medical Devices*, *9*(5), 491–500. DOI: 10.1586/erd.12.42 PMID: 23116076

Osisanwo, F. Y., Akinsola, J. E., Awodele, O., Hinmikaiye, J., Olakanmi, O., & Akinjobi, J. (2017). Supervised machine learning algorithms: Classification and comparison. *International Journal of Computer Trends and Technology, 48*(3), 128–139. DOI: 10.14445/22312803/IJCTT-V48P126

Pai, F. Y., & Huang, K. I. (2011). Applying the technology acceptance model to the introduction of healthcare information systems. *Technological Forecasting and Social Change, 78*(4), 650–660.

Paleyes, A., Urma, R. G., & Lawrence, N. D. (2022). Challenges in Deploying Machine Learning: A Survey of Case Studies. *ACM Computing Surveys, 55*, 1–29.

Pal, S.. (2024). Bio-inspired electronic sensors for healthcare applications. *Chemical Engineering Journal, 499*, 155894. DOI: 10.1016/j.cej.2024.155894

Paluszkiewicz, C., Pięta, E., Woźniak, M., Piergies, N., Koniewska, A., Ścierski, W., Misiołek, M., & Kwiatek, W. M. (2020). Saliva as a first-line diagnostic tool: A spectral challenge for identification of cancer biomarkers. *Journal of Molecular Liquids, 307*, 112961. DOI: 10.1016/j.molliq.2020.112961

Pandey, S. K., & Sharma, V. (2019). Robotics and ophthalmology: Are we there yet? *Indian Journal of Ophthalmology, 67*(7), 988–994. DOI: 10.4103/ijo.IJO_1131_18 PMID: 31238393

Pandit, P., Crewther, B., Cook, C., Punyadeera, C., & Pandey, A. K. (2024). Sensing methods for stress biomarker detection in human saliva: A new frontier for wearable electronics and biosensing. *Materials Advances, 5*(13), 5339–5350. DOI: 10.1039/d3ma00937h

Pang, Y., Wang, W., Tay, F. E. H., Liu, W., Tian, Y., & Yuan, L. (2022). Masked autoencoders for point cloud self-supervised learning. In *Computer vision – ECCV 2022* (pp. 604–621). Springer. DOI: 10.1007/978-3-031-19821-2_35

Papernot, N., McDaniel, P., Jha, S., Fredrikson, M., Celik, Z. B., & Swami, A. (2016). The limitations of deep learning in adversarial settings. In: Proceedings of 2016 IEEE European Symposium on Security and Privacy (EuroS&P); Saarbruecken, Germany. p. 372–87.

Paramasivam, G., Sanmugam, A., Palem, V. V., Sevanan, M., Sairam, A. B., Nachiappan, N., Youn, B., Lee, J. S., Nallal, M., & Park, K. H. (2023). Nanomaterials for detection of biomolecules and delivering therapeutic agents in theragnosis: A review. *International Journal of Biological Macromolecules, 254*, 127904. DOI: 10.1016/j.ijbiomac.2023.127904 PMID: 37939770

Park, J., Kwak, I.-Y., & Lim, C. (2021). A deep learning model with self-supervised learning and attention mechanism for COVID-19 diagnosis using chest X-ray images. *Electronics (Basel), 10*(16), 1996. Advance online publication. DOI: 10.3390/electronics10161996

Park, S.-W., & Others. (2021). Review on generative adversarial networks: Focusing on computer vision and its applications. *Electronics (Basel), 10*(10), 1216. Advance online publication. DOI: 10.3390/electronics10101216

Park, Y. R., Lee, Y., Kim, J. Y., Kim, J., Kim, H. R., Kim, Y. H., Kim, W. S., & Lee, J. H. (2018). Managing patient-generated health data through mobile personal health records: Analysis of usage data. *JMIR mHealth and uHealth, 6*, e9620. PMID: 29631989

Park, Y., & Chen, J. V. (2007). Acceptance and adoption of the innovative use of smartphone. *Industrial Management & Data Systems, 107*(9), 1349–1365.

Parthasarathi, J., & Sheri, B. P. (2025, June). Integrating AI robotics in healthcare: Reducing medical costs and enhancing patient experience through automated diagnosis, treatment, and administrative workflows. *EAI Endorsed Transactions on AI and Robotics.*

Patel, S. K., Surve, J., Parmar, J., Armghan, A., Aliqab, K., Altahan, B. R., Ahmed, K., Bui, F. M., & Al-Zahrani, F. A. (2023). Graphene-based H-shaped biosensor with high sensitivity and optimization using ML-based algorithm. *Alexandria Engineering Journal, 68*, 15–28. DOI: 10.1016/j.aej.2023.01.002

Patel, V., Bhatt, S., Daspoddar, A., Shirsekar, V., Kumari, R., Chandra, P., & Srivastava, R. (2024). Evolution of materials, geometries, and fabrication of sweat patches and their use in high-throughput point-of-care/onsite sensing. *Microchemical Journal, 204*, 111165. DOI: 10.1016/j.microc.2024.111165

Pathak, D., Girshick, R., Dollár, P., Darrell, T., & Hariharan, B. (2016). Learning features by watching objects move. arXiv. https://arXiv.org/abs/1612.06370

Pathak, D., Krahenbuhl, P., Donahue, J., Darrell, T., & Efros, A. A. (2016). Context encoders: Feature learning by inpainting. *Proceedings of the IEEE Conference on Computer Vision and Pattern Recognition (CVPR)*, 2536–2544. DOI: 10.1109/CVPR.2016.278

Pavlou, P. A. (2003). Consumer acceptance of electronic commerce: Integrating trust and risk with the technology acceptance model. *International Journal of Electronic Commerce*, *7*(3), 101–134.

Pearman, C. D. (2023). *Tai Chi Enhanced Workplace Health and Wellness: A Systematic Literature Review for a Program Design, Implementation, and Evaluation* (Doctoral dissertation, University of Arizona Global Campus).

Pei, S., Ji, W., Yang, Y., Yang, S., Liu, T., Dai, J., Fu, C., Wu, J., Yin, Y., Wu, Q., Zheng, B., & Li, L. (2025). An enzyme-free wearable sweat sensor based on a Cu metal-organic frame composite material for monitoring lactate metabolism. *Sensors and Actuators. B, Chemical, 137512*. Advance online publication. DOI: 10.1016/j.snb.2025.137512

Pei, X., & Zuo, K. (2023). A review of the application of multi-modal deep learning in medicine: Bibliometrics and future directions. *International Journal of Computational Intelligence Systems, 16*(1), 44. Advance online publication. DOI: 10.1007/s44196-023-00225-6

Peter, J., & Ryan, M. (1976). An investigation of perceived risk at the brand level. *JMR, Journal of Marketing Research, 13*, 184–188.

Petersen, C. (2021). Use of patient-generated health data for shared decision-making in the clinical environment: Ready for prime time. *mHealth, 7*, 39. PMID: 34345616

Petersen, C., & DeMuro, P. (2015). Legal and regulatory considerations associated with use of patient-generated health data from social media and mobile health (mHealth) devices. *Applied Clinical Informatics, 6*, 16–26. PMID: 25848410

Pham, J. C., Aswani, M. S., Rosen, M., Lee, H., Huddle, M., Weeks, K., & Pronovost, P. J. (2012). Reducing medical errors and adverse events. *Annual Review of Medicine, 63*(1), 447–463.

Pikkarainen, T., Pikkarainen, K., Karjaluoto, H., & Pahnila, S. (2004). Consumer acceptance of online banking: An extension of the technology acceptance model. *Internet Research, 14*(3), 224–235.

Pinto, H. S., & Martins, J. P. (2004). Ontologies: How can They be Built? *Knowledge and Information Systems, 6*, 441–464.

Pisarchik, A. N., Maksimenko, V. A., & Hramov, A. E. (2019, October). From Novel technology to novel applications: Comment on "An Integrated Brain-Machine Interface Platform With Thousands of Channels" by Elon Musk and Neuralink. *Journal of Medical Internet Research, 21*(10).

Pitikultham, P., Putnin, T., Pimalai, D., Sathirapongsasuti, N., Kitiyakara, C., Jiang, Q., Ding, B., & Japrung, D. (2023). Ultrasensitive detection of MicroRNA in human saliva via rolling circle amplification using a DNA-Decorated graphene oxide sensor. *ACS Omega*, *8*(17), 15266–15275. DOI: 10.1021/acsomega.3c00411 PMID: 37151566

Pokhrel, G., Wang, Z., Cui, J., Jin, B., Zheng, H., Tao, J., & Zhang, X. (2025). Initial experience with the novel modular robotic system Carina in urology: A prospective study on safety feasibility and surgical settings. *Scientific Reports*, *15*(1), 12686. DOI: 10.1038/s41598-025-97411-7 PMID: 40221629

Polat, B., Rafeedi, T., Becerra, L., Chen, A. X., Chiang, K., Kaipu, V., Blau, R., Mercier, P. P., Cheng, C., & Lipomi, D. J. (2023). External measurement of swallowed volume during exercise enabled by stretchable derivatives of PEDOT:PSS, graphene, metallic nanoparticles, and machine learning. *Advanced Sensor Research*, *2*(4). Advance online publication. DOI: 10.1002/adsr.202200060

Ponemon Institute. (2016). *Sixth Annual Benchmark Study on Privacy & Security of Healthcare Data; Technical Report*. Ponemon Institute.

Popescu, M. C., & Sasu, L. M. (2014). Feature extraction, feature selection and machine learning for image classification: A case study. *2014 International Conference on Optimization of Electrical and Electronic Equipment (OPTIM)*, 968–973. DOI: 10.1109/OPTIM.2014.6850947

Power, D. (2024). Ethical considerations in the era of AI, automation, and surgical robots: There are plenty of lessons from the past. *Discover Artificial Intelligence*, *4*(1). Advance online publication. DOI: 10.1007/s44163-024-00166-9

Prabakaran, A., & Rufus, E. (2021). Review on the wearable health-care monitoring system with robust motion artifacts reduction techniques. *Sensor Review*, *42*(1), 19–38. DOI: 10.1108/sr-05-2021-0150

Pradhan, R. K., & Kumar, U. (Eds.). (2021). *Emotion, well-being, and resilience: Theoretical perspectives and practical applications*. CRC Press.

Promphet, N., Akgönüllü, S., Moonla, C., Nandhakumar, P., Tanglertsampan, P., Laochai, T., Laichuthai, N., Wang, J., & Rodthongkum, N. (2025). Non-Invasive Fingertip Sweat biosensor for early kidney disease biomarker screening. *Sensors and Actuators. B, Chemical*, *441*, 137967. DOI: 10.1016/j.snb.2025.137967

Promphet, N., Thanawattano, C., Buekban, C., Laochai, T., Lormaneenopparat, P., Sukmas, W., Rattanawaleedirojn, P., Puthongkham, P., Potiyaraj, P., Leewattanakit, W., & Rodthongkum, N. (2024). Smartphone based wearable sweat glucose sensing device correlated with machine learning for real-time diabetes screening. *Analytica Chimica Acta, 1312*, 342761. DOI: 10.1016/j.aca.2024.342761 PMID: 38834276

Pugliese, R., Regondi, S., & Marini, R. (2021). Machine learning-based approach: Global trends, research directions, and regulatory standpoints. *Data Science and Management, 4*, 19–29. DOI: 10.1016/j.dsm.2021.12.002

Qian, R., Meng, T., Gong, B., Yang, M.-H., Wang, H., Belongie, S., & Cui, Y. (2020). Spatiotemporal contrastive video representation learning. arXiv. https://arXiv.org/abs/2008.03800

Qi, Y., Xu, M., Lu, H., Wang, X., Peng, Y., Wang, Z., Liang, F., Jiang, X., & Du, B. (2024). Hepatic biotransformation of renal clearable gold nanoparticles for noninvasive detection of liver glutathione level via urinalysis. *Angewandte Chemie International Edition, 63*(36). Advance online publication. DOI: 10.1002/anie.202409477 PMID: 38877855

R.M. (2020). An Effective Feature Engineering for DNN Using Hybrid PCA-GWO for Intrusion Detection in IoMT Architecture. *Computer Communications, 160*, 139–149.

Radford, A., Metz, L., & Chintala, S. (2015). Unsupervised representation learning with deep convolutional generative adversarial networks. arXiv. https://arXiv.org/abs/1511.06434

Ragavendran, L. T. P, A. P., & P, A. P. P. (2024). 1D Topological Photonic Crystal based Nanosensor for Tuberculosis Detection. *Nanotechnology*. Advance online publication. DOI: 10.1088/1361-6528/ad61ec

Raghu, M., Zhang, C., Kleinberg, J., & Bengio, S. (2019). Transfusion: Understanding transfer learning for medical imaging. *Advances in Neural Information Processing Systems, 32*, 3347–3357.

Rahimi, B., Nadri, H., Afshar, H. L., & Timpka, T. (2018). A systematic review of the technology acceptance model in health informatics. *Applied Clinical Informatics, 9*(03), 604–634. PMID: 30112741

Rahi, P., Sood, S. P., Bajaj, R., & Kumar, Y. (2021). Air quality monitoring for Smart eHealth system using firefly optimization and support vector machine. *International Journal of Information Technology : an Official Journal of Bharati Vidyapeeth's Institute of Computer Applications and Management, 13*, 1847–1859.

Rahman, M. A., Bristi, S. A., Yesmin, T., & Islam, M. T. (2025). *Application of robotics in modern surgery and critical operations: Current status, challenges, and future directions*. ITPS. DOI: 10.36922/itps.4664

Rahman, S., Hasan, M., Sarkar, A. K., & Khan, F. (2023). Classification of Parkinson's Disease using Speech Signal with Machine Learning and Deep Learning Approaches. *European Journal of Electrical Engineering and Computer Science*, *7*(2), 20–27. DOI: 10.24018/ejece.2023.7.2.488

Rajan, A., Vishnu, J., & Shankar, B. (2024). Tear-Based Ocular Wearable biosensors for human health monitoring. *Biosensors (Basel)*, *14*(10), 483. DOI: 10.3390/bios14100483 PMID: 39451696

Ramanathan, K., Jenefa, L., & Radhi, A. R. A. H. (2024). Redesigning of Marketing Mix Elements Affecting Medical Tourism Through Artificial Intelligence (AI). In *Reskilling the workforce for Technological Advancement* (pp. 222–240). IGI Global.

Ram, P. R., Jeyaraman, M., Jeyaraman, N., Yadav, S., & Venkatasalam, R. (2023). Revolutionizing Orthopedic Healthcare: The Role of Robotics. *Cureus*, *15*(9), e44820. DOI: 10.7759/cureus.44820 PMID: 37809251

Rashid, A. B. (2024). AI revolutionizing industries worldwide: A comprehensive overview of its diverse applications. *Hybrid Advances*, *7*, 100277. DOI: 10.1016/j.hybadv.2024.100277

Rawat, D., Sharma, S., & Bhadula, S. (2025b). CT Imaging-Based Deep Learning System for Non-Small Cell Lung Cancer Detection and Classification. *International Journal of Advanced Computer Science and Applications*, *16*(5). Advance online publication. DOI: 10.14569/ijacsa.2025.0160561

Rawat, R., Goyal, H. R., & Sharma, S. (2024b). Hofstede's Cultural Dimension Driven Artificial Narrow Intelligence IDFIS for Industry 5.0 Empowered Digital Society. *Recent Patents on Engineering*, *19*. Advance online publication. DOI: 10.2174/0118722121334543241001050846

Rawat, R., Goyal, H. R., Sharma, S., & Kotiyal, B. (2025b). SQRCD: Building Sustainable and Customer Centric DFIS for the Industry 5.0 ERA. *International Journal of Advanced Computer Science and Applications*, *16*(2). Advance online publication. DOI: 10.14569/ijacsa.2025.0160293

Rawstorne, P., Jayasuriya, R., & Caputi, P. (2000) Issues in predicting and explaining usage behaviors with the technology acceptance model and the theory of planned behavior when usage is mandatory. *Proceedings of the 21st international conference on information systems*, 35–44.

Reddy, K.. (2023). Advancements in robotic surgery: A comprehensive overview of current utilizations and upcoming frontiers. *Cureus*, *15*(12), e50415. DOI: 10.7759/cureus.50415 PMID: 38222213

Reed, C. J. (2022). Self-supervised pre-training improves self-supervised pre-training. *Proceedings of the IEEE/CVF Winter Conference on Applications of Computer Vision (WACV)*, 2584–2594. DOI: 10.1109/WACV51458.2022.00263

Ren, Z., Guo, Y., Yu, S. X., & Whitney, D. (2021). Improve image-based skin cancer diagnosis with generative self-supervised learning. *2021 IEEE/ACM Conference on Connected Health: Applications, Systems and Engineering Technologies (CHASE)*, 23–34. DOI: 10.1109/CHASE52844.2021.00012

Richert, A., Shehadeh, M. A., Müller, S. L., Schröder, S., & Jeschke, S. (2016). Socializing with robots: Human-robot interactions within a virtual environment. Paper presented at the 2016 IEEE Workshop on Advanced Robotics and its Social Impacts (ARSO).

Rivero-Moreno, Y., Echevarria, S., Vidal-Valderrama, C., Pianetti, L., Cordova-Guilarte, J., Navarro-Gonzalez, J., & Acero-Alvarracín, K. (2023). Robotic Surgery: A Comprehensive Review of the Literature and Current Trends. *Cureus*, *15*(7), e42370. DOI: 10.7759/cureus.42370 PMID: 37621804

Rizvi, S. A., Tang, R., Jiang, X., Ma, X., & Hu, X. (2023). Local contrastive learning for medical image recognition. arXiv. https://arXiv.org/abs/2303.14153

Rodziewicz, T. L., & Hipskind, J. E. (2020). *Medical error prevention. StatPearls*. StatPearls Publishing.

Rogers, E. M. (1995). *Diffusion o f Innovations*. The Free Press.

Rojas Burbano, J. C., Ruiz, N. I., Rojas Burbano, G. A., Guacho Inca, J. S., Arragan Lezama, C. A., & González, M. S. (2025). Robot-Assisted Surgery: Current Applications and Future Trends in General Surgery. *Cureus*, *17*(4), e82318. DOI: 10.7759/cureus.82318 PMID: 40376327

Rony, M. K. K.. (2024). The role of artificial intelligence in enhancing nurses' work-life balance. *Journal of Medicine, Surgery, and Public Health*, *3*, 100135. DOI: 10.1016/j.glmedi.2024.100135

Roppelt, J. S., Kanbach, D. K., & Kraus, S. (2023). Artificial intelligence in healthcare institutions: A systematic literature review on influencing factors. *Technology in Society*, *76*, 102443. DOI: 10.1016/j.techsoc.2023.102443

Rosa, M., Liu, R., Pitruzzello, G., & Tortora, G. (2022). A smart modular IoT sensing device for enhancing sensory feedbacks in surgical robotics. *Applied Sciences (Basel, Switzerland), 12*(16), 8083. DOI: 10.3390/app12168083

Rossi, F., Trakoolwilaiwan, T., Gigli, V., Tortolini, C., Lenzi, A., Isidori, A. M., Thanh, N. T. K., & Antiochia, R. (2024). Progress in Nanoparticle-based Electrochemical Biosensors for Hormone detection. *Nanoscale, 16*(39), 18134–18164. DOI: 10.1039/d4nr02075h PMID: 39254475

Rossor, A. M., & Reilly, M. M. (2022). Blood biomarkers of peripheral neuropathy. *Acta Neurologica Scandinavica, 146*(4), 325–331. DOI: 10.1111/ane.13650 PMID: 35611606

Roth, S. C., Hinton, E. G., & Jivanelli, B. (2023). Impact of COVID-19 on Parents/Guardians in the Library Profession: A Narrative Review and Shared Experiences. *Library Leadership & Management (Online), 37*(2), 1–72.

Ruan, J., Chen, C., Shen, J., Zhao, X., Qian, S., & Zhu, Z. (2017). A gelated colloidal crystal attached lens for noninvasive continuous monitoring of tear glucose. *Polymers, 9*(4), 125. DOI: 10.3390/polym9040125 PMID: 30970805

Rubin, K. I. (2022). *The Great Balancing Act: Women Seeking Work-Life Balance during COVID-19* (Doctoral dissertation, University of Southern California).

Rudolph, S. (2011). Foundations of Description Logics. In. Lecture Notes in Computer Science: Vol. 6848. *Reasoning Web. Semantic Technologies for the Web of Data. Reasoning Web 2011*. Springer.

Saba, T. (2020). Intrusion Detection in Smart City Hospitals Using Ensemble Classifiers. *Proceedings of the 2020 13th International Conference on Developments in eSystems Engineering (DeSE),* 418–422.

Sadee, W.. (2023). Pharmacogenomics: Driving personalized medicine. *Pharmacological Reviews, 75*(4), 789–814. DOI: 10.1124/pharmrev.122.000810 PMID: 36927888

Saedi, Z., Masroor, M. J., Jahangiri-Manesh, A., Rezaei, A., Siskova, K., & Nikkhah, M. (2024). A Label-Free sensor array based on carbon quantum dots for detection of A-Synuclein oligomers in saliva. *Analytical Chemistry*. Advance online publication. DOI: 10.1021/acs.analchem.4c00874 PMID: 39034918

Sakhare, N. S. A., Kale, N. a. A., More, N. D. G., Kumkar, N. P. A., Mirase, N. J. M., & Sahu, N. U. S. (2023a). Smart wearable safety jacket. *International Journal of Advanced Research in Science Communication and Technology*, 8–14. DOI: 10.48175/ijarsct-9311

Salman, M., Ahmed, A. W., Khan, A., Raza, B., & Latif, K. (2017). Artificial intelligence in biomedical domain an overview of ai based innovations in medical. *International Journal of Advanced Computer Science and Applications*, *8*, 319–327.

Sarker, I. H. (2021). Machine learning: Algorithms, real-world applications and research directions. *SN Computer Science*, *2*(3), 160. Advance online publication. DOI: 10.1007/s42979-021-00592-x

Satyapanich, T., Ferraro, F., & Finin, T. (2020). CASIE: Extracting Cybersecurity Event Information from Text. *Proceedings of the Thirty-Fourth AAAI Conference on Artificial Intelligence, AAAI 2020, the Thirty-Second Innovative Applications of Artificial Intelligence Conference, IAAI 2020*, 8749–8757.

Sawik, B.. (2023). Robots for elderly care: Review, multi-criteria optimization model and qualitative case study. *Healthcare (Basel)*, *11*(9), 1286. DOI: 10.3390/healthcare11091286 PMID: 37174828

Schaper, L. K., & Pervan, G. P. (2007). ICT and OTs: A model of information and communication technology acceptance and utilisation by occupational therapists. *International Journal of Medical Informatics*, *76*, S212–S221. PMID: 16828335

Schork, N. J.. (2019). Artificial intelligence and personalized medicine. *Cancer Treatment and Research*, *178*, 265–283. DOI: 10.1007/978-3-030-16391-4_11 PMID: 31209850

Schütz, A. E., Fertig, T., & Weber, K. (2021). Defining a Core Ontology for Medical Devices in Germany to Ensure Semantic Interoperability. In Simian, D., & Stoica, L. F. (Eds.), *Modelling and Development of Intelligent Systems. MDIS 2020. Communications in Computer and Information Science* (Vol. 1341). Springer.

Seppänen, A., Vepsäläinen, J., Ojala, R., & Tammi, K. (2022). Comparison of Semi-autonomous Mobile Robot Control Strategies in Presence of Large Delay Fluctuation. *Journal of Intelligent & Robotic Systems*, *106*(1), 28. DOI: 10.1007/s10846-022-01711-3

Seth, I., Lim, K., Chang, E., Rozen, W. M., & Ng, S. K.-H. (2025). Evaluating the Clinical Utility of Robotic Systems in Plastic and Reconstructive Surgery: A Systematic Review. *Sensors (Basel)*, *25*(10), 3238. https://www.mdpi.com/1424-8220/25/10/3238 PMID: 40432030

Setiadi, R. N., Umar, L., & Arfianti, A. (2024). Low noise signal processing for electrochemical biosensor using narrow bandwidth filter. *Journal of Physics: Conference Series*, *2866*(1), 012032. DOI: 10.1088/1742-6596/2866/1/012032

Shah, S.. (2025). The evolution of brain surgery: Exploring the impact of continuum robotics. *Brain Hemorrhages*, *6*(1), 38–56. DOI: 10.1016/j.hest.2024.11.002

Shan, L. L., & Zhang, Y. (2024). Preparation and application of ZnO-Ecoflex composite sensors for lactate detection during physical training. *Journal of Ovonic Research*, *20*(6), 763–778. DOI: 10.15251/jor.2024.206.763

Shanmugasundaram, A., & Lee, D. (2022). SnO2/rGO nanocomposite for the detection of biomarkers of lung cancer. *Micro and Nano Systems Letters*, *10*(1). Advance online publication. DOI: 10.1186/s40486-022-00154-7

Sharma, S., Tyagi, R., & Mohan, S. (2024). Generative Artificial Intelligence-Enabled climate change and Deep-Sea food webs. In Advances in environmental engineering and green technologies book series (pp. 199–224). https://doi.org/DOI: 10.4018/979-8-3693-6670-7.ch009

Sharma, S., Tyagi, R., & Mohan, S. (2025a). Artificial intelligence and optimized computational modelling against climate crisis. In Elsevier eBooks (pp. 1–14). https://doi.org/DOI: 10.1016/b978-0-443-21905-4.00006-7

Sharma, S., Tyagi, R., & Mohan, S. (2025b). Blockchain-Based Security and Privacy in Digital Healthcare Recommender Systems. In In Healthcare Recommender Systems (pp. 221–237). https://doi.org/DOI: 10.1007/978-3-031-80056-6_10

Sharma, A., & Singh, B. (2022). Measuring Impact of E-commerce on Small Scale Business: A Systematic Review. *Journal of Corporate Governance and International Business Law*, *5*(1).

Sharmile, N., Chowdhury, R. R., & Desai, S. (2025). A comprehensive review of quality control and reliability research in Micro–Nano technology. *Technologies*, *13*(3), 94. DOI: 10.3390/technologies13030094

Shetty, K. H., Desai, D. T., Patel, H. P., Shah, D. O., Willcox, M. D., & Maulvi, F. A. (2024). Contact lens as an emerging platform for non-invasive bio-sensing: A review. *Sensors and Actuators a Physical*, *376*, 115617. DOI: 10.1016/j.sna.2024.115617

Shevchenko, N. (2018). *Threat Modeling: 12 Available Methods*. Carnegie Mellon University.

Shi, Q., Yang, Y., Sun, Z., & Lee, C. (2022). Progress of advanced devices and internet of things systems as enabling technologies for smart homes and health care. *ACS Materials Au*, *2*, 394–435. PMID: 36855708

Showrov, A. A. (2024). Generative adversarial networks (GANs) in medical imaging: Advancements, applications and challenges. *IEEE Access : Practical Innovations, Open Solutions*, *12*, 11805–11816. DOI: 10.1109/ACCESS.2024.3357685

Shreef, A., Shah, M., Habashy, A., & Mohamed, M. (2023). The Association of Microalbuminuria with Severity of Coronary Artery Disease Detected by Angiography in Type II Diabetes. *Zagazig University Medical Journal*. DOI: 10.21608/zumj.2023.224417.2830

Shurrab, S., & Duwairi, R. (2022). Self-supervised learning methods and applications in medical imaging analysis: A survey. *PeerJ. Computer Science*, *8*, e1045. Advance online publication. DOI: 10.7717/peerj-cs.1045

Si-Ahmed, A., Al-Garadi, M. A., & Boustia, N. (2023). Survey of Machine Learning Based Intrusion Detection Methods for Internet of Medical Things. *Applied Soft Computing*, *140*, 110227.

Siganidou, S. (2020). Work-related employee stress in 4* & 5* hotels in Greece. A study about the city of Thessaloniki. Acad4emic Press.

Sigeman, H., & Adolfsson, M. (2021). Maintaining well-being when working remotely: Work habits of employees at a geographical IT office in Sweden during the COVID-19 pandemic, their perceived well-being and productivity.

Sindhwani, N., Anand, R., George, A., & Pandey, D. (Eds.). (2024). *Robotics and Automation in Industry 4.0: Smart Industries and Intelligent Technologies* (1st ed.). CRC Press.

Singh, B. (2023). Blockchain Technology in Renovating Healthcare: Legal and Future Perspectives. In *Revolutionizing Healthcare Through Artificial Intelligence and Internet of Things Applications* (pp. 177-186). IGI Global.

Singh, B. (2024). Lensing Legal Dynamics for Examining Responsibility and Deliberation of Generative AI-Tethered Technological Privacy Concerns: Infringements and Use of Personal Data by Nefarious Actors. In Ara, A., & Ara, A. (Eds.), *Exploring the Ethical Implications of Generative AI* (pp. 146–167). IGI Global. DOI: 10.4018/979-8-3693-1565-1.ch009

Singh, B. (2024). Social Cognition of Incarcerated Women and Children: Addressing Exposure to Infectious Diseases and Legal Outcomes. In Reddy, K. (Ed.), *Principles and Clinical Interventions in Social Cognition* (pp. 236–251). IGI Global. DOI: 10.4018/979-8-3693-1265-0.ch014

Singh, P. (2024). Role Of Automation And Robotics In Transforming The Food Industry. *Revista Electrónica de Veterinaria, 25*(1), 1119–1125. DOI: 10.69980/redvet.v25i1.809

Singh, P., Gaba, G. S., Kaur, A., Hedabou, M., & Gurtov, A. (2023). Dew-Cloud-Based Hierarchical Federated Learning for Intrusion Detection in IoMT. *IEEE Journal of Biomedical and Health Informatics, 27*, 722–731. PMID: 35816521

Singh, R. P., Hom, G. L., Abramoff, M. D., Campbell, J. P., & Chiang, M. F. (2020). Current challenges and barriers to real-world artificial intelligence adoption for the healthcare system, provider, and the patient. *Translational Vision Science & Technology, 9*(2), 45–45.

Society for Brain Mapping and Therapeutics. (2024, December 18). *Role of nanotechnology in modern surgical techniques - Society for Brain Mapping and Therapeutics*. Society for Brain Mapping and Therapeutics - Breaking Boundries of Science, Technology, Medicine, Art & Healthcare Policy. https://www.worldbrainmapping.org/courses/lessons/role-of-nanotechnology-in-modern-surgical-techniques

Soomro, T. A., Zheng, L., Afifi, A. J., Ali, A., Yin, M., & Gao, J. (2022). Artificial intelligence (AI) for medical imaging to combat coronavirus disease (COVID-19): A detailed review with direction for future research. *Artificial Intelligence Review*, •••, 1–31.

South, C., Megafu, O., Moore, C., Williams, T., Hobson, L., Danner, O., & Johnson, S. (2025). Robotic surgery in Safety-Net Hospitals: Addressing health disparities and improving access to care. *The American Surgeon*. Advance online publication. DOI: 10.1177/00031348241312121 PMID: 39749432

Spitzer, H., Kiwitz, K., Amunts, K., Harmeling, S., & Dickscheid, T. (2018). Improving cytoarchitectonic segmentation of human brain areas with self-supervised siamese networks. In *MICCAI 2018* (pp. 663–671). Medical image computing and computer-assisted intervention. Springer. DOI: 10.1007/978-3-030-00931-1_76

Sreepada, A., Khasanov, R., Elkrewi, E. Z., De La Torre, C., Felcht, J., Abdulqader, A. A., Martel, R., Hoyos-Celis, N. A., Boettcher, M., Wessel, L. M., Schäfer, K., & Tapia-Laliena, M. Á. (2025). Urine miRNA signature as potential non-invasive diagnostic biomarker for Hirschsprung's disease. *Frontiers in Molecular Neuroscience, 17*. Advance online publication. DOI: 10.3389/fnmol.2024.1504424 PMID: 39872605

Stahl, B. C., & Coeckelbergh, M. (2016). Ethics of healthcare robotics: Towards responsible research and innovation. *Robotics and Autonomous Systems, 86*, 152–161. DOI: 10.1016/j.robot.2016.08.018

Stoumpos, A. I., Kitsios, F., & Talias, M. A. (2023). Digital transformation in healthcare: Technology acceptance and its applications. *International Journal of Environmental Research and Public Health, 20*(4), 3407. PMID: 36834105

Stuart, C. M., Meguid, R. A., & Rove, J. Y. (2025). Noteworthy in Cardiothoracic Surgery 2024. *Seminars in Cardiothoracic and Vascular Anesthesia, 29*(2), 126–133. DOI: 10.1177/10892532251332455 PMID: 40198923

Suarez-Ortegón, M. F., Del Pilar Zea-León, M., Astudillo-Gironza, A. M., Garzón, S., Portela, G. F., & Villarreal-Nieto, O. D. (2024). Sweat rate, sweat sodium losses, and body composition in professional male soccer players in Southwest Colombia. *Medicina, 60*(1), 113. DOI: 10.3390/medicina60010113 PMID: 38256373

Subramanian, H. (2023). A Decentralized Marketplace for Patient-Generated Health Data: Design Science Approach. *Journal of Medical Internet Research, 25*, e42743. PMID: 36848185

Sulaiman, N. b., binti Mahmud, N. P. N., Nazir, U., binti Abdul Latib, S. K. K., Muhammad Hafidz, H. F. b., & Abid, S. K. (2021). The Role of Autonomous Robots in Fourth Industrial Revolution (4IR) as an Approach of Sustainable Development Goals (SDG9): Industry, Innovation and Infrastructure in Handling the Effect of COVID-19 Outbreak. *IOP Conference Series. Earth and Environmental Science, 775*(1), 012017. DOI: 10.1088/1755-1315/775/1/012017

Sun, S., Reagan, K., Seker, E., & Vega, K. (2024). GLUCAT: a feline Biofluids IoT hub for electrochemical glucose biosensing. *TEI '24: Proceedings of the Eighteenth International Conference on Tangible, Embedded, and Embodied Interaction*, 70. DOI: 10.1145/3623509.3635250

Sun, T. Q., & Medaglia, R. (2019). Mapping the challenges of Artificial Intelligence in the public sector: Evidence from public healthcare. *Government Information Quarterly, 36*(2), 368–383.

Sutyak, K. M., & Tsao, K. (2024). Pedi-Bots: Innovations and progress in robotic pediatric general surgery. *Journal of Pediatric Surgery Open, 7*, 100156. DOI: 10.1016/j.yjpso.2024.100156

Swarnkar, A. (2025). Medical device: Development of next-generation devices from an engineering perspective. In *Targeted therapy for the central nervous system* (pp. 405–422). Academic Press. DOI: 10.1016/B978-0-443-23841-3.00018-2

Szegedy, C., Toshev, A., & Erhan, D. (2013). Deep neural networks for object detection. *Advances in Neural Information Processing Systems, 26*, 2553–2561.

Szeredi, P., Lukácsy, G., & Benkő, T. (2014). *Description Logic. The Semantic Web Explained The Technology and Mathematics behind Web 3.0.* Cambridge University Press.

Taha, B. A., Addie, A. J., Haider, A. J., & Arsad, N. (2025). Nanosensors Based on Breathomics for Human Disease Diagnosis: A New Frontier in Personalized Healthcare. *BioNanoScience*, *15*(2). Advance online publication. DOI: 10.1007/s12668-025-01876-9

Tajbakhsh, N., Shin, J. Y., Gurudu, S. R., Hurst, R. T., Kendall, C. B., Gotway, M. B., & Liang, J. (2016). Convolutional neural networks for medical image analysis: Full training or fine tuning? *IEEE Transactions on Medical Imaging*, *35*(5), 1299–1312. DOI: 10.1109/TMI.2016.2535302

Taleb, A., Kirchler, M., Monti, R., & Lippert, C. (2022). ContIG: Self-supervised multimodal contrastive learning for medical imaging with genetics. *2022 IEEE/CVF Conference on Computer Vision and Pattern Recognition (CVPR)*, 20876–20889. DOI: 10.1109/CVPR52688.2022.02024

Taleb, A., Lippert, C., Klein, T., & Nabi, M. (2021). Multimodal self-supervised learning for medical image analysis. In *Information processing in medical imaging* (pp. 661–673). Springer. DOI: 10.1007/978-3-030-78191-0_51

Talukder, M. S., Sorwar, G., Bao, Y., Ahmed, J. U., & Palash, M. A. S. (2020). Predicting antecedents of wearable healthcare technology acceptance by elderly: A combined SEM-Neural Network approach. *Technological Forecasting and Social Change*, *150*, 119793.

Tang, Z., Pei, S., Peng, X., Zhuang, F., Zhang, X., & Hoehndorf, R. (2022). TAR: Neural Logical Reasoning across TBox and ABox. arXiv:2205.14591.

Tang, L., & Mahmoud, Q. H. (2021). A Survey of Machine Learning-Based Solutions for Phishing Website Detection. *Mach. Learn. Knowl. Extr.*, *3*, 672–694.

Tania, M. H., Lwin, K. T., Shabut, A. M., Najlah, M., Chin, J., & Hossain, M. (2019). Intelligent image-based colourimetric tests using machine learning framework for lateral flow assays. *Expert Systems with Applications*, *139*, 112843. DOI: 10.1016/j.eswa.2019.112843

Tasnim, T., Sugireng, S., Imran, I., & Akib, N. I. (2024). Analysis of differences in early detection of chronic kidney disease with urine creatinine, proteins and individual health status based on behavioural, stress and genetic factors in Kendari City, Indonesia. *Public Health of Indonesia*, *10*(2), 203–213. DOI: 10.36685/phi.v10i2.801

Taylor, J. (1974). The role of risk in consumer behavior. *Journal of Marketing, 38*, 54–60.

ten Brummelhuis, L. L., ter Hoeven, C. L., & Toniolo-Barrios, M. (2021). Staying in the loop: Is constant connectivity to work good or bad for work performance? *Journal of Vocational Behavior, 128*, 103589.

Tenorio, J. L., & Vu, H. T. (2021). *A Cross-sectional Study during the COVID-19 Pandemic: Work Events and Affective Reactions as Predictors of Loss of Productivity and Intention to Leave* (Master's thesis, Handelshøyskolen BI).

Thakkar, A. (2024). Artificial intelligence in positive mental health: A narrative review. *Frontiers in Digital Health, 6*, 1280235. DOI: 10.3389/fdgth.2024.1280235 PMID: 38562663

Thakur, A., & Thakur, G. K. (2024). Developing GANs for synthetic medical imaging data: Enhancing training and research. *International Journal of Advanced Multidisciplinary Research, 11*(1), 70–82. DOI: 10.22192/ijamr.2024.11.01.008

Thapa, C., & Camtepe, S. (2021). Precision Health Data: Requirements, Challenges And Existing Techniques For Data Security And Privacy. *Computers in Biology and Medicine, 129*, 104130. PMID: 33271399

Tian, L., Jiang, M., Su, M., Cao, X., Jiang, Q., Liu, Q., & Yu, C. (2022). Sweat cortisol determination utilizing MXene and multi-walled carbon nanotube nanocomposite functionalized immunosensor. *Microchemical Journal, 185*, 108172. DOI: 10.1016/j.microc.2022.108172

Tiase, V. L., Hull, W., McFarland, M. M., Sward, K. A., Del Fiol, G., Staes, C., Weir, C., & Cummins, M. R. (2020). Patient-generated health data and electronic health record integration: A scoping review. *JAMIA Open, 3*, 619–627. PMID: 33758798

Tikhomirov, M., Loukachevitch, N. V., Sirotina, A., & Dobrov, B. V. (2020). Using BERT and Augmentation in Named Entity Recognition for Cybersecurity Domain. *Proceedings of the Natural Language Processing and Information Systems—25th International Conference on Applications of Natural Language to Information Systems, NLDB, 12089*, 16–24.

Topol. E. J. (2018). High-performance medicine: The Convergence of human of human and artificial intelligence.

Tricoli, A., Nasiri, N., & De, S. (2017). Wearable and miniaturized sensor technologies for personalized and preventive medicine. *Advanced Functional Materials, 27*, 1605271.

Trifan, A., Oliveira, M., & Oliveira, J. L. (2019). Passive sensing of health outcomes through smartphones: Systematic review of current solutions and possible limitations. *JMIR mHealth and uHealth, 7*, e12649. PMID: 31444874

Trivino, G., Mengual, L., & van der Heide, A. (2009). Towards an architecture for semiautonomous robot telecontrol systems. *Information Sciences, 179*(23), 3973–3984. DOI: 10.1016/j.ins.2009.08.007

Turhan, G. (2012). An assessment towards the acceptance of wearable technology to consumers in Turkey: The application to smart bra and t-shirt products. *Journal of the Textile Institute, 104*(4), 375–395.

TytoCare. (n.d.). *Home*. https://www.tytocare.com/

Uddin, M. S., Alam, J. B., & Banu, S. (2017, September). Real time patient monitoring system based on Internet of Things. In *2017 4th International conference on Advances in Electrical Engineering (ICAEE)* (pp. 516-521). IEEE.

Ueda, D., Kakinuma, T., Fujita, S., Kamagata, K., Fushimi, Y., Ito, R., Matsui, Y., Nozaki, T., Nakaura, T., Fujima, N., Tatsugami, F., Yanagawa, M., Hirata, K., Yamada, A., Tsuboyama, T., Kawamura, M., Fujioka, T., & Naganawa, S. (2024). Fairness of artificial intelligence in healthcare: Review and recommendations. *Japanese Journal of Radiology, 42*(1), 3–15. DOI: 10.1007/s11604-023-01474-3 PMID: 37540463

Umapathy, V. R., Raj, R. D. S., Yadav, S., Munavarah, S. A., Anandapandian, P. A., Mary, A. V., & Mary, V. (2023). Perspective of artificial intelligence in disease diagnosis: A review of current and future endeavours in the medical field. *Cureus, 15*(9).

Unnissa, Z., Unissa, M., & Khan, S. (2024). A Comprehensive Review of Medication Errors in Modern Healthcare. *Journal of Drug Delivery and Therapeutics, 14*(5).

Urrea, C., & Kern, J. (2025). Recent Advances and Challenges in Industrial Robotics: A Systematic Review of Technological Trends and Emerging Applications. *Processes (Basel, Switzerland), 13*(3), 832. https://www.mdpi.com/2227-9717/13/3/832

Van De Sande, N., Ramakers, I. H. G. B., Visser, P. J., Verhey, F. R. J., Verbraak, F. D., Bouwman, F. H., Berendschot, T. T. J. M., Nuijts, R. M. M. A., Webers, C. B., & Gijs, M. (2023). Tear biomarkers for Alzheimer's disease screening and diagnosis (the TearAD study): Design and rationale of an observational longitudinal multicenter study. *BMC Neurology, 23*(1). Advance online publication. DOI: 10.1186/s12883-023-03335-y PMID: 37543602

Vanderstappen, M., van Ochten, J. H. M., & Verborgt, O. (2025). Robotics in arthroplasty: How good are they? *JSES International*, *9*(3), 968–973. DOI: 10.1016/j.jseint.2024.09.005 PMID: 40486812

Venkatesh, V., & Davis, F. D. (2000). A theoretical extension of the technology acceptance model: Four longitudinal field studies. *Management Science*, *46*(2), 186–204.

Venkatesh, V., Morris, M. G., Davis, G. B., & Davis, F. D. (2003). User acceptance of information technology: Toward a unified view. *Management Information Systems Quarterly*, 425–478.

Vincent, P., Larochelle, H., Bengio, Y., & Manzagol, P.-A. (2008). Extracting and composing robust features with denoising autoencoders. *Proceedings of the 25th International Conference on Machine Learning*, 1096–1103. DOI: 10.1145/1390156.1390294

Vo, D. K.. (2024). Advances in wearable biosensors for healthcare: Current trends, applications, and future perspectives. *Biosensors (Basel)*, *14*, 560. DOI: 10.3390/bios14110560 PMID: 39590019

Vrazhnov, D. A., Ovchinnikova, D. A., Kabanova, T. V., Paulish, A. G., Kistenev, Y. V., Nikolaev, N. A., & Cherkasova, O. P. (2024). Terahertz Time-Domain spectroscopy of blood serum for differentiation of glioblastoma and traumatic brain injury. *Applied Sciences (Basel, Switzerland)*, *14*(7), 2872. DOI: 10.3390/app14072872

Wachter, R. M. (2010). Patient safety at ten: Unmistakable progress, troubling gaps. *Health Affairs*, *29*(1), 165–173.

Wah, J. N. K. (2025). Revolutionizing surgery: AI and robotics for precision, risk reduction, and innovation. *Journal of Robotic Surgery*, *19*(1), 47. DOI: 10.1007/s11701-024-02205-0 PMID: 39776281

Wali, R., Moulaee, K., Qasymeh, M., Maalej, R., & Neri, G. (2024). Atomic layer deposition of NiO-Coated CNT nanocomposites: Tailoring electrochemical properties for salivary lactate detection. *Journal of Electroanalytical Chemistry (Lausanne, Switzerland)*, *971*, 118594. DOI: 10.1016/j.jelechem.2024.118594

Wang, F., & Liu, H. (2021). Understanding the behaviour of contrastive loss. *Proceedings of the IEEE/CVF Conference on Computer Vision and Pattern Recognition (CVPR)*, 2495–2504. DOI: 10.1109/CVPR46437.2021.00250

Wang, G., Tang, Y., Lin, L., & Torr, P. H. S. (2022). Semantic-aware auto-encoders for self-supervised representation learning. *Proceedings of the IEEE/CVF Conference on Computer Vision and Pattern Recognition (CVPR)*, 9664–9675. DOI: 10.1109/CVPR52688.2022.00944

Wang, T., Huang, X., Huang, H., Luo, P., & Qing, L. (2022). Nanomaterial-based optical- and electrochemical-biosensors for urine glucose detection: A comprehensive review. *Advanced Sensor and Energy Materials*, *1*(3), 100016. DOI: 10.1016/j.asems.2022.100016

Warnecke, H. J., & Schiele, G. (1985). Performance Characteristics and Performance Testing of Industrial Robots — State of the Art. Academic Press.

Wartenberg, C., Elden, H., Frerichs, M., Jivegård, L. L., Magnusson, K., Mourtzinis, G., & Vallo Hult, H. (2025). Clinical benefits and risks of remote patient monitoring: An overview and assessment of methodological rigour of systematic reviews for selected patient groups. *BMC Health Services Research*, *25*(1), 133. PMID: 39849519

Wasilewski, T., Kamysz, W., & Gębicki, J. (2024). AI-Assisted detection of biomarkers by sensors and biosensors for early diagnosis and monitoring. *Biosensors (Basel)*, *14*(7), 356. DOI: 10.3390/bios14070356 PMID: 39056632

Weber, M. B., & De Fino, M. (2022). *Virtual technical services: a handbook.* Rowman & Littlefield.

Weerarathna, I. N., Kumar, P., Dzoagbe, H. Y., & Kiwanuka, L. (2025). Advancements in Micro/Nanorobots in Medicine: Design, actuation, and Transformative Application. *ACS Omega*, *10*(6), 5214–5250. DOI: 10.1021/acsomega.4c09806 PMID: 39989765

Weerarathna, I. N., Raymond, D., & Luharia, A. (2023). Human-Robot Collaboration for Healthcare: A Narrative Review. *Cureus*, *15*(11), e49210. DOI: 10.7759/cureus.49210 PMID: 38143700

Wei, K., Li, J., Ding, M., Ma, C., Yang, H. H., Farokhi, F., Jin, S., Quek, T. Q., & Poor, H. V. (2020). Federated Learning With Differential Privacy: Algorithms And Performance Analysis. *Ieee Trans. Inf. Forensics Secur.*, *15*, 3454–3469.

WellMed Medical Management. (2023). Staying hydrated is especially important for older adults. https://www.wellmedhealthcare.com/staying-hydrated-is-especially-important-for-older-adults

Wiewiora, M., Jopek, J., Świętochowska, E., Sławomir, G., Piecuch, J., Gąska, M., & Piecuch, J. (2023). Blood-based protein biomarkers and red blood cell aggregation in pancreatic cancer. *Clinical Hemorheology and Microcirculation*, *85*(4), 371–383. DOI: 10.3233/ch-231814 PMID: 37718785

Williams, M. A., McVeigh, J., Handa, A. I., & Lee, R. (2020). Augmented reality in surgical training: A systematic review. *Postgraduate Medical Journal*, *96*(1139), 537–542. DOI: 10.1136/postgradmedj-2020-137600 PMID: 32229513

Wilson, J., Heinsch, M., Betts, D., Booth, D., & Kay-Lambkin, F. (2021). Barriers and facilitators to the use of e-health by older adults: A scoping review. *BMC Public Health*, *21*, 1–12. PMID: 34399716

World Health Organization. (2021). *Decade of healthy ageing: baseline report*. World Health Organization. UNIVERSAL, M. P. T. Health at a Glance: Asia/Pacific 2022.

World Health Organization. (2024, October 1). *Ageing and health*. https://www.who.int/news-room/fact-sheets/detail/ageing-and-health

Wu, D. T., Xin, C., Bindhu, S., Xu, C., Sachdeva, J., Brown, J. L., & Jung, H. (2020). Clinician perspectives and design implications in using patient-generated health data to improve mental health practices: Mixed methods study. *JMIR Formative Research*, *4*, e18123. PMID: 32763884

Wu, D., Guo, P., & Wang, P. (2020). Malware Detection based on Cascading XGBoost and Cost Sensitive. *Proceedings of the 2020 International Conference on Computer Communication and Network Security (CCNS)*, 201–205.

Wu, I., & Wu, K. (2005). A hybrid technology acceptance approach for exploring e-CRM adoption in organizations. *Behaviour & Information Technology*, *24*(4), 303–316.

Wu, J. H., & Wang, S. C. (2005). What drives mobile commerce?: An empirical evaluation of the revised technology acceptance model. *Information & Management*, *42*(5), 719–729.

Wu, J.-H., Wang, S.-C., & Lin, L.-M. (2007). Mobile computing acceptance factors in the healthcare industry: A structural equation model. *International Journal of Medical Informatics*, *76*, 66–77. PMID: 16901749

Wu, L., Zhuang, J., & Chen, H. (2024). Voco: A simple-yet-effective volume contrastive learning framework for 3D medical image analysis. *Proceedings of the IEEE/CVF Conference on Computer Vision and Pattern Recognition (CVPR)*, 25628–25638.

Wu, W., Yang, J., Zhou, Y., Zheng, Q., Chen, Q., Bai, Z., & Niu, J. (2023). Chemometrics-based signal processing methods for biosensors in health and environment: A review. *Electroanalysis, 36*(7). Advance online publication. DOI: 10.1002/elan.202300207

Wu, Z., Qiao, Z., Chen, S., Fan, S., Liu, Y., Qi, J., & Lim, C. T. (2024). Interstitial fluid-based wearable biosensors for minimally invasive healthcare and biomedical applications. *Communications Materials*, *5*(1). Advance online publication. DOI: 10.1038/s43246-024-00468-6

Wu, Z., Zheng, Y., & Zhang, X. (2024). Safety and efficacy of orthopedic robots in total hip arthroplasty: A network meta-analysis and systematic review. *Journal of Orthopaedic Surgery and Research*, *19*(1), 846. DOI: 10.1186/s13018-024-05279-6 PMID: 39696343

Xu, C., Wu, F., Duan, Z., Rajbanshi, B., Qi, Y., Qin, J., Dai, L., Liu, C., Jin, T., Zhang, B., & Zhang, X. (2025). Microneedle-aided nanotherapeutics delivery and nanosensor intervention in advanced tissue regeneration. *Journal of Nanobiotechnology*, *23*(1). Advance online publication. DOI: 10.1186/s12951-025-03383-1 PMID: 40319333

Xu, L. D., Xu, E. L., & Li, L. (2018). Industry 4.0: State of the art and future trends. *International Journal of Production Research*, *56*(8), 2941–2962. DOI: 10.1080/00207543.2018.1444806

Xu, R., Zi, Y., Dai, L., Yu, H., & Zhu, M. (2024). Advancing Medical Diagnostics with Deep Learning and Data Preprocessing. *International Journal of Innovative Research in Computer Science & Technology*, *12*(3), 143–147. DOI: 10.55524/ijircst.2024.12.3.24

Xu, Y., Xu, G., Liu, Y., Liu, Y., & Shen, M. (2024). A Survey Of The Fusion Of Traditional Data Security Technology And Blockchain. In *Expert Systems With Applications* (p. 124151). Elsevier.

Yadav, N., Narang, J., Chhillar, A. K., Rana, J. S., Siddique, M. U. M., Kenawy, E., Alkahtani, S., Ahsan, M. N., Nayak, A. K., & Hasnain, M. S. (2023). Diagnostic methods employing kidney biomarkers clinching biosensors as promising tools. *Sensors International*, *5*, 100253. DOI: 10.1016/j.sintl.2023.100253

Yammouri, G., & Lahcen, A. A. (2024). AI-Reinforced wearable sensors and intelligent Point-of-Care tests. *Journal of Personalized Medicine*, *14*(11), 1088. DOI: 10.3390/jpm14111088 PMID: 39590580

Yang, G. Z., Cambias, J., Cleary, K., Daimler, E., Drake, J., Dupont, P. E., & Taylor, R. H. (2017). Medical robotics-Regulatory, ethical, and legal considerations for increasing levels of autonomy. *Science Robotics*, *2*(4). Advance online publication. DOI: 10.1126/scirobotics.aam8638 PMID: 33157870

Yang, P., & Xu, L. (2018). The Internet of Things (IoT): Informatics methods for IoT-enabled health care. *Journal of Biomedical Informatics*, *87*, 154–156.

Yang, Y., Sheng, C., Dong, F., & Liu, S. (2024). An integrated wearable differential microneedle array for continuous glucose monitoring in interstitial fluids. *Biosensors & Bioelectronics*, *256*, 116280. DOI: 10.1016/j.bios.2024.116280 PMID: 38603840

Yao, A. C. (1982). Protocols For Secure Computations. *Proceedings Of The Ieee 23rd Annual Symposium On Foundations Of Computer Science (Sfcs 1982)*, 160–164.

Yarbrough, A. K., & Smith, T. B. (2007). Technology acceptance among physicians: A new take on TAM. *Medical Care Research and Review : MCRR*, *64*(6), 650–672. PMID: 17717378

Yeboah-Ofori, A., Mouratidis, H., Ismai, U., Islam, S., & Papastergiou, S. (2021). Cyber Supply Chain Threat Analysis and Prediction Using Machine Learning and Ontology. *Proceedings of the Artificial Intelligence Applications and Innovations—17th IFIP WG 12.5 International Conference, AIAI 2021*, *627*, 518–530.

Ye, H., Chen, X., Huang, X., Li, C., Yin, X., Zhao, W., & Wang, T. (2024). Patterned gold nanoparticle superlattice film for wearable sweat sensors. *Nano Letters*, *24*(35), 11082–11089. DOI: 10.1021/acs.nanolett.4c03254 PMID: 39171663

Yin, S., Chen, X., Li, R., Sun, L., Yao, C., & Li, Z. (2024). Wearable, biocompatible, and Dual-Emission ocular multisensor patch for continuous profiling of fluoroquinolone antibiotics in tears. *ACS Nano*, *18*(28), 18522–18533. DOI: 10.1021/acsnano.4c04153 PMID: 38963059

Yousuf, H., Lahzi, M., Salloum, S. A., & Shaalan, K. (2020). Systematic Review On Fully Homomorphic Encryption Scheme And Its Application. In *Recent Advances In Intelligent Systems And Smart Applications* (pp. 537–551). Springer.

Yuan, X., Ouaskioud, O., Yin, X., Li, C., Ma, P., Yang, Y., Yang, P., Xie, L., & Ren, L. (2023). Epidermal wearable biosensors for the continuous monitoring of biomarkers of chronic disease in interstitial fluid. *Micromachines*, *14*(7), 1452. DOI: 10.3390/mi14071452 PMID: 37512763

Yurt, M., Dar, S. U., Erdem, A., Erdem, E., Oguz, K. K., & Çukur, T. (2021). mustGAN: Multi-stream generative adversarial networks for MR image synthesis. *Medical Image Analysis, 70*, 101944. Advance online publication. DOI: 10.1016/j.media.2021.101944

Yu, W., Mou, S., Zhang, X., Sun, J., Xue, Y., Xiong, H., Hsia, K. J., Wan, H., & Wang, P. (2024). Application of sensing devices in the detection of oral, pulmonary, and gastrointestinal diseases. *Chemosensors (Basel, Switzerland), 12*(4), 57. DOI: 10.3390/chemosensors12040057

Zenati, M. A., & Mahvash, M. (2012). 4 - Robotic systems for cardiovascular interventions. In Gomes, P. (Ed.), *Medical Robotics* (pp. 78–89). Woodhead Publishing.

Zeng, N., & Gao, Z. (2017). Health wearable devices and physical activity promotion. In *Technology in Physical Activity and Health Promotion* (pp. 148–164). Taylor & Francis.

Zeng, Z., Li, W., Zhang, J., Hu, Z., Wu, J., Ye, G., & Luo, Y. (2024). Highly sensitive and specific graphene oxide-based FRET aptasensor for quantitative detection of human soluble growth stimulating gene protein 2. *Talanta, 271*, 125629. DOI: 10.1016/j.talanta.2024.125629 PMID: 38245955

Zhang, B., & Dafoe, A. U. S. (2020). Public opinion on the governance of artificial intelligence. In: *AIES 2020—Proceedings of the AAAI/ACM Conference on AI, Ethics, and Society*. New York, NY, USA: Association for Computing Machinery, Inc; 187–193.

Zhang, R., Isola, P., & Efros, A. (2017). Split-brain autoencoders: Unsupervised learning by cross-channel prediction. *Proceedings of the IEEE Conference on Computer Vision and Pattern Recognition (CVPR)*, 433–441. DOI: 10.1109/CVPR.2017.514

Zhang, K.. (2024). Concepts and applications of digital twins in healthcare and medicine. *Patterns (New York, N.Y.), 5*(8), 101028. DOI: 10.1016/j.patter.2024.101028 PMID: 39233690

Zhang, M., Wang, Y., You, B., Qi, Z., Wang, Y., & Zhang, Z. (2024). Nickel oxide decorated popcorn derived biochar as a non-invasive electrochemical sensor for sensitive detection of glucose in saliva. *Journal of Alloys and Compounds, 1010*, 177427. DOI: 10.1016/j.jallcom.2024.177427

Zhang, Y., Bi, K., Zhou, L., Wang, J., Huang, L., Sun, Y., Peng, G., & Wu, W. (2024). Advances in blood biomarkers for Alzheimer's Disease: Ultra-Sensitive Detection Technologies and Impact on clinical diagnosis. *Degenerative Neurological and Neuromuscular Disease, 14*, 85–102. DOI: 10.2147/dnnd.s471174 PMID: 39100640

Zhang, Y., Liu, X., Qiao, X., & Fan, Y. (2023). Characteristics and Emerging Trends in Research on Rehabilitation Robots from 2001 to 2020: Bibliometric Study. *Journal of Medical Internet Research*, *25*, e42901. DOI: 10.2196/42901 PMID: 37256670

Zhang, Y., Yang, X., Liu, Y., Zhou, J., Huang, Y., Li, J., Zhang, L., & Ma, Q. (2024). A Time-Series Neural Network For Pig Feeding Behavior Recognition And Dangerous Detection From Videos. *Computers and Electronics in Agriculture*, *218*, 108710.

Zhang, Y., Yan, P., Tang, H., & Zhang, J. (2023). Rapid detection of tear lactoferrin for diagnosis of dry eyes by using fluorescence polarization-based aptasensor. *Scientific Reports*, *13*(1). Advance online publication. DOI: 10.1038/s41598-023-42484-5 PMID: 37704755

Zhang, Z., Hamadi, H. A., Damiani, E., Yeun, C. Y., & Taher, F. (2022). Explainable Artificial intelligence Applications in Cyber Security: State-of-the-Art in Research. *IEEE Access : Practical Innovations, Open Solutions*, *10*, 93104–93139. DOI: 10.1109/access.2022.3204051

Zhang, Z., Li, Z., Wei, K., Cao, Z., Zhu, Z., & Chen, R. (2024). Sweat as a source of non-invasive biomarkers for clinical diagnosis: An overview. *Talanta*, *273*, 125865. DOI: 10.1016/j.talanta.2024.125865 PMID: 38452593

Zhao, H., Zhao, H., Wang, J., Ren, J., Yao, J., Li, Y., & Zhang, R. (2023). Bovine OMASUM-Inspired Interfacial Carbon-Based nanocomposite for saliva metabolic screening of gastric cancer. *Analytical Chemistry*, *95*(30), 11296–11305. DOI: 10.1021/acs.analchem.3c01358 PMID: 37458487

Zhao, L. (2023). China's aging population: A review of living arrangement, intergenerational support, and wellbeing. *Health Care Science*, *2*(5), 317–327. DOI: 10.1002/hcs2.64 PMID: 38938584

Zhao, M., Hoti, K., Wang, H., Raghu, A., & Katabi, D. (2021). Assessment of medication self-administration using artificial intelligence. *Nature Medicine*, *27*(4), 727–735.

Zheng, X., Wang, Y., Wang, G., & Liu, J. (2018). Fast and robust segmentation of white blood cell images by self-supervised learning. *Micron (Oxford, England)*, *107*, 55–71. DOI: 10.1016/j.micron.2018.01.010

Zheng, Z.. (2024). Wearable and implantable biosensors: Mechanisms and applications in closed-loop therapeutic systems. *Journal of Materials Chemistry. B*, *12*(35), 8577–8604. DOI: 10.1039/d4tb00782d PMID: 39138981

Zhong, H. (2021). A self-supervised learning based framework for automatic heart failure classification on cine cardiac magnetic resonance image. *2021 43rd Annual International Conference of the IEEE Engineering in Medicine & Biology Society (EMBC)*, 2887–2890. DOI: 10.1109/EMBC46164.2021.9630910

Zhuang, X., Li, Y., Hu, Y., Ma, K., Yang, Y., & Zheng, Y. (2019). Self-supervised feature learning for 3D medical images by playing a Rubik's cube. In *MICCAI 2019* (pp. 420–428). Medical image computing and computer-assisted intervention. Springer. DOI: 10.1007/978-3-030-32245-8_47

Zhu, X., Liu, B., Zhu, C., Ding, Z., & Yao, L. (2023). Approximate Reasoning for Large-Scale ABox in OWL DL Based on Neural-Symbolic Learning. *Mathematics*, *11*, 495.

Zong, S., Ritter, A., Mueller, G., & Wright, E. (2019). Analyzing the Perceived Severity of Cybersecurity Threats Reported on Social Media. In *Proceedings of the 2019 Conference of the North American Chapter of the Association for Computational Linguistics: Human Language Technologies*. Association for Computational Linguistics.

Zou, M. (2022). *Market Manipulation: Identification, Characteristics And Prevention* [Ph.D. Thesis]. Macquarie University, Macquarie Park, Australia.

About the Contributors

Ben Othman Soufiene is an Assistant Professor of computer science at the Applied College, King Faisal University, Saudi Arabia. He received his Ph.D. degree in computer science from Manouba University in 2016 for his dissertation on "Secure data aggregation in wireless sensor networks. He also holds M.S. degrees from the Monastir University in 2012. My research interests focus on the Internet of Medical Things, Wireless Body Sensor Networks, Wireless Networks, Artificial Intelligence, Machine Learning and Big Data. Dr. Ben Othman has published more than 120 papers at reputed international journals, conferences, and book chapters. He is an Editorial Board Member in the different Journals and Conferences. He serves as an associate editor/academic editor for international journals including IEEE Access, IEEE Sensors, IEEE Internet of Things, Elsevier, Springer, Taylor & Francis, IGI, IET, Telecommunication Computing Electronics and Control, and Wiley. Dr. Ben Othman is a Technical Program Committee Member for more than a dozen of international conferences.

* * *

Saurabh Chandra is an accomplished legal scholar and currently serves as an Associate Professor & Assistant Dean at the School of Law, Bennett University, India. With a robust academic foundation, he earned his Bachelor of Arts and Bachelor of Laws (B.A. LL.B.) from the prestigious Aligarh Muslim University (A.M.U.). He further specialized in Business Laws, completing his Master of Laws (LL.M.) at the renowned National Law School of India University (NLSIU), Bangalore. Dr. Chandra's academic journey culminated in a Doctorate in Law (Ph.D.) from the esteemed National Law University (NLU) Delhi. In addition to his impressive legal education from some of India's most prestigious institutions, Dr. Chandra also holds a master's degree in Management with specialization in Human Resources in Management and another in Journalism and Mass Communication. With more than sixteen years of teaching experience, he has numerous publications to his credit. His expertise is complemented by a robust portfolio of scholarly publications. By bridging the gap between theoretical insights and real-world applications, Dr. Chandra's work serves as a valuable resource for academics, legal practitioners, and industry professionals alike. Dr. Chandra brings a wealth of experience in Academic Administration, having successfully held various key administrative positions. His diverse qualifications and extensive experience make him a distinguished figure in the academic and legal communities.

Juhi Kangkana Baruah completed B.Tech degree from North Eastern Hill University in 2016 and M.Tech from Gauhati University in 2019. Currently pursuing PhD from Gauhati University. Her research interests include- Biomedical, Sinal Processing, IoT and Artificial Intelligence.

Leena Jenefa, working as an Associate Professor in Hindustan Institute of Technology and Science, Chennai India, Prior that she worked in Vel Tech Rangarajan Dr Sagunthala R&D Institute of Science and Technology, Avadi, Chennai. She is having 19 years of experience in the teaching field. Prior to joining to Vel Tech -Chennai, she worked in Tecnia Institute of Advanced Studies-Delhi, DMI- St. Eugene University-Zambia, Linton University affiliated to University of East London-Malaysia.

Suphan Nasir received her BS degree in Sociology from Bogaziçi University and her PhDdegree in Marketing from Istanbul University, Turkey. She is currently Professor at Istanbul University and she has been the Chair of Marketing since 2009. She was the chief editor of the International Journal of E-Entrepreneurship and Innovation between 2010 and 2014, and also she was the editor of the International Journal of Higher Education between 2010-2023. Her articles have been published in reputable books and international academic journals. Customer relationship management as well as consumer behavior, sustainability, voter behavior, and higher education issues are the scope of her interest area. She attended some major international conferences as keynote speaker. Dr. Nasir received several scientific publications and best presenter awards. She worked as a mentor, evaluator and team leader at institutional external evaluation and institutional accreditation programs for the Higher Education Quality Board between 2016 and 2021; and also served as a member of the Advisory Board for TÜBİTAK Scientist Support Program between 2019-2022.

Anisur Rahman is an Associate Professor in the Department of Computer Science and Engineering at East West University, Bangladesh, where he also serves as Proctor. He holds a B.S. from Middle East Technical University (METU), Turkey, an M.S. from the University of Phoenix, USA, and a Ph.D. in Information and Communication Technology from Griffith University, Australia, with a research focus on underwater communication and localization. With a strong international academic background and over four years of administrative experience, Dr. Rahman is dedicated to advancing research and education in ICT.

Sachin Sharma is currently working as a Professor, Amity School of Engineering and Technology, Amity University, Punjab, Mohali, India. He also worked as Associate Dean, International Affairs and Professor, Department of Computer Science and Engineering at Graphic Era Deemed to be University, Dehradun, Uttarakhand, India. He has experience of 15+ years in industry and academia. He is also Co-founder and Chief Technology officer (CTO) of IntelliNexus LLC, Arkansas, USA based company. He also worked as a Senior Systems Engineer at Belkin International, Inc., Irvine, California, USA. He received his Philosophy of Doctorate (Ph.D.) degree in Engineering Science and Systems specialization in Systems Engineering from University of Arkansas at Little Rock, USA with 4.0 out 4.0 GPA and M.S. degree in Systems engineering from University of Arkansas at Little Rock with 4.0 out 4.0 GPA. Dr. Sharma has authored/coauthored over 300+ publications in the form of books, patents, and papers in refereed journals and conference proceedings. He holds 100+ US, Indian and international patents in the area of IoT, wireless communication and AI. He has also served as a Guest Reviewer for several Special issues of IEEE/ACM Transactions. His research interests include 6G wireless communication networks, Cloud Computing, Artificial Intelligence, Quantum Computing, IoT, Vehicular ad hoc networking and Cyber security.

Bhupinder Singh is working as Professor at Sharda University, India. Also, Honorary Professor in University of South Wales UK and Santo Tomas University Tunja, Colombia. His areas of publications as Smart Healthcare, Medicines, fuzzy logics, artificial intelligence, robotics, machine learning, deep learning, federated learning, IoT, PV Glasses, metaverse and many more. He has 3 books, 139 paper publications, 163 paper presentations in international/national conferences and seminars, participated in more than 40 workshops/FDP's/QIP's, 25 courses from international universities of repute, organized more than 59 events with international and national academicians and industry people's, editor-in-chief and co-editor in journals, developed new courses. He has given talks at international universities, resource person in international conferences such as in Nanyang Technological University Singapore, Tashkent State University of Law Uzbekistan; KIMEP University Kazakhstan, All'ah meh Tabatabi University Iran, the Iranian Association of International Criminal law, Iran and Hague Center for International Law and Investment, The Netherlands, Northumbria University Newcastle, UK.

Mohammad Salah Uddin is an Associate Professor in the Computer Science and Engineering Department at East West University Dhaka, Bangladesh. Before this, he worked as a researcher (Tradr - European project) at the Sapienza University of Rome. After completing his B.Sc in Computer Science and Engineering from East West University in 2012, he joined as a Lecturer at Central Women's University, Bangladesh. In October 2013, he enrolled in Sapienza University of Rome, Italy, to pursue his PhD. Degree and received the PhD degree in Robotics in July 2017. His research mainly focuses on Heterogeneous Robotics systems, Task planning/ Allocation for Multi-Robotics systems, IoT-Robotics, Sensors and Systems, Embedded Systems, Internet of Things, Computer Vision, etc. He published several research papers in peer-reviewed conferences/journals from his research work. In 2018, He delivered a speech at Maker Faire Shenzhen 2018 as a forum speaker. He is a member of the IEEE Robotics and Automation Society and holds the IEEE professional membership. He also has some other National and International membership.

Index

A

B

C

D

E

F

G

H

I

M

N

P

R

S

T

V

W

www.ingramcontent.com/pod-product-compliance
Lightning Source LLC
LaVergne TN
LVHW062334300926
849161LV00007B/1692